"Written by a group of clinical experts, this brilli[...] and evidenced-based strategies to help anxious yo[...] all clinicians. The authors demystify one of the m[...] [...]ponents of treatment for pediatric anxiety disorders—namely, conducting exposures—and provide helpful, step-by-step guidance for clinicians. This book contains a wealth of clinical wisdom, creative suggestions, case examples, and sample scripts that will be indispensable for clinicians who work with anxious youth."

> —**Golda S. Ginsburg, PhD**, professor in the department of psychiatry at the University of Connecticut School of Medicine

"*Exposure Therapy for Treating Anxiety in Children and Adolescents* is a must-read for every therapist working with anxiety and related disorders. This incredibly well-organized guide will become every new and experienced cognitive behavioral therapy (CBT) clinician's go-to resource for creative and effective exposure planning. Brimming with innovative, specific, and easy-to-implement exposure ideas, the authors have teamed up to create a one-of-a-kind book that contains every essential piece of information that a clinician needs to successfully plan and implement exposure-based treatment for childhood anxiety. Based on the most empirically supported approach to addressing anxiety, this guidebook will empower and fuel clinicians to provide the most effective treatment possible."

> —**Bonnie Zucker, PsyD**, author of *Anxiety-Free Kids* and *Take Control of OCD*

"Anxiety disorders are among the most common and interfering mental health problems affecting children and adolescents, but too few therapists are adequately equipped to provide quality care. Raggi and colleagues have done an absolutely terrific job of providing practical and easy-to-understand guidance for trainees and seasoned clinicians alike in proper treatment methods. This very welcome resource strikes a needed balance in covering both the science and the art of exposure therapy, and offers invaluable 'tips from the trenches' for flexibly applying evidence-based strategies. *Exposure Therapy for Treating Anxiety in Children and Adolescents* is sure to become a go-to desk reference in the offices of many clinicians and trainees working to improve the lives of kids suffering from anxiety and related problems."

> —**Jonathan S. Comer, PhD**, professor of psychology and psychiatry at Florida International University; director of the Mental Health Interventions and Technology (MINT) Program; president-elect of the Society of Clinical Psychology; and associate editor of *Behavior Therapy*

"Conducting exposures for anxious youth is deceptively straightforward, so when treatment fails, practitioners are often unsure how to proceed. Therapists' own anxieties about creating child distress or making fears worse can further derail treatment. This essential book walks therapists through the subtle yet critical nuances of effective exposure, providing evidence-based guidance for designing individualized treatments that work. The wealth of creative examples all but ensures this resource will be used again and again."

> —**Candice A. Alfano, PhD**, licensed psychologist, professor of psychology, and director of the Sleep and Anxiety Center of Houston (SACH) at the University of Houston

"Although instinctively, everyone knows that to get over your fear of a dog, you have to be around a dog, successfully getting over fears is not just a matter of rushing into the feared situation. Were it that simple, therapists would be out of jobs and this book would be unnecessary. Full of helpful information about how to conduct exposure therapy properly with children and adolescents, this book contains the necessary and useful information to engineer and implement exposure therapy. Thoughtfully written to address all the issues that therapists face, this book will be an invaluable resource for anyone who works with children with anxiety disorders."

—**Deborah C. Beidel, PhD, ABPP**, trustee chair, Pegasus Professor of psychology and medical education, and director of UCF RESTORES at the University of Central Florida

"The authors of this excellent book provide abundant, detailed illustrations on how to apply the exposure principle in creative, flexible, and diverse ways to help children and adolescents overcome anxiety and obsessive-compulsive disorders. Their book is essential reading for any clinician working with these young clients."

—**Richard J. McNally, PhD**, professor and director of clinical training in the department of psychology at Harvard University, and author of *What Is Mental Illness?*

"Mental health professionals now have their 'consultant on a shelf' for conducting exposures with anxious youth. The book goes beyond elucidating basic elements of exposures and considerations regarding their implementation, and provides mental health professionals with the ingredients for carrying out successful exposures with youths presenting with a range of anxiety concerns. The authors walk you through a number of options for conducting exposures, and as a reader I felt like I was meeting with an experienced professional who I sought to give me advice on how to use exposure to meet the needs of one of my clients."

—**Andres De Los Reyes, PhD**, associate professor of psychology and director of clinical training at University of Maryland, College Park; director of The Comprehensive Assessment and Intervention Program; and editor of the *Journal of Clinical Child & Adolescent Psychology (JCCAP)*

Exposure Therapy *for* Treating Anxiety *in* Children *and* Adolescents

A COMPREHENSIVE GUIDE

Veronica L. Raggi, PhD
Jessica G. Samson, PsyD
Julia W. Felton, PhD
Heather R. Loffredo, PsyD
Lisa H. Berghorst, PhD

New Harbinger Publications, Inc.

Publisher's Note

This publication is designed to provide accurate and authoritative information in regard to the subject matter covered. It is sold with the understanding that the publisher is not engaged in rendering psychological, financial, legal, or other professional services. If expert assistance or counseling is needed, the services of a competent professional should be sought.

Distributed in Canada by Raincoast Books

Copyright © 2018 by Veronica Raggi, Julia Felton, Lisa Berghorst, Heather Loffredo, and Jessica Samson
New Harbinger Publications, Inc.
5674 Shattuck Avenue
Oakland, CA 94609
www.newharbinger.com

Cover design by Amy Shoup

Acquired by Wendy Millstine

Edited by Susan LaCroix

Indexed by James Minkin

All Rights Reserved

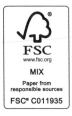 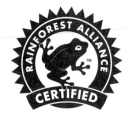

Library of Congress Cataloging-in-Publication Data on file

20   19   18

10   9   8   7   6   5   4   3   2   1   First Printing

Dedication

We would like to express immense gratitude to our loved ones, both family and friends. This project would not have been possible without their support.

With our love, admiration, and respect, we dedicate this book…

To my daughter, Avery; to Tom, my parents, and my family

—Veronica

To my parents, Rhona and Joel; and my sister, Sara

—Jessica

To Brian, Sydney, Brody, my parents, the Mejia family, and the Loffredo family

—Heather

To my parents and Andy, Alice, Rory, Adrian, and Tom

—Julia

To my parents, Ted and Debbie; and my husband, Dan

—Lisa

Contents

Foreword

Exposure therapy, a technique that introduces gradual approaches for facing one's fears, is backed by strong empirical evidence. Yet this technique is underutilized by clinicians. Exposures can seem complicated and difficult because they arouse *the* very anxieties and sensations of discomfort the client is looking to overcome. Sometimes clinicians wonder, "Are we being cruel to elicit such distress? Will it make the client get worse? Will it induce trauma or retraumatize the client? What about our ethical obligation to do no harm?" These are questions asked by clinicians, even those who are trained in cognitive behavioral therapy (CBT) and exposure. Despite these concerns, when exposure therapy is done thoughtfully and in conjunction with the underlying principles that guide it, it works, and often quickly! Further, sometimes it can be logistically difficult to target certain core fears. What type of exposure tasks would address a fear of dying? How about vomit? By offering practical, specific suggestions, this book targets these logistical concerns that may otherwise prevent clinicians from engaging in exposures with their clients.

This is the first book I am aware of that describes the basic principles of CBT and exposure for youth and expands these concepts fully—in terms of how to prepare children, teens, and families for exposure therapy, and how to design and implement practical, specific, and engaging exposure ideas for children and teens. It is written by clinicians, for clinicians. The ideas contained herein have been tried, tweaked, and implemented in an outpatient therapy practice. The inspiration for this book came about through peer consultation groups held by Alvord, Baker, & Associates. We hold several small groups which clinicians can join in-person or via video. All clinicians are solidly trained in evidence-based principles, including exposure, for anxiety disorders. Each week, questions are addressed as to what specific, detailed steps on a hierarchy would be effective for a specific problem, or how one would enhance a particular exposure for a client with obsessive-compulsive disorder (OCD) or anxiety issues. Prior to the inception of this book, we were unable to find a single source that provided guidance on the best ways to approach children, teens, and their families, and which also described varied and creative exposure ideas for children and teens.

Many clinicians within the practice made contributions to this book. The team effort was led by Veronica Raggi, PhD, who developed it from an initial idea, to the organization of its content, to solicitation of the authors, to the final product! The book is filled with pragmatic ideas that were elicited from real-world practice experiences.

This book helps get into the nitty-gritty of what clinicians should do, why they should do it, and how they should do it. In addition, for those who treat children and teens, you know that successful therapeutic strategies must be tailored to the developmental level of the child or teen. The strategies must be relevant, must make sense to children and teens, and, most importantly, should be introduced at a pace at which they can be tolerated. Each chapter focuses on a specific childhood anxiety disorder. Clinicians are guided through all the steps in the detail necessary for properly implementing the strategies. Also discussed are typical obstacles encountered and suggestions for how to overcome barriers and troubleshoot.

If you currently practice exposure therapy with children and teens, you are probably always looking for better ways to creatively and effectively encourage their participation and "ownership" of the exposure treatment. For those of you who might be just starting to do this work or have been hesitant up to this point, this book provides a treasure chest of practical, implementable, realistic, and clinician-tested exposures. Examples are included with sample dialogues between clinicians and clients to help you implement the exposure session from start to finish and, when necessary, make adjustments. This book is comprehensive; it provides specific procedures for a breakdown of what and how to do exposures all under one cover!

—Mary Karapetian Alvord, PhD

Acknowledgments

We would like to give special thanks to Dr. Mary Alvord for her unwavering support and encouragement of our project. She has provided steadfast mentorship to each of us throughout the years at Alvord, Baker, & Associates, LLC, and has furthered our commitment to providing high-quality, evidence-based care for our clients. We also sincerely appreciate the writing and editing contributions of Colleen Cummings, PhD; Betsy Carmichael, LCSW; Michelle Gryczkowski, PhD; and Nina Shiffrin, PhD. Thank you to Melissa Zarger, MA, for her editing support. Drs. Loffredo, Samson, Felton, and Berghorst are also especially grateful to Dr. Raggi for initiating and spearheading this project.

Finally, thank you to the many children and families we have been so fortunate to work with over the years. We are inspired by your strength and resilience in the face of life's challenges, your willingness to allow us to share in your journey, and your leaps of faith in trying something new.

CHAPTER 1

The Nature of Childhood Anxiety and Why Exposure Works

The purpose of this chapter is to provide you with an overview of the nature of child and adolescent anxiety and help you gain a general understanding of why exposure therapy is a powerful and effective treatment approach. We review the nature of childhood anxiety, risk factors associated with its development and maintenance, and how exposure therapy specifically targets the behavioral, cognitive, and physiological underpinnings of the disorder. We broadly review research on exposure-based cognitive behavioral therapy (CBT) in the treatment of various child and adolescent anxiety disorders. Throughout this chapter, we make reference to generalized anxiety disorder (GAD), separation anxiety disorder (SAD), social phobia (SoP), selective mutism (SM), obsessive-compulsive disorder (OCD), panic disorder (PD), and specific phobia (SP). Please refer to the specific chapter on each disorder for detailed definitions and descriptions.

The Nature of Childhood Anxiety

Let's start by looking at the natural course of childhood anxiety disorders and comparing typical developmental manifestations of fear to clinical forms of anxiety. Then we'll discuss common risk factors that predict clinical anxiety in childhood and adolescence. This section will set the stage for our later discussion of how effective treatment specifically targets the behavioral, physiological, and cognitive processes underlying anxiety in youth as well as common components of these treatment approaches.

Prevalence, Age of Onset, and Gender Differences

Anxiety disorders are the most common psychiatric diagnoses among youth, with prevalence rates ranging from 10% to 20% (Costello, Egger, & Angold, 2005; Merikangas et al., 2010). The onset of anxiety disorders typically occurs in childhood (Kessler et al., 2005), although age of onset varies for each specific anxiety disorder (Beesdo, Knappe, & Pine, 2009). SAD and SP have the earliest age of onset among the anxiety disorders, with most cases emerging prior to the age of 12 (Wittchen et al., 2003). In contrast, the core risk period for the emergence of SoP is late childhood through early adolescence (Beesdo et al., 2007; Wittchen & Fehm, 2003); PD and GAD tend to emerge in late adolescence or early adulthood (Beesdo, Pine, Lieb, & Wittchen, 2010), though some research studies note earlier childhood onsets (Rapee, Schniering, & Hudson, 2009).

Although there are no remarkable gender differences in age of onset of childhood anxiety disorders, they typically occur approximately two times as often in girls than boys, and this trend continues into adolescence (Costello et al., 2003; McLean & Anderson, 2009; Merikangas et al., 2010). OCD is the only anxiety-related disorder found to be more prevalent in boys than in girls during childhood (Castle, Deal, & Marks, 1995), although the gender distribution equalizes by adulthood (Mancebo et al., 2008).

The Natural Course of Childhood Anxiety

Without treatment, the majority of children diagnosed with anxiety disorders are likely to continue to meet diagnostic criteria for anxiety or other psychiatric disorders over time (Gregory et al., 2007; Kendall, Safford, Flannery-Schroeder, & Webb, 2004). Associations have been found between childhood and adolescent SAD as well as childhood and adolescent SoP (Bittner et al., 2007). Further, untreated anxiety conditions in youth lead to more complicated and pervasive problems over time. For example, childhood GAD is linked to the development of depression in adulthood (Copeland, Shanahan, Costello, & Angold, 2009); adolescent anxiety is a predictor of adult depression and substance abuse or dependence disorders (Essau, Lewinsohn, Olaya, & Seeley, 2014; Pine et al., 1998). There are also high rates of comorbidity between child anxiety disorders and other mental health conditions, including attention deficit/hyperactivity disorder (ADHD) and oppositional defiant disorder (Costello et al., 2003; Christophersen & Vanscoyoc, 2013; Kendall et al., 2010). All of these findings underscore the importance of early intervention to prevent the continuation (and exacerbation) of impairment into adulthood.

Developmental vs. Pathological Fears and Anxieties

It can be challenging to separate normal developmental fears from anxiety that is pathological in nature. Fear and anxiety are a part of a child's normal developmental trajectory: separation fears occur normatively in children around 12 to 18 months of age; fear of thunder and lightning around 2 to 4 years of age; fear of death around 4 to 5 years of age; fear of germs, natural disasters, and monsters around 5 to 7 years of age; and fear of rejection from peers around 12 to 18 years of age (Beesdo et al., 2009).

In contrast, children and adolescents are diagnosed with anxiety disorders when their fears or anxieties are excessive, last beyond a developmentally appropriate time range, and lead to significant impairment in daily functioning. Impairment may include difficulties in the following areas: sleep (for example, trouble falling or staying asleep; Alfano, Ginsburg, & Kingery, 2007), social life (loneliness, rejection, isolation), academic performance (difficulty concentrating, poor school attendance), family (increased parental stress, parent-child conflict), or emotional functioning (negative self-concept; Beidel & Alfano, 2011). The physical symptoms of anxiety (such as stomach pain or headaches) can lead to increased avoidance of anxiety-provoking situations, further compounding the problem.

The need for intervention is determined predominantly by the severity and quality of impairment in functioning (for example, when getting through the daily routine becomes extremely challenging due to the impact the child's anxiety is having on the entire family system). Additionally, youth may seek treatment when they are no longer able to engage in activities or experiences they would otherwise find enjoyable. As such, a primary goal of treatment is to provide them with strategies that will improve their quality of life so they no longer feel their lives are controlled by their anxiety.

Risk Factors for Childhood Anxiety

Below we present several risk factors that relate to the development and maintenance of child anxiety disorders. We review the factors that are important for consideration as you develop a case conceptualization and exposure hierarchy for each client.

Negative Affectivity

Affective reactivity (negative and positive affectivity) is an individual's response to stress and an important construct in anxious children. Negative affectivity (NA) is a temperamental factor comprising a greater proclivity toward the experience of distressing emotions (such as sadness, anger, or frustration) in response to environmental stressors (Rothbart & Rueda, 2005). In other words, children with high levels of NA tend to become upset, scared, or worried more easily and more frequently than children with lower levels of NA. NA is related to depression and anxiety and may partially explain the overlap between these types of internalizing pathology (see discussions of the Tripartite Model, Clark, & Watson, 1991; Mineka, Watson, & Clark, 1998). For the current discussion, we focus on the relationship between NA and anxiety in youth.

The inability to regulate negative emotions is related to difficulties in multiple domains (Langley et al., 2014). It is well established that anxious youth demonstrate difficulties managing NA (Suveg, Sood, Comer, & Kendall, 2009; Suveg, Hoffman, Zeman, & Thomassin, 2009). NA is posited to play a role in all types of anxiety disorders, including SoP (Anderson, Veed, Inderbitzen-Nolan, & Hansen, 2010), worry/GAD (McLaughlin, Borkovel, & Sibrava, 2007; Brown, Chorpita, & Barlow, 1998), panic (Hayward, Killen, Kraemer, & Taylor, 2000), and OCD and SAD (Dia & Bradshaw, 2008). Empirical data in older youth suggest that NA may be comprised of two components, fear and distress (Ebesutani, Okamura, Higa-McMillan, & Chorpita, 2011). Not surprisingly, individuals are motivated to avoid stimuli that result in NA (Rothbart & Rueda, 2005).

Cognitive Biases

Youth with anxiety also exhibit biased cognitive processing (Chorpita, Albano, & Barlow, 1996; Marques, Pereira, Barros, & Muris, 2013; Muris & Field, 2008). This faulty processing may take the form of an attention or interpretation bias (Muris & Field, 2008). Attention bias, which occurs during the encoding stage of information processing, involves hyperfocusing on potentially threatening material (Daleiden & Vasey, 1997). Interpretation bias, appearing during the conceptual stage of information processing, refers to the tendency to interpret ambiguous stimuli as threatening, overestimate the probability of a threatening incident occurring, and express intent to avoid the feared situation (Chorpita et al., 1996). There is also preliminary evidence to suggest that cognitive biases are activated in situations relevant to the specific anxiety disorder (Bögels, Snieder, & Kindt, 2003). For example, children with SAD or SoP exhibit more cognitive biases in response to separation or social situations.

Anxiety Sensitivity

Anxiety sensitivity (AS) is a key risk factor for the development of clinical anxiety in youth (Allan et al., 2014; Nöel & Francis, 2011). In other words, anxiety symptoms are harmful in and of themselves, leading to negative physical, social, or cognitive consequences (Reiss, Peterson, Gursky, & McNally, 1986). The concept of AS was developed by Reiss and McNally (1985) and originates from the concept of "the fear of fear" as posited by Goldstein and Chambless (1978). For instance, a child may worry that she will "go crazy" from anxiety, a racing heart may lead to a heart attack, or others will judge her for shaking during a class presentation. As a result, she may avoid situations that would put her at risk of experiencing anxiety symptoms in order to avoid perceived negative consequences.

In their meta-analysis, Nöel and colleagues (2011) described the clinical presentation of AS in youth. First, they found that AS is higher among youth with an anxiety disorder compared to community controls. Second, they determined that the relationship between AS and anxiety increases with age. Third, AS may be highest among youth with panic disorder, although this finding is preliminary. Interestingly, AS is currently thought to be transdiagnostic in nature (Knapp et al., 2016) and a unifying factor among all anxiety disorders (Boswell et al., 2013). For instance, worry may be related to the fear of experiencing anxiety, as individuals may worry in an effort to minimize uncomfortable feelings. Indeed, increases in fear of anxiety are associated with increases in worry (Buhr & Dugas, 2009). Adolescents who assume that anxiety is uncontrollable and damaging to their health may be more susceptible to worry. Finally, AS has important treatment implications for anxious youth. For example, AS was found to moderate the relationship between fear of spiders and avoidance of spider images among clinically anxious youth (Lebowitz et al., 2015): that is, children with spider phobias and higher AS ratings were more likely to avoid spider images than those with lower AS ratings. Thus, reducing AS may be a key treatment target.

Intolerance of Uncertainty

Individuals who present with intolerance of uncertainty (IUC) demonstrate negative beliefs about uncertainty and struggle to cope in situations that involve ambiguity (Dugas & Robichaud, 2007). IUC is purported to involve two dimensions (McEvoy & Mahoney, 2011): a cognitive (prospective) dimension (example: "I am upset by situations that are uncertain") and a behavioral (inhibitory) dimension ("I must avoid situations where the outcome is ambiguous"). Not surprisingly, IUC is higher in children with anxiety disorders as compared to non-anxious youth (Comer et al., 2009; Donovan, Holmes, & Farrell, 2016) and is associated with worry among children as young as 7 years old (Fialko, Bolton, & Perrin, 2012). A 5-year longitudinal study reported a reciprocal relationship between IUC and worry among adolescents (Dugas, Laugesen, & Bukowski, 2012). IUC may increase worry through cognitive (interpretation of ambiguous information as threatening) and behavioral (avoidance) means. Conversely, worry may increase IUC via negative reinforcement: adolescents may incorrectly assume that because they worried, they were prepared and the feared outcome did not occur (Greco, Lambert, & Baer, 2008; Hadwin, Garner, & Perez-Olivas, 2006).

While the negative perception of ambiguous situations is an important factor across all anxiety disorders, some evidence suggests that IUC may be most strongly associated with GAD (Read, Comer, & Kendall, 2013) and OCD (Lind & Boschen, 2009). Preliminary data suggest the cognitive dimension of IUC is more heavily associated with OCD and GAD, whereas the behavioral dimension is more closely linked to social anxiety, panic, and agoraphobia (McEvoy & Mahoney, 2011). Given the strong link between IUC and anxiety, targeting IUC in treatment is strongly recommended.

Environmental Factors

In addition to temperamental factors, the development of anxiety in children is also influenced by environmental factors. The interaction between one's temperament and life experiences contributes to shaping a child's view of the world and the likelihood of developing an anxiety disorder (Barlow, 2000). Below we discuss life experiences that may contribute to a child's risk of developing an anxiety disorder.

Parenting Factors

Specific parenting behaviors are linked to higher levels of child anxiety. Anxious children are more likely to have been exposed to parenting styles characterized by excessive use of control, overprotection, intrusiveness, lack of emotional warmth, increased criticism, or modeling of anxious behavior (see review by Drake & Ginsburg, 2012).

Adverse Life Experiences and Perception of Control

Further, children with anxiety disorders often perceive a lack of personal control over external threats as well as internal emotional and body reactions (Barlow, 2002; Weems, Silverman, Rapee, & Pina, 2003). This perception may, in part, stem from negative experiences early in childhood, in which they felt they had little control (such as parental divorce, parental psychopathology, neglect, or abuse) (Chorpita & Barlow, 1998; Chorpita, 2007).

There is also evidence that the interaction between specific life experiences and a child's temperament can increase vulnerability to a particular type of anxiety disorder (Barlow, 2002; Phillips et al., 2005). For example, if a child demonstrating high levels of NA and AS has a parent with a chronic illness, GAD may be likely to develop; excessive teasing may lead to social phobia; a bad experience with a blood draw may lead to a specific phobia of needles/blood (Chorpita, 2007). These early experiences may contribute to increasingly negative reactions to threatening events in the future, as well as the perception of a lack of control in problem solving and lack of influence in the external world.

Conceptualization of the Maintenance of Anxiety

The risk factors as described above predispose youth to the development and maintenance of clinical anxiety. These factors impact the behavioral patterns, cognitions, and physiological states that develop in youth. Below we describe how cognitive, physiological, and behavioral factors interact with one another to maintain abnormal levels of anxiety.

First, it is important to understand anxiety in its adaptive form. Anxiety is an individual's response to his lack of control over a potentially threatening event or situation (Barlow, 2002). In its adaptive—or "normal"—form, anxiety serves the useful purpose of alerting an individual to danger and motivating him to engage in adaptive behaviors to avoid negative consequences (such as studying for a test, or looking both ways before crossing the street; Albano & Kendall, 2002). This "fight-or-flight" response is a built-in protective system that enables us to respond to the perceived threat: oxygen and blood flow is increased, stimulating muscles and increasing heart rate and breathing; attention is focused on the source of danger to respond to threat cues. The fight-or-flight response occurs simultaneously on physiological, cognitive, and behavioral levels with the goal of priming the individual to react to the perceived threat and move toward safety (Abramowitz, Deacon, & Whiteside, 2011).

There are times, however, when the fight-or-flight response is unnecessarily triggered by a "false alarm," or the clinical manifestation of anxiety or fear (Barlow, 2002). There is no actual danger, or the likelihood of actual danger is low; however, our mind believes there is danger or threat, our body reacts as such, and we are then motivated to avoid the feared situation. There are three core components of clinical anxiety: physiological responses (such as shallow breathing, rapid heart rate, and stomachaches), cognitions (such as cognitive distortions and maladaptive belief systems), and behavioral responses (such as avoidance and ritual behaviors). It is the interaction of these components that contributes to the maintenance of anxiety disorders (Lang, 1968; Barlow, Raffa, & Cohen, 2002).

To illustrate this conceptualization, let's use an example: A child with GAD has her first swim meet of the season (feared situation). The morning of the event she complains that her stomach hurts (physiological response). She then tries to convince her parents that she cannot attend the meet (behavioral response). Some of her worries include: *What if I mess up and let my team down?* and *I don't know what to expect since this isn't the pool I usually swim at* (cognitions). The physiological and cognitive responses of this child fuel her desire to avoid the feared situation. Over time, avoidance of anxiety-provoking stimuli that are not actually dangerous can lead to impairment in daily functioning. If her parents allow her to miss this swim meet, a pattern may be initiated in which avoidance of the anxiety-provoking situation and subsequent physiological reaction strengthen the anxiety. Avoidance of the situation takes away her opportunity to recognize that the feared outcomes may not occur and that even if they do, they are tolerable or temporary (Mowrer, 1947; Beidel & Alfano, 2011). Therefore, through avoidance, this child will likely develop additional maladaptive cognitions that further reinforce the fear over time. She may believe that she is safe and okay only because she missed the swim meet; that is, if she had gone, something terrible or disastrous would have happened and she would not have been able to handle her anxiety. Her absence at the meet only reinforces these cognitions and the thought that her anxiety is lessened through avoidance. This is called negative reinforcement. It is the principle by which the absence of a negative outcome serves to reinforce the behavior (such as avoidance).

Exposure Therapy for Youth with Anxiety

In the treatment of anxiety, there are a wide variety of options available. It can be an overwhelming process to sift through competing philosophies and approaches, many of which have unclear research support. Fortunately, you can take solace in the fact that exposure therapy has emerged as a critical component in anxiety disorder treatment and is widely supported by research. Exposure tasks are important therapeutic ingredients in the overall treatment of anxiety as a result of their ability to directly target the negative reinforcement cycle that maintains anxiety (Bouchard, Mendlowitz, Coles, & Franklin, 2004; Foa & Kozak, 1986; Kazdin & Weisz, 1998; Kendall et al., 2005).

Exposure therapy involves helping the client to approach, and repeatedly come in contact with, a previously avoided, feared stimuli. Thus, the client learns to face and experience, rather than avoid, their anxiety. Exposure typically takes place in a series of graduated, increasingly challenging exercises that allow the client to face her fears and reduce avoidance in stages or steps. The feared stimulus may be internal (for example, scary images or intrusive thoughts) or situational (objects, people, or places). Exposures may involve direct ("in vivo") confrontation with the stimulus, imaginal or visualization activities, video or audio exposures, modeling or observation, or exposures to the physiological sensations themselves (interoceptive).

By participating in exposure tasks, the client typically experiences habituation, or a weakening of the physiological fear response with repeated and prolonged presentation of the feared stimulus. Habituation has historically been considered a central mechanism of change in exposure therapy (Lader & Matthews, 1968; Watson, Gaind, & Marks, 1972). It is the disconnection between the presence of a fearful stimulus and its ability to elicit a fearful response. However, recent research suggests that habituation during a task may be a temporary change, and that more long-term, sustained change requires the reprocessing of the feared event, object, or other stimuli post exposure.

Therefore, emotional processing also plays a major role in anxiety reduction during exposure therapy. It involves activation of "fear structures" stored in one's memory. Fear structures are defined as maladaptive beliefs about feared stimuli, responses, and their meaning. These structures are stored in one's memory and associate the feared stimuli with danger (Foa & Kozak, 1986; Abramowitz et al., 2011). Through repeated and prolonged exposure tasks, clients with anxiety learn that they can respond to the originally feared stimuli in a more adaptive manner that is incompatible with the information present in the fear structure. This experience leads to an awareness that the dreaded outcome does not occur and the unpleasant feelings they experience are often short-lived and tolerable. Once they achieve an awareness that the anticipated consequence does not occur with one particular stimulus, through the process of generalization they gradually apply this more adaptive way of evaluating other unrelated fear stimuli.

Perceived self-efficacy is another important cognitive factor in exposure work and specifically targets avoidance behavior (Bandura, 1983, 1997). Self-efficacy is one's attitude toward his ability to successfully handle a specific situation or accomplish a particular task (Bandura, 1983). According to the self-efficacy theory, it is the perceived inability to cope with the feared stimulus that maintains the anxiety. Self-efficacy can be accomplished through behavioral mastery over the potentially aversive stimulus. Therefore, exposure therapy allows young people with anxiety to strengthen their self-efficacy (in other words, belief in their ability to handle the fear), which ultimately reduces avoidance behavior.

History of Exposure Therapy

Exposure therapy dates back to the behavior therapy movement of the 1950s. One of the first forms of exposure therapy was systematic desensitization (SD). Joseph Wolpe, a psychiatrist oriented in learning theory and experimental psychology, was one of the first to conduct laboratory research using this technique (Wolpe, 1958). SD involves a graduated approach of pairing a phobic stimulus with a physiological state that is incompatible with anxiety. The goal of this intervention is that the client becomes relaxed through the use of progressive muscle relaxation while in the presence of his phobic stimuli. There is substantial clinical and experimental research to demonstrate the efficacy and effectiveness of SD for specific phobias, social phobia, and agoraphobia (Abramowitz et al., 2011).

Clinical interest and research on SD declined as flooding and implosive therapy emerged in the 1970s and 1980s (McGlynn, Smitherman, & Gothard, 2004). These treatment interventions were derived from the behavioral principal of extinction: repeated presentation of the feared stimulus in the absence of the feared consequence or any escape or avoidance behavior results in the reduction of the fear. Flooding involves prolonged exposure to the most feared stimuli without escape from the feared situation until the anxiety subsides. Implosive therapy was a variation of flooding with a psychodynamic component, involving exposure only to imagined, and often exaggerated, feared stimuli (Stampfl & Levis, 1967). The 1970s and 1980s also led to the development and testing of contemporary exposure therapy without the relaxation component of SD, the rapid exposure of flooding, or the psychodynamic component of implosive therapy. The focus became conducting exposure in a series of graduated or increasingly challenging steps. Further, increased understanding of the importance of cognitive processes in the development and maintenance of psychological disorders also led to the gradual merging of cognitive and behavioral therapies into cognitive behavioral therapy (CBT; Benjamin et al., 2011).

Exposure Within the Context of Cognitive Behavioral Therapy

While exposure therapy is a strong and powerful treatment approach, it is rarely used in isolation. Typically, it is integrated within a larger CBT treatment protocol. CBT is a goal-oriented, skills-focused therapy that targets patterns of thinking, physiological sensations, and behaviors that maintain maladaptive functioning. It is often manual-based, with common treatment protocols consisting of approximately 12 to 20 sessions. CBT offers youth specific guidance and active strategies for managing anxiety. These strategies are typically taught through the use of concrete and engaging activities and exercises. Youth actively participate and take ownership for their treatment. They complete homework between sessions to hone their therapeutic skills and enhance the generalization of skill use to multiple settings and domains.

Common components of CBT include psychoeducation, cognitive restructuring, behavioral exposure, relaxation training, parent training, contingency management, role-play, modeling, and problem solving (Kendall, Peterman, & Cummings, 2015). In the context of CBT, behavioral exposure is typically a heavily emphasized component. It is often delivered in a series of focused sessions following psychoeducation, cognitive restructuring and/or relaxation skills, and development of a contingency management or reward system. While this book is primarily focused on delineating exposure-based techniques, chapter 4 will highlight this broader treatment framework.

CBT can be provided in individual, group, or family-based modalities, with varying levels of parental involvement. When considering which modality to use, clinicians may consider the various advantages of each. Individual CBT, the most common approach, optimizes the ability to personalize treatment. Group treatment increases your "reach" by working with multiple youth at a time and allows them to complete exposure tasks with the support of peers. As described in chapter 13, this can be particularly helpful for clients with social anxiety. Additionally, group CBT can reduce the isolation often felt by children with anxiety disorders, as they have the opportunity to connect with peers who have similar difficulties. Family-based CBT can target maladaptive familial patterns and parenting practices that may be maintaining the anxiety.

When developing a treatment plan, consideration is also given to how frequently to include parents or caregivers (hereafter referred to solely as "parents") in the therapy process. Available treatment protocols typically include some form of parental involvement, which can vary from a few parent sessions (e.g., Coping Cat; Kendall & Hedtke, 2006) to parent-focused treatment (e.g., the Cool Little Kids Program; Kennedy, Rapee, & Edwards, 2009). Overall, the degree to which parents participate in their children's treatment depends on several factors, including child age, parental mental health, and maladaptive parenting behaviors (for example, high levels of criticism or parental accommodation; Barmish & Kendall, 2005; Creswell & Cartwright-Hatton,

2007). CBT with active parental involvement, emphasizing contingency management and transfer of intervention control from provider to parents or teachers, is associated with long-term maintenance of treatment gains (Manassis et al., 2014).

Finally, CBT for youth anxiety can vary regarding the number of sessions and intensity of treatment. Although treatment often involves 12 to 20 sessions, brief treatments are available for clients who present with mild anxiety (e.g., Beidas, Mychailyszyn, Podell, & Kendall, 2013). Treatment may even involve a single extended exposure session for youth with specific phobias such as fear of spiders (Ollendick et al., 2009). In contrast, clients with severe, pervasive anxieties may benefit from exposure-based CBT provided in a more intensive fashion, such as intensive outpatient treatment (e.g., for OCD; Lewin et al., 2005; Rudy et al., 2014) or camp-based programs (e.g., Ehrenreich-May & Bilek, 2011; Kurtz, 2009; Santucci et al., 2009; Santucci & Ehrenreich-May, 2010).

Addressing Risk Factors Through Exposure-Based CBT

Exposure-based CBT addresses each of the anxiety risk factors discussed earlier in this chapter: NA, distorted thinking processes (such as IUC, AS, and faulty perceptions related to control), and environmental factors. For example, NA is an important treatment target in CBT for anxious youth. Instruction in relaxation and other coping skills through broad-based CBT skills give youth strategies for regulating their emotional responses. In addition, exposure tasks give them the opportunity to practice regulating and tolerating NA within the context of feared stimuli.

Another goal of treatment is challenging or reframing the distorted thinking that anxious children experience, via cognitive restructuring. As a result of greater adaptive thinking, youth are often more open than adults to approaching, rather than avoiding, feared situations. Exposure work can facilitate cognitive change in youth by providing corrective experiences that challenge faulty assumptions. For AS specifically, exposure-focused CBT serves a critical role by allowing youth to challenge the faulty assumption that anxiety is inherently harmful. An adolescent boy, for example, may learn during public speaking exposures that his increased heart rate and shakiness is tolerable and will eventually subside. Further, interoceptive exposures (see chapter 7) target the physical component of AS through activities specifically designed to generate the physical sensations of anxiety, with the goal of habituation during, and cognitive reprocessing after, these exercises.

IUC can be targeted through uncertainty exposures (see chapter 12). These exposures allow youth to face, rather than avoid, ambiguous situations, thereby challenging the notion that these situations are dangerous or intolerable. Similarly, exposure work in general is designed to facilitate a greater sense of control by teaching people to "master" their fears. Clients will develop a higher perception of control as they learn to differentiate between real versus imaginary threat, and systematically face their fears.

Exposure-based CBT also addresses environmental factors that may be maintaining a child's anxiety symptoms. It is generally important to include parents in the treatment process, particularly those parents who present with anxiety disorders or parenting styles that may inadvertently increase a child's anxiety symptoms. This approach includes coaching parents to help them become more aware of their parenting style, make adjustments to reduce accommodation of their child's anxiety (see chapter 3), and facilitate exposure exercises. Through these goals, parents can effectively support their child in treatment.

There are times when exposure to traumatic life experiences will lead to emotional and behavioral symptoms that may need to take precedence in treatment over the co-occurring anxiety disorder. Trauma-focused CBT (TF-CBT) is an evidence-based treatment approach for treating traumatized children (Jensen et al., 2014). The trauma narrative and cognitive processing of the traumatic experience differentiate this exposure-based treatment approach from the CBT model for other anxiety disorders. See Cohen, Mannarino, & Deblinger (2006) for a detailed description of this treatment approach.

Evidence Base for CBT with Exposure

CBT with an exposure focus has a long history of empirical support that demonstrates its ability to reduce the symptoms and impairment associated with a wide variety of mental health disorders, including anxiety (Barlow, 2002). In fact, a wealth of large, well-controlled clinical trials and numerous research studies have led to CBT emerging as the treatment of choice for anxiety disorders. In particular, CBT with exposure has been deemed a well-established treatment for child and adolescent anxiety disorders based on a large body of literature that supports its efficacy (Hollon & Beck, 2013). As a result, it has become a prominent and frequently utilized therapeutic modality in the treatment of youth anxiety. It is outside of the scope of this chapter to discuss all available CBT protocols for child anxiety, but we mention several below. Further, we review a number of protocols within future chapters and also refer the reader to the website www.effectivechildtherapy.org as a resource.

One of the most studied empirically-supported CBT protocols for youth is the Coping Cat program, designed for children and adolescents with GAD, SAD, and SP (Kendall & Hedtke, 2006). Several randomized controlled trials (RCTs) support its efficacy (e.g., Kendall, 1994; Walkup et al., 2008) with gains maintained at one-year to seven-year follow-ups (Kendall et al., 2004; Puleo, Conner, Benjamin, & Kendall, 2011). Other programs with demonstrated efficacy include a group treatment for adolescents with SP (Stand Up, Speak Out; Albano & DiBartolo, 2007), Panic Control

Treatment for youth with PD (Pincus et al., 2010), and the Cool Kids program for children with various anxiety disorders (Hudson et al., 2009; Rapee et al., 2006). Newer protocols, including modular CBT (e.g., Building Confidence Program; Wood, McLeod, Hiruma, & Phan, 2008; Chiu et al., 2013) and computer-assisted programs (e.g., Camp Cope-A-Lot; Khanna & Kendall, 2008; and Cool Teens; Cunningham, Rapee, & Lyneham, 2007), show promising initial results in treating child anxiety disorders.

Although OCD is now classified in a chapter separate from other anxiety disorders in the *Diagnostic and Statistical Manual of Mental Disorders, Fifth Edition* (DSM-5; American Psychiatric Association, 2013), exposure therapy—called exposure and response prevention (ERP) in the context of OCD—is considered an efficacious treatment for youth with OCD (Barrett et al., 2008; Weisz et al., 2013). Indeed, exposure-based CBT is currently considered the first-line treatment for children and adolescents with OCD, with higher rates of treatment response and symptom/diagnostic remission than medication alone or combined treatment (e.g., Ivarsson et al., 2015; McGuire et al., 2015; Öst et al., 2016).

Despite the strong support for exposure-focused CBT, there is evidence that exposure is underutilized among community clinicians in their practice with anxious youth (Becker, Zayfert, & Anderson, 2004; Chu et al., 2015; Whiteside, Deacon, Benito, & Stewart, 2016). For example, a study of sessions conducted for anxious youth within a clinical practice at a large medical center indicated that in-session exposure was used less frequently (35% of sessions) than non-CBT supportive therapy (45% of sessions) (Whiteside et al., 2016). Over half of the anxious children in the study were never introduced to exposure. This underutilization may occur for a number of reasons: therapists may lack specific training in implementing exposure work, or may feel intimidated by aspects of exposure work, including the need to collect materials, leave the clinic to implement exposures, or extend the length of sessions as needed. Clinicians may also experience their own discomfort with the idea of generating anxiety or discomfort in their clients during the exposure process, or may not understand the underlying rationale for exposure-based work.

Despite the underutilization of exposure therapy in clinical practice, the evidence supporting exposure tasks as an essential ingredient of CBT for youth cannot be overstated. Research studies of CBT among youth with anxiety suggest that meaningful gains do not occur until exposure tasks are implemented (Kendall et al., 1997). In the largest RCT for youth with anxiety, the Child Anxiety Multimodal Study (CAMS), the introduction of exposure tasks in treatment was shown to accelerate the rate of improvement on measures of symptom severity and global functioning (Peris et al., 2014). In a second CAMS study, improvements in coping efficacy played a key role in treatment gains, and exposure tasks were believed to be largely responsible for improved coping efficacy (Kendall et al., 2016). Additionally, a study utilizing a modular CBT treatment manual for children (MCBT, Chorpita, 2007) demonstrated that exposure was the key element for decreasing both anxiety symptoms and cognitive errors (Nakamura, Pestle, & Chorpita, 2009). Variations in procedures for implementing exposure tasks (such as the amount of preparation, execution, and processing of the experience) have been examined, with post-exposure processing (and modification of maladaptive cognitive beliefs) significantly predicting greater improvement at post-treatment (Tiwari et al., 2013). Indeed, after conducting a meta-analysis, Ale, McCarthy, Rothschild, and Whiteside (2015) concluded that the potency of current treatment protocols for childhood anxiety disorders could be increased by offering exposure and post-exposure processing *earlier* and more *often*, with *less* time spent on general anxiety management strategies (such as relaxation and cognitive restructuring).

Conclusion

Anxiety disorders in children and adolescents are associated with significant distress and impairment. When left untreated, these impairments often persist into adulthood and are associated with comorbidities including substance use and mood disorders. As such, early intervention is critical. CBT, a well-established treatment for childhood anxiety disorders, targets maladaptive patterns of thinking and behaving. Exposure is the hallmark component of CBT for anxiety, directly targeting the negative reinforcement cycle that maintains anxiety. Despite its effectiveness, exposure therapy is unfortunately underutilized in the community.

Through this book, we strive to demystify exposure tasks and bolster their use among clinicians who treat pediatric anxiety disorders. To achieve this goal, beginning chapters offer detailed information and guidance in how to prepare children, adolescents, and their families for exposure work. This includes how to conduct a functional assessment, introduce the rationale for exposure to the client, coach and encourage parental involvement, and teach basic cognitive behavioral techniques to target faulty thinking and physiological reactivity. After exploring these foundations, we provide the basic principles and specific details for implementing exposure therapy, encompassing all steps from the initial design of an exposure hierarchy to managing session length and frequency, and utilizing reward systems. For those already well-versed in the use of exposure, we offer clinically meaningful suggestions to enhance the application of exposure tasks. Later chapters consist of disorder-specific guides that highlight important considerations for each condition and provide comprehensive lists of exposure ideas. We provide an array of creative and constructive suggestions for developing unique and effective exposures. We hope that you will utilize our book as a reference guide for implementing successful exposure therapy in your clinical practice.

CHAPTER 2

Clinical Assessment of Child Anxiety

Assessment is the cornerstone of exposure-based treatments. Understanding child and adolescent anxiety requires completing two distinct, but related, types of evaluations. The first, a *diagnostic assessment*, is intended to capture the clinical picture of the child's symptoms and impairments, including all necessary components for establishing a diagnosis. The second, a *functional behavioral analysis* (or functional assessment), is meant to gather information specific to the child's anxieties and fears. While the former evaluates how the youth is functioning compared to typical peers, the latter assesses the client's symptoms from a patient-centered perspective. This chapter will review both types of assessment methods as well as helpful self-reporting and clinician-administered assessment tools to aid therapists in establishing a diagnosis of anxiety, tracking symptoms over time, and establishing specific targets for exposure work.

Diagnostic Assessment

The purpose of the diagnostic assessment is to determine how a child is functioning and to assign (when appropriate) a diagnosis. Diagnostic assessment should happen both at the beginning of treatment and throughout the therapeutic process to measure changes in symptomology. Most diagnostic tools aim to assess the frequency, intensity, and duration of youths' anxiety symptoms; however, there are a number of procedures for attaining this information. Clinical interviews and rating scales are two of the most common methods in diagnostic assessment. While many therapists use both interviews and rating scales, a rating scale alone may be preferable if there is very limited time. Clinicians may also choose to conduct a school observation in which they assess the context and triggers of the anxiety within the school setting and track specific anxiety-related behaviors. For a child with frequent emotional meltdowns, this might involve identifying the triggers of these meltdowns and the response of school staff. Further, clinicians may consider "challenge tasks," such as observing the child directly in a feared situation. For example, in the case of a child with separation anxiety, the therapist may observe whether she is able to separate from her parent in the waiting room or play with the clinician alone.

Alongside any diagnostic approach, therapists should also include a thorough history of the presenting problem to evaluate possible organic causes of anxiety symptoms in children. For instance, pediatric autoimmune neuropsychiatric disorders (PANDAS) are believed to be caused by strep bacteria and can manifest in a variety of anxiety symptoms, including behaviors that look like OCD, tic disorder, or separation anxiety. A medical evaluation may also assess for conditions that trigger anxiety or physical sensations that can be misinterpreted as anxiety. These conditions may have potential implications for subsequent exposure work. For example, thyroid or adrenal gland problems, asthma, hypoglycemia, seizures, and tics are just a few examples of medical conditions that may result in physical sensations mimicking anxiety or exacerbate an anxious response. Clients should be encouraged to seek a medical evaluation or talk to their primary care doctors alongside a psychological assessment.

Eliciting information on developmental history is also necessary to rule out other conditions that may lead to avoidance or reduced social interaction—such as autism, aphasia, and cognitive disability (Viana, Beidel, & Rabian, 2009). For children with a developmental history of speech problems, a speech and language assessment is often an important part of the diagnostic process (Manassis et al., 2007). For example, many children with selective mutism (SM) display deficits in phonemic awareness, receptive language, and grammar ability.

Careful consideration should also be given to who provides information about the child's symptoms. Most diagnostic approaches utilize both child and caregiver reports in order to develop a complete picture of the child's problems in a variety of contexts. Other adults in the child's life (such as teachers, coaches, school nurse, pediatrician, school counselor, and extended family members) may also be important sources of information.

Given the number of possible avenues for assessing anxiety symptoms, selecting the right diagnostic tool can be a challenge. Time, resources, and feasibility should all be considered. Below, we review two of the most common methods for assessing symptomology: clinical interviews and rating scales.

Clinical Interviews

Diagnostic clinical interviews can take a number of forms, from fully structured to semistructured to unstructured. Each approach offers both advantages and disadvantages; however, research suggests that even highly skilled clinicians may disagree on diagnoses, especially when using unstructured diagnostic methods (Miller et al., 2001). In order to increase clinicians' ability to reliably and adequately diagnose anxiety disorders among youth, the use of structured or semistructured interviews is recommended. These "gold standard" clinical interviews have the advantage of being both comprehensive and flexible in their administration, and widely available for use in clinical practice.

One of the most common clinical interviews for children is the Kiddie Schedule for Affective Disorders and Schizophrenia—Present and Lifetime Version (K-SADS-PL). The K-SADS-PL is a semistructured interview that covers both current and past symptomology and includes a timeline to help the evaluator chronicle episodic disorders and understand recurrence and remittance of symptoms (Kaufman, Birmaher, Brent, & Rao, 1997). The K-SADS-PL begins with a screener that allows the therapist to quickly "rule out" some disorders and flag others for follow-up questioning. Parents and children are interviewed separately and a summary score is used to determine whether a child meets criteria for a specific disorder.

Another evidence-based option is the Anxiety Disorders Interview Schedule for DSM-IV for Children (ADIS-IV: C), developed by Silverman and Albano (1996), to assess a variety of anxiety symptoms as well as related disorders, including disruptive behaviors, substance use, disordered eating behaviors, and mood symptoms. The ADIS-IV: C guides the clinician through administering a series of questions, allowing him to administer related follow-up questions and skip irrelevant items where appropriate. Interviews are conducted with the parent and child individually, allowing the clinician to consider multiple sources of information to determine a diagnosis.

Rating Scales

Rating scales provide the advantage of being quickly and easily administered, allowing for easy charting of anxiety symptoms, as well as changes in specific anxious thoughts and avoidance behaviors associated with anxiety disorders. While a plethora of rating scales exist and a comprehensive review is beyond the scope of the current chapter, we have highlighted a few of the widely utilized scales below.

The Multidimensional Anxiety Scale for Children, 2nd Edition (MASC 2) is composed of 50 items that assess a variety of anxiety symptoms. Youth are asked to rate how true each item is for them on a 4-point scale, ranging from 0 (*never true about me*) to 3 (*often true about me*). The measure was developed by March et al. (1997) and is appropriate for use with youth between the ages of 8 and 19. A brief (10-item) version is also available and takes approximately 5 minutes for children to complete.

The Screen for Childhood Anxiety Related Emotional Disorders (SCARED) assesses behavioral, cognitive, and physical symptoms of a variety of disorders, including generalized anxiety, separation anxiety, social anxiety, and school refusal. This measure was created by Birmaher and colleagues (1997) for use with children over the age of 7, and consists of 41 items that the child rates on a 0-to-2 scale. Clinicians can choose to administer the entire measure or select specific, relevant modules.

The Spence Children's Anxiety Scale (SCAS) was written by Spence (1998). The measure consists of two parallel forms. The first is a 34-item form completed by the parent and is intended to assess symptoms in preschoolers, ages 2.5 to 6.5 years old. The second is a 45-item self-report measure for children ages 8 to 12. Each item is ranked on a 4-point scale, ranging from 0 (*never*) to 3 (*always*). The SCAS assesses separation anxiety, social anxiety, OCD, panic disorder, generalized anxiety, and concerns regarding physical injury.

The Children's Yale-Brown Obsessive Compulsive Scale (CY-BOCS) was developed by Scahill and colleagues (1997) to assess youths' OCD symptoms. Clinicians rate each of 10 pediatric OCD symptoms on five criteria, including: (1) how time consuming the OCD symptoms are, (2) how much symptoms interfere with daily functioning, (3) how much distress the symptoms cause, (4) how easily the child can resist the compulsions, and (5) how much control the child feels over each symptom. The measure is validated for children ages 6 to 14 and a number of adaptations for special populations (such as OCD symptoms in children with autism spectrum disorders) are available.

The Social Phobia and Anxiety Inventory for Children (SPAI-C) is a youth-report measure created by Beidel, Turner, and Morris (1995). The measure is 26 items long and assesses thoughts, behaviors, and specific physical complaints common to social anxiety. The child reports how often she experiences symptoms related to social phobia on a scale from 0 (*never or hardly ever*) to 2 (*most of the time or always*).

Functional Behavioral Assessment

The second critical target for assessment is an understanding of the internal and external factors that play a role in the initiation and maintenance of anxiety in the youth's life. As opposed to the diagnostic assessment, which seeks to gather concrete data on symptom severity, impairment, and duration, the functional behavioral analysis (FBA), or functional assessment, is intended to understand the larger context of the anxiety-related problems. The FBA will therefore provide the foundational information the therapist will use to craft his specific exposure-based treatment plan.

To that end, the purpose of the FBA is to understand the specific factors or stimuli (objects, images, people, and situations) that trigger anxiety, and their association with the thoughts, feelings, and behaviors that happen before, during, and after the anxiety-producing situation. Just like the diagnostic assessment, an FBA should be completed in the beginning of treatment, but also at various points during treatment to ascertain any changes in the context of the child's anxiety.

By the end of the FBA, the clinician should be able to identify most (if not all) of the following components of the youth's anxiety:

- What situations or triggers are associated with the child feeling anxious?

- What does the child think will happen if she is made to stay in the anxiety-producing situation? What does she think will happen if she can't immediately reduce her own anxiety?

- What types of behaviors does the child do to avoid either the situation or the resulting distress or negative feelings? What are her safety behaviors?

- How are these safety behaviors maintained? What role do others (her parents, siblings, or other trusted adults) play in maintaining these actions?

- How do these behaviors affect her life? What is she missing out on?

The FBA will likely take one or more sessions to complete. We've mapped out a six-step plan to conducting an FBA with an anxious child below. While we suggest that a clinician follow the general outline below, there may be times where it makes sense to move some of the steps around. For instance, sometimes it's easier for the child to identify the anxious behaviors she engages in first, and then identify the situations and thoughts that surround those behaviors. Being flexible in this approach will allow the clinician to collect rich information that will form the basis of effective exposure therapy.

Develop the Rationale for the FBA

The therapist should start by introducing the rationale for the FBA to the child and (where applicable) guardian.

Therapist: Today, I'd like us to put our heads together to dive a bit deeper and understand a little more about what makes [whatever the client's fears are] so scary. We are going to try to understand more about some of the times you felt afraid or worried and your fears got in the way of you doing something. In order to really understand what happened, I want to know what happened before, during, and after the situation. So, your job is to be a sportscaster and describe the play by play of what happened, just as if we were describing each moment in a game. I also want you to tell me about the thoughts and feelings going on inside of you during this time. I will help by asking you questions as we go. Sharing all of this information will help us come up with a plan to help you feel better. How does that sound?

The most important thing is to help the child understand that he and the therapist will be working together to better understand his anxiety. While the therapist may be the expert in treating anxiety, it is important to underscore for the child that he is the expert in his own thoughts, feelings, and behaviors.

Generate a List of Anxiety-Triggering Situations

The child will work with the therapist to generate a list of situations that he or his parents find challenging. Understanding what situations trigger anxiety is critical not only for gaining a better understanding of how the child's anxiety manifests, but also for creating the exposure hierarchy in the following sessions. Therefore, careful attention should be paid to making sure the therapist has developed a comprehensive understanding of what the youth identifies as anxiety producing and, relatedly, what things spur the child's problematic behaviors. Triggers of anxiety are often called "fear cues" and fall largely into one of three categories: environmental stimuli, bodily or physiological sensations, and intrusive anxious thoughts.

ENVIRONMENTAL STIMULI

Environmental stimuli can include any specific external situation, object, or environmental context. For example, for a child with a dog phobia, coming across a dog in the street would likely constitute a fear cue. Seeing a dog in a photograph or in a movie may also elicit similar levels of anxiety. The therapist should take care to understand both the central trigger (in this case, a dog) and the related, generalized triggers (the photo or movie).

BODILY OR PHYSIOLOGICAL SENSATIONS

Changes in bodily or physiological sensations may also serve as a trigger for anxiety. Children may point to specific physical complaints that are associated with the onset of anxiety, such as stomachaches, headaches, fatigue, dizziness, and increased heart rate. While it is important to help the child understand that these sensations are related to her anxiety, it is also critical (especially at this stage of the evaluation) to validate the child's experience of these somatic symptoms and ensure that she doesn't feel that the therapist is accusing her of "faking" illness.

INTRUSIVE ANXIOUS THOUGHTS

Finally, distressing thoughts, images, or flashbacks may trigger anxiety in a child. These may be thoughts that the child finds embarrassing or upsetting. For example, a child may have repetitive, intrusive thoughts about engaging in sexual acts with a peer. Or a child with a sexual abuse history may have "flashbacks" to images from the assault. Often these thoughts are experienced as so distressing that children may be reluctant to share them with the therapist. As with other fear triggers, the therapist should seek to validate the child's feelings and convey that the therapist is not disgusted or distressed by the content of these thoughts.

Given the distressing nature of these triggers, it is often difficult for children to identify and share what immediately precedes their anxiety. For younger children it may be helpful to have the parent or guardian in the room to help elicit examples of problematic situations. For older children who are self-conscious of these triggers, it may be preferable to meet without the parent present.

The therapist may ask questions like:

What are some of the hardest things for you to do because you feel nervous?

What are some of the things that make you feel the most afraid?

What are you doing when your [stomach/head/chest] starts to really hurt [feel funny]?

What are some of the scary thoughts or pictures that pop into your head before you feel very nervous [uncomfortable/upset/disgusted]?

What do to you try to avoid doing or get out of because it feels too scary?

What are the things that you are doing [not doing] that frustrate your parents?

In cases where the child is having trouble identifying specific problems, the therapist may incorporate information gathered from the clinical interview to guide the child toward identifying problematic behaviors. Let's take the example of a 12-year-old girl with social anxiety. The clinician asked her a series of questions regarding situations that made her feel nervous and she generated the following list:

1. Going to the bathroom at school

2. Eating lunch at school

3. Hearing my stomach make gurgling noises

4. Feeling butterflies in my stomach

5. Talking to people I don't know well

6. Talking during class

7. Picturing people making fun of the way I talk

8. Changing into gym clothes in the locker room

Evaluate Anxious Attitudes and Beliefs

Once a list of anxiety-triggering situations has been generated, the therapist will assess the dysfunctional attitudes and beliefs that go along with these fear cues. One way to identify these thoughts is to ask a series of "what would happen if this happened" questions. This approach allows the therapist to gently query the child to uncover the core beliefs underlying her concern with being exposed to the anxiety-provoking stimuli. For example, this may be a fear of death or bodily injury, separation from loved ones, or ridicule and rejection from peers. The script below demonstrates the use of this technique with a 10-year-old with separation anxiety:

Therapist: So the problem you mentioned was walking from your mom's car into the school building in the morning. Can you tell me a little more about why that is so scary?

Child: I don't know; I just don't like to go in. I hate having to walk past all of those other kids in the hallway. And sometimes I get lost and I can hear them laughing at me.

Therapist: I see—that does sound kind of scary! So, just so I'm sure I understand, what do you think would happen if you got lost on your way to class in the morning?

Child: All the kids would laugh at me.

Therapist: Ah, they would laugh. What would that mean, if they laughed at you?

Child: That they're making fun of me. That they don't like me or want to be my friend.

Therapist: Huh, I see. And what would happen if those kids weren't your friends?

Child: Then I wouldn't have any friends, and everyone would know I'm a loser.

Therapist: And if everyone knew you were a loser?

Child: I wouldn't have anyone to hang out with and I would be all alone.

During this initial evaluative period the therapist will primarily use this technique to understand the child's dysfunctional thoughts and attitudes. As the therapy progresses to conducting exposures, however, the therapist will return to these beliefs and attempt to challenge them using evidence from the exposure practices.

Understand Safety Behaviors

Once the therapist understands the child's fear cues and their related dysfunctional attitudes, the therapist should next seek to understand the behaviors that serve to maintain or exacerbate these anxious symptoms. These actions are often called "safety behaviors" because, paradoxically, the child believes that by engaging in them, he is keeping himself safe. Some common types of safety behaviors are described below.

AVOIDANCE

Avoidance behaviors may take the form of active or passive avoidance of activities or situations that are associated with fear cues. For instance, a child with a water phobia may avoid going to camp because he knows that he will have to participate in a swim test. Another child may keep her face covered with her hands when she watches a movie in order to avoid inadvertently seeing something she is scared of. Other forms of avoidance may be difficult to immediately notice. For example, a child may hold his breath every time he drives past a graveyard because he is afraid of ghosts. In some cases, a child may avoid objects or situations that have become associated in her mind with the given fear. For example, an adolescent with a vomit phobia refuses to wear purple nail polish after vomiting repeatedly one day when she had on purple polish.

REASSURANCE SEEKING

Anxious children may excessively seek reassurance from adults and other trusted individuals to confirm specific information about their fears. While all children seek out some level of assurance from their caregivers, maladaptive reassurance seeking can be differentiated from more adaptive support seeking in that it: (1) doesn't provide new information for the child and (2) does not result in the child feeling more confident in the face of the fear cue. For instance, a child with a severe weather phobia may repeatedly ask his mother to look at a weather map and confirm that a storm is not approaching. Or, a youth with OCD may ask her teacher repeatedly if her hands are clean after she touches various objects. These children are not using their own problem-solving and coping skills to manage the worry and self soothe. In contrast, they are over-relying on adult responses for continued and excessive reassurance.

CHECKING, COUNTING, AND OTHER COMPULSIVE RITUALS

Anxious youth may create and compulsively engage in specific rituals that they have come to believe will help them gain a sense of control over their distress. These rituals are often excessive (such as washing hands for 15 minutes after using the bathroom) or not realistically related to the desired outcome (such as having to sing a specific song while driving in the car in order to keep the family from crashing). Other examples include a child with OCD who may insist on arranging objects in his bedroom in a specific manner before going to sleep or a youth with a choking phobia who insists on chewing her food a specified number of times before swallowing.

SAFETY OBJECTS

Children may believe that a specific object can keep them safe while in its presence. These objects can range from a good luck charm to antianxiety medication. While the child may not always use the object in any purposeful way when faced with a fear cue, he may believe that the presence of the object decreases or negates the feared outcome. For example, a child may need to always have a cell phone on him in case he has a medical emergency and needs to call an ambulance. A child with a vomit phobia may insist that a garbage pail be next to her bed each night. An adolescent with fear of panic and bodily sensations may carry his water bottle with him wherever he goes.

MENTAL RITUALS

Anxious children may engage in a variety of mental rituals to decrease their feelings of distress. These rituals typically decrease the child's distress in the short term; however, they are ultimately maladaptive because the child is using the ritual to actively avoid any attention to or experience with the fearful stimuli. Sometimes these rituals will be difficult to identify because they resemble coping techniques that the therapist has taught the child. The important distinction here is that the child is using the technique to avoid an experience with the fearful stimulus, rather than to manage her anxiety in an adaptive way while she approaches or experiences the fear. For instance, one child may seek to repress all negative thoughts and images regarding the fear and refuse to acknowledge them. Another child may use deep breathing techniques during an exposure exercise to avoid feeling any physical sensations of distress.

When talking with the child about which safety behaviors he engages in, it is also important to understand the larger context of why he performs these actions. For instance, a child may refuse to use the bathroom at school because he is afraid that other children will overhear embarrassing noises. By understanding why the child is avoiding use of the bathroom, the therapist can use this information to design effective exposures that seek to help the child learn that he can manage his embarrassment at school. The therapist may say:

When we are feeling scared we often do things to try to make that feeling go away. For instance, we might try to leave the room or run away. Or we might do little things that we think will help calm us down—like we might stay really close to our mother, or put our head down so that no one can see us or we cannot see what is scaring us. We call these things 'safety behaviors' because they make us feel safe at the time. I want to understand some of the things you do to feel safe and why you think these things help you. Can you think of any safety behaviors that you use?

Identify Accommodating Behavior

Next, the therapist should seek to understand the role of family members and other important people in the youth's life. Sometimes even well-meaning parents behave in ways that allow their child to continue to engage in behaviors that maintain or increase anxiety. This is called "parental accommodation" and includes any behaviors that the parent engages in that support the child's safety behaviors. For instance, for a child with a germ phobia who engages in excessive hand washing, the parents' choice to continue buying excessive amounts of soap could be seen as an accommodating behavior. Alternatively, the parent of a child with social phobia may accommodate this anxiety by writing notes excusing the child's absence from school on days when she has to give a presentation.

Most parents find themselves engaging in these behaviors because they experience their child's distress as overwhelming. This topic will be addressed in considerable detail in chapter 3. It is important to ask the parent directly about these behaviors. The therapist may consider asking questions like:

You mentioned that [your child] often refuses to go to school. How have you handled that with the teachers in the past?

It must be hard to have your child constantly seeking your reassurance. What do you do when he asks you for assurance?

You mentioned that your child asks you to always have her bottle of antianxiety medication with you. How do you handle that?

It sounds like your child gets pretty upset when he can't sit in the seat that he wants to in the car. What do you do when it is time for the entire family to go somewhere together?

Understand the Consequences of Anxiety

Finally, the therapist should seek to understand the consequences of engaging in safety behaviors. Given that the child may be focusing on the proximal outcomes of these actions, including the immediate relief of distress, the distal negative impact of avoiding anxiety may not be immediately obvious to her. In this section, the therapist will attempt to understand how this anxiety, and its related avoidance behaviors, have impacted the child's life.

Specifically, clinicians should gather information on how avoidance behaviors may have gotten in the way of: (1) school and academic outcomes, (2) social opportunities and interpersonal relationships, (3) family functioning, (4) extracurricular and athletic pursuits, and (5) taking part in important and valued activities. The therapist may ask questions like:

In what ways does being anxious make it hard for you to do things?

How does your fear or anxiety affect your relationship with your parents/friends/teachers? Do they get upset/annoyed with you because of certain things you do when you are scared or anxious?

What would you be able to do if you weren't so afraid of [fear cue]?

How would your life change if you didn't have to [engage in the safety behavior]?

Identifying the consequences of avoidance behavior not only provides rich information on how anxiety has impacted the child's life, but also sets the stage for creating the motivation to change these anxious behaviors. This section is the starting point for engaging the child in the difficult work of exposure therapy and allows the therapist to set the expectation that, by challenging these dysfunctional beliefs and actions, the child can master his own anxiety.

Conclusion

Assessment is the foundation of providing effective therapy and a critical piece in the development of a successful exposure-based intervention. Without a clear understanding of both the child's diagnostic picture and the role of anxiety in her life, it is difficult to formulate an accurate case conceptualization and plan for structuring subsequent exposure sessions. While we often think of evaluating symptoms as the first step in therapy, it is important to remember that assessment should happen at regular intervals throughout the therapeutic process. We need to establish a clear picture of how the child is currently functioning, as well as how her symptoms are changing over the course of therapy. We will use this information to develop a fear hierarchy, or step-by-step plan, for challenging the fear.

CHAPTER 3

Parental Involvement and Accommodation

Parents are key figures in successfully treating children with anxiety disorders. Relationship dynamics between the parent and child, parental psychopathology, and parental knowledge and skills are all significant factors in both the development and treatment of anxiety in youth. This chapter will explore how the dynamic relationship between parent and child factors into the development and maintenance of child anxiety. We will look at the common traps parents fall into when attempting to help their child with anxiety. Finally, we will discuss techniques to teach parents to effectively guide their child in facing fears. These skills will prepare them for the more specific exposure protocol discussed with the parent and child in chapter 5. These approaches will also prepare caregivers for subsequently tolerating their child's discomfort as he works on fear-related goals, encouraging his persistence with difficult tasks, and refraining from behaviors that reinforce his anxiety.

Parental Anxiety and Accommodation

A number of factors contribute to the development of childhood anxiety. In particular, research suggests that parental mental health may play an important role. Indeed, the likelihood that a child develops an anxiety disorder increases by a factor of six if her parent is also diagnosed with an anxiety disorder (Burstein, Ginsburg, & Tein, 2010). Research also suggests that this relationship can proceed in the opposite direction: higher levels of child anxiety can affect parental behavior, leading parents to engage in more overprotective and controlling parenting behaviors (e.g. Gouze, Hopkins, Bryant, & Lavigne, 2016). In other words, symptoms of anxiety in parents and their children influence each other in a bidirectional manner, such that as one increases, so does the other. Consider, for instance, a kindergartener going to school for the first time. The child displays some natural hesitation about walking into a classroom full of strangers for the first time. He then looks to his mother, who sees that he is afraid and becomes anxious herself, imagining how frightened her child is. Her posture begins to stiffen and she breathes quickly, grabbing her child's hand. The child interprets these cues to mean that his mother doesn't believe the situation is safe, thus increasing his own level of anxiety. In this case, the child's anxiety cued his mother's anxious response that, in turn, served to increase his own level of fear. Thus, we can think of the relationship between parent and child anxiety as part of a larger cycle, one in which each individual implicitly or explicitly engages in behaviors that serve to elevate the level of anxiety in the other.

Indeed, in many cases, parents of anxious children pay more attention to their children's anxiety-driven behaviors than their brave acts. This *positive reinforcement* both provides something that the child craves (attention) and serves to increase the likelihood that the child will engage in the anxious behavior again. For instance, a child who screams and hides behind her parents when meeting a new adult is likely to receive a reassuring hug, whereas the child who bravely says "hello" to the stranger is unlikely to be noticed. Again in this instance, the child's anxiety propels the parent to react in an anxious manner herself, trying to comfort, soothe, or remove the child from the situation. Many parents are uncomfortable with the idea of allowing the child space to struggle with and manage his own anxiety. Giving excess attention to anxious behaviors may serve to inadvertently reinforce them, causing these responses to increase over time. As another example, parents with poor frustration tolerance skills may come across as reactive and angry in stressful situations, modeling maladaptive coping strategies for their child and increasing child anxiety due to the perception that their environment is out of control, unsafe, or unstable. Alternatively, a child's extreme or aggressive reactions may lead to increased parental anxiety and harsher responses on the part of parents.

How Do Parents Accommodate?

While this book spends considerable time exploring the role of child avoidance in increasing anxiety, parents also often *accommodate* their children in the avoidance of stressful or anxiety-provoking experiences and feelings. Parental accommodation is defined as any parental behavior that attempts to reduce a child's exposure to distressing situations that are, in fact, safe or age appropriate, or parental behavior that supports the child's avoidance of distressing feelings. Unfortunately, attempting to shield and protect their child from experiencing and working through feelings in the moment does a major disservice to their child (e.g. Thompson-Hollands, Kerns, Pincus, & Comer, 2014). It teaches the child that distressing feelings are too overwhelming for her to handle on her own and that it is better to avoid situations that produce strong negative feelings. This message often leads children to connect perceived safety with their avoidance of the situation over time.

Most accommodating behaviors fall into one of three categories. First, parents may engage in a cyclical pattern that results when they provide excessive reassurance to their child. Specifically, anxious children may turn to their parents to provide certainty about what will happen in any given situation. However, the relief the child feels from having a parent reassure him that he is safe provides only a short-term, immediate decrease in anxiety. Soon after, the child beings to feel distress again and attempts to gain additional parental reassurance, thus creating a negative cycle that ultimately serves to *increase* negative emotions.

Second, parents may escalate their child's anxiety by allowing or encouraging their avoidance of feared situations. For instance, for a child who is nervous about going to a swimming lesson, the parent may allow her to skip the practice session (*direct avoidance*), tell the teacher to not make her get into the pool if she is nervous (*requiring others to accommodate the child's avoidance*), or physically get into the pool with her child (*engaging in overprotective behaviors*).

Third, parents may increase their child's anxiety by minimizing the child's perceived ability to control his own feelings or behaviors. For instance, a parent may tell a child that he is an "anxious person" or that these feelings "run in the family." Labeling a child in this way displaces the child's internal locus of control or self-efficacy (the child's belief in his ability to have control over himself and influence on the world around him). This behavior also implies that anxious feelings are stable and uncontrollable. Similarly, parents may be overly permissive in their tolerance for their child's emotion-driven negative or destructive behaviors. Excusing anxiety-related irritability or aggression as outside of the child's responsibility sends a clear signal to the child that these behaviors are acceptable and that the child isn't expected (or able) to control his own impulses. Alternatively, parents may tell the child exactly what to do in each situation, preventing the child from developing his own coping strategies and learning how to problem solve in a variety of life situations. Children may misinterpret these signals and instructions as the parent's belief that they do not have the coping capacity to handle or develop solutions to their own problems.

EXAMPLES OF ACCOMMODATING BEHAVIORS

Below are some examples of typical parental accommodation:

Driving the child back home after she refuses to engage in an anxiety-producing activity

Allowing the child to cancel activities that she is afraid of

Writing notes that excuse the child from taking part in activities she fears

Going with the child into feared situations when it is inappropriate for parents to join the activity

Purchasing items for the child that are needed to complete ritualistic behaviors, or agreeing to participate in the ritual

Why Do Parents Accommodate?

Parental accommodation of children's behavior may happen for a number of reasons. For instance, parents may believe that anxiety is harmful to their child or that their child cannot tolerate distress. Thus, they accommodate their child's avoidant behaviors in an effort to reduce uncomfortable feelings. Alternatively, parents may experience their own anxiety when observing their child in distress and seek to relieve these negative emotions by colluding in their child's avoidance. Or, parents may find the child's reaction to anxious situations (especially aggressive or destructive behaviors) too hard to cope with and may choose to accommodate their anxiety as the "path of least resistance." Unresolved concerns from their own childhoods can also play a role in parental accommodation. For example, a parent who experienced harshness or abuse as a child may swing in the opposite direction as an adult; that is, he may now be reluctant to set limits or boundaries, including appropriate and reasonable ones, on his own child's behavior.

Assessment of Parental Accommodation

Teasing apart appropriate parental reactions to anxiety (including validating feelings and scaffolding difficult behaviors) from accommodating behaviors (including providing excessive reassurance and taking over difficult tasks for the child) can be challenging at times. Approaches to assessing parental accommodation are discussed in greater detail in chapter 2. In particular, conducting a functional behavior assessment is a helpful tool in identifying specific parental behaviors in response to child anxiety. For instance, the therapist helps the parent map out what behaviors she engages in immediately following her child's display of anxiety, how the child responds, what the parent does next, and whether this serves to increase or decrease the child's anxiety in the long run.

Further, self-report questionnaires, such as the Family Accommodation Scale—Anxiety (FASA; Lebowitz et al., 2013) may be useful for evaluating specific accommodating behaviors, as well as for helping parents better understand their own roles in the maintenance of their children's anxiety.

Parental Emotion Regulation and Anxiety Management

In many cases, it makes good sense for anxious parents to seek individual therapy concurrent with their child's therapy. This can arm them with tools for managing their own anxiety and addressing their own vulnerabilities. Alternatively, parents can be taught basic CBT skills for anxiety management in small doses, integrated throughout child-focused sessions. For example, the topic of the week can be discussed with both parent and child together, or parents can be given similar homework to practice the in-session skills taught during the week. While the teaching of adult anxiety management is beyond the scope of this book, we highlight below a few important concepts related to parental awareness and modeling of emotions that we feel are critical topics to address with parents during the therapy process.

Parent Self-Monitoring

Having parents engage in self-monitoring, such as recording their thoughts, feelings, and behaviors during stressful situations with their child, can increase their awareness of how those thoughts, feelings, and behaviors, in turn, impact their child's level of anxiety. We recommend that parents keep a simple tracking form during the week, with columns for *Trigger Situation, Emotion Intensity, My Response,* and *Child Response.* The tracking form helps them observe which situations typically trigger strong emotions, rate the intensity of those emotions (such as on a 1-to-10 scale), record their verbal and nonverbal responses, and observe their child's responses. Through this process, they can better understand how their responses are connected to their child's responses and brainstorm adjustments they can make in their approach that will facilitate reductions in their child's anxiety and increases in confidence and brave behavior.

Parents as Coping Models

We strongly recommend that you support parents in working toward healthy emotion regulation and resilience in their own lives and particularly in the presence of their child. They should not be expected or encouraged to be infallible cookie cutter parents devoid of negative emotion, but rather, "coping beings" who think and feel, manage and regulate their emotions in the moment, problem solve, and flexibly adjust to changes in their environment. We encourage parents to share emotions with their child within appropriate limits given the child's age and development. That is, we feel it is helpful for children to observe their parents successfully managing emotions regarding minor situations or events that they can reasonably tolerate hearing about. In contrast, children should not be burdened with adult problems or made to feel responsible for fixing their parents' problems. Further, observing parents feeling helpless, out of control, or stuck in an emotional experience can be detrimental to youth.

Imagine two contrasting scenarios: In the first, a mother locks her keys in the car. She immediately feels a rush of panic, and as a result, shakes and looks disoriented. She repeats nervous statements such as, "What are we going to do now?" "I can't believe this happened," "We will never get to the party on time," or "I don't know what to do." She remains stuck and unable to take action. As she is lost in her own negative, anxiety-provoking thoughts and unable to regulate her own physiological response, the child's anxiety levels increase. The child perceives the situation as dangerous and expects a negative outcome, given his mother's strong response and nervous statements. He observes her as unable to cope with the given situation, which results in considerable uncertainty, anxiety, and helpless feelings on the part of the child.

In contrast, imagine this same mother again locks her keys in the car, but she has now learned skills to effectively manage her response. Upon recognition of the keys in her car, her heart rate immediately speeds up and she notices panic sensations. She tells her child that she is feeling anxious and needs a moment to calm down. She proceeds to sit down and regulate her breathing by taking long, slow belly breaths. She verbalizes her approach to her child: "When Mommy feels nervous, I take long, slow breaths. This helps my body slow down." She then uses her experience and practice with challenging negative thoughts and managing uncertainty to model this behavior for her child. This time, the parent demonstrates coping actions in an effort to solve the problem, and conveys to the child that she can handle the situation despite her nervousness: "I am feeling worried about us being locked out of the car, but I know we can handle this. I am going to call our car insurance company to get help. We might have to wait a little bit, but that is the worst of it. I am not sure whether we will get to the party on time, but if we're late I bet we can stay a little later to make up for it. If not, we will plan another get-together with our friends soon." All of these messages teach the child that anxiety and difficult situations can be tolerated and managed successfully.

Parents as Models for Managing Change, Uncertainty, and Failure

Along these same lines, it can be beneficial to have parents explore in therapy their personal needs for order, perfection, and certainty, and their adherence or rigidity to certain routines or outcomes, and whether they may be modeling these behaviors for their child. For example, do the parents keep their home cleaned to perfection, demonstrating frustration or agitation when anything is out of place? Do they avoid any risk taking for fear of failure? Do they search for 100% certainty before making a decision? Do they become overwhelmed when the schedule or routine does not go as planned? Do they demonstrate negative self-talk in the presence of their child? In what ways are these temperamental styles impacting their child? As the therapist, you can facilitate the parents' exploration of how their own anxiety and behavioral tendencies impact their child. What are they teaching and modeling for their child through their own behavior? What skills and techniques can they utilize to move toward flexibility in the face of uncertain, unexpected, or unwanted situations; acceptance of their own mistakes; regulation of their emotional states; an ability to approach fearful situations; and healthy decision making?

Effective and Empathic Responding to Child Anxiety

We thus far have been discussing how parents can become more aware of their own internal emotional experiences and behavioral response patterns with the goal of learning to model adaptive emotion regulation. Similarly, parents are also best served when we can aid them in developing specific skills to respond effectively when their child demonstrates fear, worry, uncertainty, or self-doubt. Below, we highlight critical guidelines for parents to consider in effectively responding to their child's anxiety. These practices also serve as a foundation for parents as they subsequently learn to become effective exposure coaches for their children.

For the clinician, there are a multitude of avenues for teaching these skills. Discussion and exploration of concepts, soliciting questions and concerns from parents, checking for understanding, and addressing perceived obstacles are a few of the most common. In addition, whenever possible, clinicians should observe parent interactions with their child and offer gentle, constructive feedback as needed. In some cases, families may be open to videotaping dialogue or interactions from the home setting for subsequent discussion in the clinic with the therapist. Role-play of skills with the therapist is another fundamental means for reinforcing and practicing the skills discussed. During family sessions, parents can practice the guidelines below as their child demonstrates anxiety during in-session exposure practice.

Occasionally parents become resistant to utilizing new techniques. In some cases, it may be that they believe the focus of therapy should be exclusively on the child. In that instance, it may be helpful to reframe these techniques as ways in which the parent can feel empowered to fill the role of the "at-home therapist." Alternatively, resistant parents may also feel that they have failed in the past and are ill equipped or unwilling to try new techniques for dealing with their distressed child. Motivational approaches are often beneficial, including statements such as: "It sounds like you've tried a lot of different methods to help your daughter that haven't worked in the past. I have some new ideas that we can try together. Even if these don't work, every time we try something new, we are gathering more information on what does and does not work for her, and we will be able to refine these techniques together to find something that is helpful."

The following section lists several principles or tools to share with parents in order to help them approach their anxious child:

Principle 1: Summarize and Validate the Child's Experience

The first principle involves teaching the parents to provide brief and calm validation of the child's feelings when the child expresses anxiety, uncertainty, worry, or panic. We encourage parents to avoid long dialogues, negotiations, or arguments with the child. That is, parents should offer a brief summary, reflection, or acknowledgement of the child's feelings (such as "I understand you are frustrated"), without attempting to alter, change, negate, or critique the child's emotional experience. Parents and other caretakers should avoid telling the child that he should not be afraid, or minimize the anxiety by telling him that he is not really that afraid—both of which may invalidate the child's experience. In contrast, they should check in with the child to ensure that they understand the nature of his feeling.

Here are some examples of validating statements:

It sounds like you are feeling uncertain about attending the soccer game today. Is that correct?

I think I understand. You are telling me that you are scared to sleep in your room alone tonight.

Principle 2: Encourage the Use of Coping Skills

It is critical to remind parents that providing all the answers and fixing problems should not be their primary goal. In contrast, we want to support them in helping their child develop an ability to appropriately seek new information and experiences and effectively cope with the feelings that arise. That is, the only way to overcome anxiety is to experience anxiety. Therapists can prompt parents to ask open-ended questions that encourage the child to take ownership of and practice use of her coping skills. Parents and other caretakers should not do the problem-solving work for the child. They should avoid telling her exactly what to do, as this may increase resistance and passivity and reduce personal responsibility. Instead, they should focus on scaffolding adaptive responses for their child. If she struggles with generating options to handle her fear, it is reasonable for parents to present some suggestions. Parents should also make sure to provide positive attention for any effort on the child's part to participate in these conversations and utilize her coping skills. To understand the rationale for this, it can be helpful to suggest to parents that: "Just as a building being constructed requires structural support until it is well developed and sturdy enough to stand on its own, your job as the parent is to provide just enough scaffolding and support to allow growth to continue."

Here are some examples of encouraging statements and questions:

"What skills can you use to handle these feelings?"

"How can you challenge that scary thought?"

"What do you think about trying _____?"

"I wonder if you have considered _____?"

"I am so proud of you for coming up with ideas to try to handle this."

Principle 3: Maintain Reasonable Boundaries

Therapy should also focus on teaching parents to reduce avoidance by setting boundaries and expectations that are consistent with the child's coping abilities, developmental level, and progress in treatment. Appropriate expectations should push children to use their coping abilities to manage a low to moderate level of anxiety in feared situations. For instance, a child afraid of being separated from his parents might not yet be expected to tolerate his parents leaving the building during gymnastics practice, but might be expected to allow his parents to leave the gymnastics floor briefly to make a phone call or use the restroom. For expectations that are too high or not yet attainable, treatment will focus on a series of goals that move the youth toward increased coping capacity in these situations.

For situations in which parents are struggling to set a reasonable limit, it may be helpful to engage with the parents in behavioral rehearsal. This is a technique in which you and the parents identify common situations that have, in the past, triggered parental accommodation, and come up with specific strategies for them to use as an alternative to accommodating. You can then role-play these situations in therapy sessions to help them manage their own behaviors during high-stress interactions. For instance, a child with social anxiety may try to avoid going to school on a day when she has to give a presentation in class. A common parental accommodation behavior may be to allow her to stay home from school and to write the teacher a note saying the child was sick. The therapist and the parents may, instead, come up with a plan to tell the child that she needs to go to school and that they will not write a note. The therapist and parents should then role-play the child's (likely) escalation of negative behaviors, as well as an empathic response to their child that allows them to manage their own anxiety without giving in to her requests.

Here are some examples:

I promise that I will not leave the building during Tae Kwon Do today. But I will need to use the bathroom and will be gone for about 5 minutes. I know you can handle this. If you feel nervous, what skills can you use?

We have to go to school today. These are the rules and I am not willing to negotiate.

I understand you are upset, but I cannot participate in your ritual. Please use your skills for challenging these thoughts. I know you can do it.

Principle 4: Avoid Reinforcing Negative Behavior

As described in detail earlier in this chapter, parents of anxious children often inadvertently give more attention to their child's anxious behaviors compared to times of bravery or confidence. For example, they may excessively reassure the child that everything will be okay, coax, negotiate, plead, lecture, or reprimand, or give excessive hugs and physical comfort. They may provide continued attention at times when their child is engaged in negative behavior such as yelling, hitting, or making demands. Parents must be educated in this key behavioral principle: children will work for adult attention, both positive and negative, and whatever parents give their attention to will be reinforced and increase in frequency over time (Forehand & Long, 1996). Further, research has found that while negative parental attention such as lecturing or reprimands might force compliance in the immediate moment, it ultimately reinforces negative child behavior in the long run. Therefore, parents should aim to remove or limit their attention for negative child behaviors such as whining, complaining, demanding, and yelling. Instead, they should provide brief validation and encourage their child's use of coping skills. Further, they should consider limiting their verbal responses to the child's attempts for repeated reassurance in anxiety-provoking situations.

In many situations, there exist natural outcomes or repercussions for avoiding a given activity or exhibiting a negative behavior. Instead of focusing on an extended verbal dialogue with the child, parents should offer brief encouragement to engage in the activity, remind him of the limits present, and allow logical or natural consequences to function for negative behavior that occurs. Reasonable consequences for yelling, hitting, or other escalated behavior may involve removing a privilege, not earning a point on a reward chart, or not being able to participate in a preferred activity. Removal of parental attention or active ignoring, in which the parents remove all attention from their child for a short period of time while yelling or aggressive behavior is occurring, should also be considered as a natural consequence. Alternatively, if parents attempt to protect their child from the natural consequences, jump in and try to fix the situation, or provide considerable positive attention for the avoidant behavior, the child will not learn how to manage his emotional responses or anxiety. Allowing him to sit with and experience anxiety in the moment without rescuing or enabling his avoidance or aggressive responding gives him the opportunity to learn to tolerate anxiety and increase self-confidence. In these moments, parental modeling of calm behavior and expression of confidence in the child's ability to handle the situation conveys to him that the situation is not a crisis, he does not need rescue, and the parent believes he has the skills to manage it.

In addition to having parents refrain from directly answering reassurance-seeking questions or engaging in behaviors that support avoidance or safety behaviors, it is helpful to give parents language to use when faced with these questions or requests. Instead of just ignoring the questions or requests, you and parents can help children recognize when questions or requests might be anxiety-driven and learn to externalize the anxiety (for example: "That sounds like the anxiety talking. I don't want to strengthen it, so I'm not going to do what you are asking me to do. This way I can help you get stronger instead."). Furthermore, you and parents can provide validation without reassurance about the specific concern at hand (for example: "I know this is challenging for you, but I am confident you can be stronger than the anxiety.").

Example Situations

Here are some examples of situations and ways to handle them:

For the child who refuses to go to school, a plan should be developed in advance. For example, a school counselor could be present at parent drop-off to walk the child into the school. The parent focuses on providing brief encouragement and subsequently ignoring the child's attempts to pull her into a negotiation or argument. If the child refuses to get into the car to go to school, a plan can be set up so that the day at home is experienced as largely nonreinforcing. For example, the day should involve no use of electronics.

When the parent refuses to participate in an OCD ritual, she should subsequently remove her attention from their child's subsequent demands and arguing. She will provide attention only for neutral or positive behavior, such as calming down or using skills to manage anxiety (such as allowing the parent to read a bedtime story to him without first going through the ritual).

For the child who refuses to engage in the next step on his hierarchy or fear ladder, the parent should not spend time engaged in long dialogues or arguments with him about engaging in the desired task. Instead, she can simply suggest an alternative bravery exposure that is somewhat easier and remind him of the potential rewards for participating in the exposure. If he does not participate, no further attention or coaxing is provided.

Principle 5: Offer Specific and Frequent Praise

Sometimes, parents are so relieved when their child is not having a meltdown or arguing about why she can't or won't do something, that they become afraid of disturbing the situation. In other words, they fail to offer positive attention or praise.

Unfortunately, this is another problem with the misuse of attention (Forehand & Long, 1996). When parents do not reinforce brave behavior with positive attention, they make it less likely the child will be motivated to continue that behavior in the future. Thus it is critical that praise be used frequently, delivered enthusiastically and sincerely, and focused on specific behaviors.

Here are some examples of positive reinforcement:

Wow, I am so proud of you for attempting to climb that wall. You were nervous but you tried anyway!

I like how you tried to use your positive thinking skills when you felt scared. You got closer to the spider today, and I am giving you a brave point for your effort.

Considering Parenting Style

It has been our clinical experience that some parents with a personal history of having their own feelings dismissed by a caregiver can be more reluctant to provide strict limits and less able to tolerate the anxiety of their child. It is understandable that these parents may focus on not repeating the mistakes of their own parents, who they may have perceived as overly authoritarian, cold, or harsh in their parenting approach. Therefore, they strive for the opposite in their approach—a nurturing, flexible style that allows their child considerable autonomy. While many aspects of this style are beneficial and positive, an overly permissive parenting style can cause considerable problems in the long term.

In these cases, it can be helpful to discuss with parents the research of Baumrind's three parenting styles: permissive, authoritarian, and authoritative (1967). It should be pointed out that the authoritative style of parenting, in which calm and empathic parenting is combined with clear and firm limits, has been demonstrated by considerable research to be the most positive and effective parenting approach. The authoritative style is not devoid of warmth; however, it is firm and maintains limits. When the child is upset, the parents do not get angry, lecture, or chastise. They validate the child's feelings, while maintaining a calm and firm demeanor that upholds reasonable boundaries.

Further, research has found that use of an authoritative parenting style leads to increased feelings of safety and security of the child in the home environment (Stassen Berger, 2011). The limits authoritative parents set are consistent and predictable, and they respond to negative behavior with a calm and measured approach. These boundaries provide a secure environment for the child. Parents with permissive tendencies may find this somewhat surprising, assuming that the flexibility and control their child is afforded in a permissive household would lead to greater feelings of comfort and safety. It is important to correct this misassumption when it occurs, as this thinking can serve as a considerable obstacle to parents serving as effective coaches of exposure work outside of the therapy office. In actuality, children in permissive households often feel increased levels of anxiety and insecurity. They often have ambivalent feelings regarding their experience of power within the family household. They may push for control and make demands to get what they want or to avoid anxiety, but paradoxically they end up feeling overwhelmed by, and unequipped to handle, the power they accrue. They may feel guilty and embarrassed regarding the negative behaviors they use to influence their parents, and wish that their parents would demonstrate a stronger presence so that they would not have the pressure of so much decision-making power. Indeed, we have encountered many children in our practice who are able to articulate these concerns quite eloquently, including their desire for their parents to provide more direction and structure within the environment.

When encouraging brave behavior by utilizing firm limits, parents can and should still come across as loving and warm. They can validate the child's concerns, encourage their belief in his abilities, and maintain a positive and calm demeanor in the midst of his angst, while simultaneously maintaining their boundaries and refusing to actively participate in and enable anxious behavior and avoidance.

Conclusion

Parental behavior plays a critical role in both the maintenance and treatment of childhood anxiety disorders. To begin with, we must pay special attention to identifying and reducing any parental behaviors that may serve to increase child anxiety symptoms (such as parental accommodation and positive reinforcement of anxious behaviors). Simultaneously, we must foster parental confidence and expertise in responding appropriately to their child's anxiety and preparing for the role of exposure coach. In this way, parents can become powerful allies in conducting exposure therapy, and critical mechanisms of change for decreasing their child's anxiety and improving his life functioning.

CHAPTER 4

Setting the Stage for Exposure Work

This chapter will focus on how to help the child or adolescent prepare for subsequent exposure work. This preparation involves education about the nature of the fear response and anxiety cycle; the connection between our thoughts, feelings and behaviors; and the rationale for facing our fears. A key goal will be to increase the child's awareness of the connection between individual thoughts, physical sensations, and behaviors, when experiencing anxiety. Thereafter, strategies will be presented to help the child challenge anxious thinking through logical analysis and calm physical sensations through the use of mindfulness and relaxation skills.

Below we provide key principles to be discussed and explored with the child or adolescent in order to set the foundation for addressing anxiety through an exposure-based CBT model. We will highlight the specific role of CBT skills in overall anxiety management as well as in subsequent exposure work. We also provide sample ideas for specific dialogue, activities, and forms that will facilitate understanding of these concepts. However, please be aware that the language, methods, and techniques that will be most effective for teaching each individual child or adolescent will vary. Clinical judgment should be utilized in adapting activities based on a number of considerations, including age, developmental maturity, cognitive ability, and temperament. While an extensive discussion of this topic is beyond the scope of this book, we hope that our ideas provide a useful starting point for the clinician in providing education on the basis of fear and the connection between our thoughts, feelings, and behavior.

Identifying Physical Responses to Fear and Anxiety

Physical sensations in the body provide us with a myriad of information. They may signal hunger, fatigue, or illness, but more often these subtle physical sensations are signs of an emotional response. All emotional responses have corresponding physical sensations. Fear and anxiety are commonly associated with increased heart rate, stomach pain, and muscle tension, among others. Thus, increasing awareness of these "cues" as they occur can facilitate emotion recognition, which can in turn enable a better understanding of why physical sensations arose and how to respond in a way that can improve feelings. Given that each individual's physical experiences differ, children should be taught how to identify their own fearful sensations. The following language can facilitate the start of this conversation:

There are changes in our body (or physical sensations) that let us know we are scared, nervous, or worried. What do you notice when you are feeling scared? How do you know you are scared?

Draw an outline of the human body and have the child color in all the spots on her body where she notices having sensations when she is scared or nervous. For children with low body awareness who cannot identify physical sensations on their own, guide them by listing some of the common sensations observed by others when anxious and ask if they have experienced any of these before. Common physical sensations associated with anxiety or fear include:

- Fast or racing heart beat

- Short, fast, or shallow breathing

- Shaking

- Sweating

- Feeling dizzy or light-headed

- Tingling sensations or numbness in arms, legs, or face

- Muscle tightness or tension

- Stomachaches, nausea, or feeling of butterflies in stomach

- Headaches

- Knot or tightness in throat

- Chest pain

Another useful exercise is to have the child practice identifying physical sensations while imagining a fearful situation. Have him close his eyes and first imagine something calming and pleasant, like petting a soft kitten's fur, lying in the sand at the beach, or being under their warm covers in bed. Ask him to notice how his body feels (for example, breathing slow, muscles relaxed, belly comfortable). Then ask him to change the channel in his mind (in other words, imagine having a remote control for the brain and going to a different channel) and imagine something that might generate fear, such as a standing next to a large snake or getting a shot at the doctor's office. Have him identify physical changes he notices in his body. It is important to make sure the child is willing and open to imagining whatever stimuli are chosen. It is best not to choose images from his primary or presenting fear, as he may not be ready for that challenge.

Education on the Nature of Fear and Anxiety

Psychoeducation is a critical and key component to effective exposure-based CBT. Youth must understand the rationale for why this treatment approach is likely to be helpful to them, what outcomes they can expect (such as fear reduction, greater confidence, and ability to cope with the fearful stimuli), and how exposure work leads to these improved outcomes. Without this knowledge, the child or adolescent may feel like a ship without a compass, following along without a sense of the purpose of these activities or confidence in the therapist's ability to help her. Proper psychoeducation can be a motivating and encouraging force, providing the client with new insights about herself and the nature of her anxiety, as well as hopefulness and renewed confidence in her ability to reduce her anxiety through a commitment to treatment. Further, it is important that parents are involved in some, if not all, of this discussion, as they must also be aware of these connections and the basis of the fear response in order to effectively serve as exposure coaches for their children.

The Nature of the Fear Response

The "fight-or-flight" fear response is the body's alarm system that alerts you to danger. It is a useful and temporary reaction to real danger. This response results in an immediate release of adrenaline within the body, which activates our energy reserves and helps us become temporarily stronger and faster (Barlow, 1988; Clark, 1996; Craske & Barlow, 2006). However, perceived danger (worry thoughts), even in the absence of actual danger, can also activate this fight-or-flight fear response. This is called a "false alarm" because there is no real danger and the fear response was not necessary (Craske & Barlow, 2006). Helping children and adolescents understand the body's natural response to danger, the usefulness of the fear response, and the temporary and harmless nature of these feelings is of critical importance. Children learn to minimize the importance of those sensations as they occur, through an understanding that they are normal, will pass, and do not harm. Below we present an illustrative sample dialogue for describing these concepts to clients. However, children vary considerably in their cognitive capacities and vocabulary, and the clinician must carefully tailor language and descriptions to meet the needs of each individual client.

> *What if a huge bear suddenly walked into this room and let out a low, throaty groan? What would happen to our bodies? What kind of sensations would we have? This fear can be helpful. It sounds the alarm when danger is present and lets our body know it is time for action. When the alarm in our body sounds, chemicals (little messengers in our body) are released that cause our heart to pump faster and our muscles to get stronger. All of those changes help prepare our body to fight or run away when we are in danger.*

So, feeling scared and nervous is actually normal and sometimes really helpful! It helps us get away from that danger fast! These feelings cannot hurt us, even though they may be very uncomfortable, and they don't last forever. As soon as the danger is no longer near us, our body starts to calm down. Our breathing slows and we begin to relax.

The same thing can happen to our bodies when we just think about something scary, or when we expect something bad to happen, even when there is no real danger. We call this a 'false alarm.' That is, our body's alarm sounds and we get lots of scared feelings, but there is no actual danger. For example, the fire alarm may sound at school, but it's most likely a fire drill and not a real fire. We feel all the same uncomfortable sensations, but there is no real danger present to use all of that energy to fight or run.

What all of this means is that the bear doesn't actually have to be in the room for us to feel scared. All we need to do is think about the bear to have these feelings. Our thoughts are powerful! The good news is that our thoughts can also help calm us down. For example, we can remind ourselves that we are safe and that the feelings in our body are temporary and cannot hurt us. I will be your coach in helping you learn how to take control of your scary thoughts and use calm thinking to help your body relax.

How Avoidance Makes Fear Stronger

When we experience the uncomfortable fear response, our natural tendency is to avoid the situation, object, or person that we fear. We behave in this way in an effort to reduce our discomfort and avoid reexperiencing the fearful response in the future. However, each time we avoid our feared stimulus and our anxiety subsequently goes down, we are making the false mental connection that we need to avoid the situation or stimulus in order to feel better and stay safe. Our overall anxiety or fear actually increases and our feelings of confidence and self-efficacy deteriorate. The pathway out of this detrimental spiral is to systematically and gradually approach the fear. There are a number of positive outcomes that result from facing our fears. Our cognitions gradually adjust to become more realistic and confident, self-efficacy in tolerating the fear increases, and the overall physical response when faced with the fear typically reduces over time. The following language is presented as a guide for explaining to youth the relationship between fear and avoidance. As always, it should be individually tailored to the specific client.

When we are scared, we often try really hard to stay far away from the things we are afraid of. If we are afraid of bees, we might avoid parks, playgrounds, and other areas where bees might be found. If we are afraid of getting an answer wrong in class, we might not raise our hand. If we are afraid of being away from our parents, we might not want to spend time with a babysitter or let parents leave our activities. When we avoid the things we are afraid of, we might feel relieved in that moment, but it actually makes those things seem even bigger and scarier over time. We don't give ourselves a chance to learn that we can handle it. We don't learn that the things we fear are not as bad as we have built them up to be in our minds.

In order to beat our fears, we must slowly get used to what we are afraid of by gradually approaching, instead of avoiding, those things. We will do this in small steps that will help you feel more confident and stronger as we go. As you face your fears, those false alarms that sound in your mind and body will get weaker and weaker! Our bodies start to relax as we get used to the things we fear. And our thoughts start to change, too! We may decide that the things we fear aren't so bad after all. We may realize we feel scared but nothing terrible happens. We might feel proud that we handled it and didn't run away.

I will be your coach in conquering your fear. We will work together step-by-step to approach the things you fear. I will encourage you and help you decide on activities that will help you overcome your fears. I will also teach you some important skills and tools that can help you stay calm. But before all of this, it is really important to become a careful observer of your feelings and the things that might cause those feelings or happen in response to them. This means that when you notice a feeling, I also want you to observe what you are thinking, your body sensations, and what you choose to do.

This dialogue sets the stage for subsequent exploration of the connection between anxious thoughts, physical sensations, and behaviors. As described above, we recommend including parents in parts of this discussion or having the child review the information with them during the last 5 to 10 minutes of session to reinforce the child's understanding and to educate the parent. Parents must be aware of these connections and the basis of the fear response in order to effectively serve as exposure coaches for their children. Consider parent-only sessions to review and assess parental accommodation as described in chapter 3, and discuss the nature of the fear response, the connection between fear and avoidance, and the rationale for exposure work.

The Role of Cognitive Behavioral Skills in Exposure Therapy

From the perspective of many clinicians, cognitive and relaxation training are an integral part of CBT and an important foundation for subsequent exposure work.

This training provides the child with tools to manage his anxiety and build confidence in his ability to face his fears. Although the use of cognitive and relaxation strategies has been found to be an important part of overall anxiety management, it is important to note that research-based CBT protocols for treating anxiety disorders in children and adolescents vary in the frequency, depth, and timing with which they incorporate these skills. For example, in many manualized CBT approaches, such as Philip Kendall's Coping Cat approach, multiple sessions are dedicated to teaching these skills prior to beginning exposure work. Coping Cat integrates these skills throughout treatment through the use of the FEAR acronym, in which the child is taught to notice his anxious feelings and thoughts in each fearful situation and determine actions and attitudes that can help (Kendall & Hedtke, 2006). Sessions typically begin with an update from parent and child regarding the week and a review of self-monitoring forms and therapy homework assigned; continue with a didactic portion in which the child is taught a specific skill through discussion, modeling, role-play, and interactive activities; and end with an assignment given to practice the CBT skill during the upcoming week.

In contrast, the Modular CBT model created by B.F. Chorpita recommends starting with psychoeducation and moving straight into the exposure module. Cognitive restructuring is incorporated through specific questions following exposure tasks to facilitate corrective learning experiences (Chorpita, 2007). That is, the child is encouraged to recognize her safety and success in each situation. Full session cognitive modules are only implemented in certain cases, such as when negative or pessimistic thoughts interfere with a child's ability to engage in, or benefit, from exposure practice.

Both approaches have demonstrated clinical effectiveness; therefore as a clinician, it is important to understand the benefits of each approach and to tailor the amount of preliminary skills work to the individual client's needs. For example, clients who are slow to build rapport or trust and demonstrate a low readiness for and motivation to change may be resistant to a speedy exposure start. These clients may benefit from a more gradual introduction to ideas and rationale for exposure prior to active work. In contrast, overall treatment duration may be reduced when moving quickly to exposure activities for clients who demonstrate a high motivation and readiness for change. The age appropriateness of conducting cognitive work should also be taken into account, as young children and those who have not yet developed abstract reasoning skills are less likely to benefit from this component. Additionally, the level of reported physiological symptoms may be important to take into account. Some clients require the use of relaxation skills for initial engagement in exposure activities, with those skills being faded out over time as the client builds confidence. Finally, it is important to consider the impact of negative thinking patterns on the client's motivation to engage in exposure work. That is, cognitive restructuring is particularly important when maladaptive beliefs interfere with the ability to engage in exposure work (for example, the belief that you will be unable to cope with the situation or outcome).

As active exposure sessions are initiated, CBT skills are incorporated in a variety of ways. For example, a child may repeat specific coping thoughts or employ a relaxation skill to manage his nervousness in preparation for approaching a fear. These skills aid him in quelling the cognitive and physical aspects of the anxiety and give him the confidence to initiate the exposure. After the exposure, children and adolescents are guided in using cognitive strategies to process the exposure—that is, to develop more adaptive ways for understanding and interpreting the stimuli or situation they experienced. In contrast, during the actual exposure, the use of these skills is generally contraindicated, as they can prevent the client from fully experiencing and attending to the exposure task, disrupt habituation to the task, and reduce the client's self-efficacy or ownership of success because of his reliance on the skills. Please refer to chapter 5 for a more expansive discussion regarding how CBT skills are utilized before, during, and after exposures.

Developing Thought Awareness and Self-Monitoring Skills

Developing greater awareness of our thought process is a key component in traditional CBT models. It allows the client the opportunity to understand the impact her automatic and fearful thoughts have on her body, mind, and actions. With this awareness, she can develop tools for accepting, managing, or challenging the thoughts as they arise. We teach children that while they may not have control over what thoughts pop into their heads, they do have control over how they choose to respond to those thoughts. Teaching thought awareness and supporting the child or adolescent in choosing the types of thoughts she wants to focus on fosters a sense of empowerment and hopefulness.

Over the course of a day, our brain never stops creating thoughts. Some thoughts are positive (*Wow, I did a great job on that test!*), some thoughts are negative (*Ugh, I hate how I look right now.*), and many thoughts are neutral (*That tree is really tall.*). In session, older and more verbal children can articulate the thoughts they observed during the day. Younger children may benefit from a concrete activity such as drawing themselves with cartoon-like thought bubbles surrounding their heads. Have the child fill in the thought bubbles with some of his most recent thoughts. These activities can be adjusted so that the child focuses on thoughts related to specific emotions (for example, writing fearful thoughts in the thought bubble).

As children begin to develop competency in identifying their thoughts, an equally important goal is an exploration of the relationship between their thoughts, physical sensations, and behavior. We want to help them understand that thoughts have the power to influence one's emotions, body, and behavior. In service of this goal, we recommend drawing a picture with three large circles that connect. (See example below.) Have the child recall a previous time she was scared. Ask her to write down in one bubble what she thought, in one bubble what she did, and in one bubble what she felt. Explore with her the relationships between these thoughts, feelings, and behaviors. For example, a child might recognize that her worry about feeling embarrassed led to a flushed or hot feeling in her face. When she noticed those physical sensations, it led to more thoughts about being embarrassed due to worry that her peers would see her red face. Therefore she chose to avoid raising her hand for fear of embarrassment.

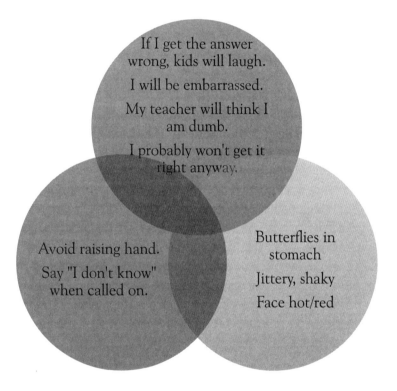

In order for the client to develop an understanding of the connection between his own feelings, thoughts, and actions, he must consistently practice the skill in daily life. A thought-feeling-action worksheet (follows) can be introduced and put into practice within the therapy session, and the client can then be assigned the worksheet as homework to practice the skill independently. Discuss with child and parent how to complete the worksheet for homework. Have the child write down at least one scary or nervous feeling each day of the week or as he notices them. (A downloadable version of this worksheet is available at http://www.newharbinger.com/39225.)

Thought-Feeling-Action Worksheet

EVENT	FEELING	THOUGHT	ACTION
Where were you? What was happening? (Example: *I didn't want mom to leave me at gymnastics.*)	How did you feel? (Example: *Scared and mad. Heart beating fast, shaking.*)	What were you thinking? (Example: *She can't make me go. Something bad could happen if she leaves. What if she doesn't come back?*)	What did you do? (Example: *I said I'm not going. I cried. I wouldn't get in the car.*)

Challenging Negative Thought Patterns

Negative thought patterns have a significant impact on a child or adolescent's perception and expectations of the world, others, and herself. This section focuses on the nuts and bolts of identifying and challenging these patterns as they relate to anxiety and exposure work, including utilizing tracking to increase awareness of the connection between thoughts and feelings, identifying and labeling thinking errors, increasing tolerance for uncertainty, engaging in thought-challenging questions, and the use of Socratic questioning in the therapy session.

Identifying Negative Thought Patterns and Thinking Errors

Before a child can begin to challenge his negative thoughts, it is helpful if he can identify the negative thought patterns or thinking errors involved (Leahy, 1996; Burns, 1980). There are many types of negative cognitions that children and teenagers may experience, and it is important to normalize negative thoughts by reminding the child that we all have intrusive thoughts or thinking errors from time to time. When introducing the types of thinking errors that are common in anxiety, it is helpful to explore characteristics and examples of each error and see if the client can identify which patterns he tends to experience the most. That way he knows which ones to watch out for!

Some creative ways to introduce thinking errors with younger children include using characters to exemplify the thinking patterns, engaging in dramatic role-plays, or using puppets. Teens may prefer discussing the negative thought patterns or thinking errors directly and engaging in more mature activities, such as trying to identify thinking errors in book characters. These imaginative approaches maintain engagement and allow the child or adolescent to begin the process of challenging thinking errors in others (external) before she begins to challenge her own thoughts (internal), as the latter may be more difficult emotionally and cognitively.

Finally, it is also important to consider the role of cognitive work, including challenging negative thought patterns, in the context of exposure treatment. As detailed below, the focus of discussion prior to exposure work should be on the most common thinking patterns that coincide with anxiety and those that are observed in your client. Core maladaptive belief patterns in anxiety generally include an overestimation of probability, magnification of risk, expectations of not being able to cope, and difficulty tolerating uncertainty. This is by no means an exhaustive list of potential thinking errors, but is limited in scope to emphasize thinking traps most likely to impact children and adolescents as they engage in exposure work. The goal of exposure exercises is to violate the client's negative expectations through new experiences, thereby creating contradictory evidence. Although the client is instructed to refrain from engaging in thought challenging during the actual exposure exercise, introducing cognitive work prior to exposure tasks prepares the child for post-exposure processing by helping him understand the difference between maladaptive and adaptive thought processes.

As follows, we review the core problematic thinking patterns that are commonly associated with exposure work and anxiety in general, including examples of specific thinking errors or traps associated with each theme, as well as specific ways to support children and adolescents in challenging those distortions.

OVERESTIMATION OF PROBABILITY

Anxiety frequently drives us to overestimate the likelihood of a negative outcome in anxiety-provoking situations. For example, a child who is fearful of bees may avoid all flowering plants because she is certain that a bee will sting her if she stands nearby. Supporting the client in separating facts from feelings can help to challenge this type of thinking error (in other words, "Just because it feels like it happens every time, does not mean it happens every time."). Jointly you could explore historical evidence and data sources that challenge the client's negative expectation of high probability, including personal experiences ("Approximately what percent of time have you seen others stand beside a flower and not get stung by a bee?"), scientific websites (search for data on frequency of bee stings or specific situations in which bees sting), or anecdotal evidence (have the client survey others about the number of times they've been stung in their lifetime). The following are specific thinking errors that often coincide with probability overestimation:

Filtering. Focusing thoughts and attention on negative experiences throughout your day allows positive experiences to slip through your memory. For example, when you have a day filled with ups and downs, you may only recall the downs. When we focus solely on negative experiences, we develop a pessimistic framework and negative expectations that lead to an overestimation of the likelihood of negative outcomes.

Example:	"I can't believe today was so terrible! First I ran out of my favorite cereal, then I stepped in a mud puddle, and *then* I left my lunch at home!"
Character:	"Frank the Filtering Phantom" is a ghost who allows positives to go right through him, but the negatives somehow get stuck. The goal is to teach him a new way to catch some positive thoughts.

Predicting the future. Based on limited information, such as one previous experience, you jump to negative conclusions or expect that future experiences or interactions will also be negative. This pattern of negative expectations skews our perception and increases our estimation of negative outcomes.

Example:	"I threw up the last time I ate in the cafeteria, so I know I'll throw up if I eat in there again."
Character:	"Felicity the Fortune Teller" is a genie who uses her crystal ball to make silly negative predictions. Have the child use his own crystal ball to make more realistic, positive predictions.

Personalizing. You assume that another person's behavior is a reaction to you. For example, your friend has a frown on her face while eating lunch, and you assume it is because she doesn't like you anymore (when in fact she is worried about her spelling test after lunch). You guess what the other person is thinking without really knowing, and you generally have an expectation that it is a negative judgment about you. This thinking error is especially common with social anxiety.

Example:	"She looked up at me when I walked into the room. I know she must be furious with me for being a minute late and probably won't want to be friends anymore!"
Character:	"All About Me Arnold" is a vampire who assumes *everything* is about him. Try having the child come up with other external explanations that challenge Arnold's point of view.

Emotional reasoning. Mistakenly interpreting one's feelings as facts can lead to an overestimation of the likelihood of a negative occurrence. For example, if a negative situation "feels" like it happens every day, then the child expects that the negative experience is the most likely outcome. As another example, if the youth feels panic sensations in a given situation, he assumes those anxious feelings indicate that danger is real or more likely.

Example:	"It feels like we hear the sirens from the fire department every second, so I know that this is a very dangerous area and we will get hurt!"
Character:	"Feeling is Believing" Fabien is a video game character who mistakes feelings for facts. To help Fabien win the game, have the child challenge the negative assumptions using logic and rational evidence, not emotions.

MAGNIFICATION OF RISK

Another common thought pattern related to anxiety is an over-prediction of the magnitude of any given negative outcome. For example, the child may not simply worry that she will be stung by a bee, but also visualize a group of killer bees joining the swarm, being stung by them 30 times, then being in severe pain and unable to breathe. In these instances, the degree of the expected negative outcome is significantly out of proportion to the given situation. Support the client in challenging this line of thinking by focusing on logic and searching for evidence that contradicts the feared outcome. In the previous example, you could question the client's earlier experiences and review scientific data related to bee sting outcomes. Below are specific thinking errors that frequently coincide with an over-prediction of risk:

Catastrophic thinking (avalanche thinking). You use "what if" worry thoughts to convince yourself that the worst-case scenario is likely to happen. This is a common thinking error with anxiety; it may start as a small worry snowball rolling downhill, but if left unchallenged, it can soon become a worry avalanche.

Example: "What if I stand up to do my presentation and I forget everything, begin to cry, and everyone laughs? I'll never be able to go to school again!"

Character: "Catastrophic Ray" is a space invader who uses his "What If" laser to turn small worries into huge worries! See if the child can identify when he is using his "What If" laser to magnify the problem and create a chain of worries that leads to prediction of catastrophe (the avalanche). Finally, use evidence to challenge the likelihood of the catastrophe and shrink the problem back down to size.

All-or-nothing thinking. This way of thinking uses extremes and rigid categories to label experiences (for example, using words such as always, never, perfect, terrible, or disaster). You fail to consider that the most likely and realistic choice or outcome is somewhere in the middle.

Example: "I can't believe I missed two problems on my math quiz! I'm always horrible at math!"

Character: The "All-or-Nothing Alligator" only talks in extremes. See if the child can challenge (or "chomp") the extreme thinking and find more balanced ideas and expectations that are in the middle.

LOW EXPECTATION OF COPING CAPACITY

Oftentimes clients do not simply fear the perceived threat, but also doubt their ability to cope with the feared outcome. For example, the child fearing bees may be afraid of being stung primarily because she is convinced she will not be able to handle the pain. This perceived helplessness leads to increased avoidance and reassurance seeking. Many children have not considered that a majority of situations, even "worst-case scenarios," are manageable even though they may be uncomfortable (physically or emotionally). The goal of challenging these thoughts is to support the child or adolescent in developing a sense of personal resilience and a "brave" stance in facing her fears. Exploring previous coping successes by asking, "Can you tell me about a time when you were able to (handle pain)?" can help the client to acknowledge her coping capacity. Additionally, noting that uncomfortable experiences are time-limited may also be helpful, as the child may be more likely to see herself as "able to handle it" when the discomfort is brief. Below are specific thinking errors that often coincide with low expectations of coping capacity:

Minimizing success and denying oneself credit. Undermining your successes, by discounting them or not giving yourself credit for them, can lead to a feeling of helplessness and perception of an inability to cope.

Example: "Sure I did well on my spelling test, but it was really easy and I'm sure everyone else got a 100% too."

Character: "Positively No Positives Pedro" goes out of his way to ignore anything he has done well. Try having the child come up with positive evidence to help Pedro take credit for his success.

"Shoulds" and "musts." Applying unrealistic personal "rules" to yourself or others in the form of "should" or "must" statements often leaves you feeling disappointed and upset when you cannot meet your own unrealistic standards, or when others do not apply the same rules or uphold the same criteria. For perfectionistic clients, there is also often a feeling that they will not be able to cope when these "rules" are violated, and an expectation that others should accommodate their rigid rules (as in, "He should not rearrange my papers because he knows it upsets me and I can't handle it.")

Examples: "I should turn in my homework 100% of the time," "Everyone should know that I sit in that chair during English class."

Character: "Should-a-Lot the Sheep" likes to share all of her silly "shoulds" and "musts," but when others don't follow her rules, she feels "baaaad." One way to challenge the "should" statement is to replace it with a "could-or" statement such as, *"People could choose to sit in the same seat, or they could choose to sit in a different seat, and I can handle it either way."*)

LOW TOLERANCE FOR UNCERTAINTY

Although most people have some uneasiness with uncertainty, high levels of intolerance for uncertainty are linked to increased symptoms of anxiety and depression, and are especially associated with GAD and OCD (Boswell, Thompson-Hollands, Farchione, & Barlow, 2013). A large part of successfully managing anxious thoughts is tolerating the possibility that the negative outcome *could* happen, even if it is unlikely. For example, you *could* get stung by a bee; you *could* be in a car accident; others *could* be thinking negative thoughts about you. Children and adolescents with anxiety may attempt to reduce this sense of uncertainty with attempts to control the environment, excessive planning, seeking reassurance, and avoidance; however, uncertainty is an unavoidable part of everyday life, and accepting the unknown requires the development of tolerance through practice.

We recommend initiating this dialogue with the client by introducing and normalizing the concept of uncertainty. It may be helpful to assist the child in weighing the pros and cons of accepting uncertainty. For example, a con may be that he will feel uncomfortable at times, but a pro may be that he saves a lot of time by not engaging in tasks geared toward reducing uncertainty. Further, it is beneficial to point out that uncertainty is not necessarily a bad thing. There are many situations where uncertainty leads to positive outcomes. Avoidance in these cases leads to fewer opportunities to reap the benefits of those positive outcomes. It is important to remind the client that, in fact, despite taking significant measures to control himself and his environment, there is still no such thing as 100% certainty.

Once the concept of uncertainty and the need for building tolerance have been addressed with the child or adolescent, it is your role as the clinician to begin to reflect uncertainty in sessions. For example, when she seeks reassurance you can warmly respond, "It is always possible that _____ could happen." The goal of this technique is to allow the child to experience and learn to tolerate the feeling of uncertainty in a safe environment. This activity can be structured as an exposure task in which she is asked to repeat these uncertainty statements verbally in session until anxiety is reduced. We also recommend recording the statements with the goal of the child listening to the recording multiple times during the week. (This technique will be discussed in additional detail in chapter 12, under Worry Loop Tapes). In addition, parents should be coached to respond similarly to reassurance seeking at home. Finally, in cases where intolerance of uncertainty is a prominent theme of the anxiety and a barrier to treatment, such as is often the case with the treatment of GAD, OCD, or separation anxiety, the intolerance may need to be addressed more thoroughly by creating a full exposure hierarchy focused specifically on practicing embracing uncertainty in worry-related situations. Detailed examples for these disorders are covered in subsequent disorder-specific chapters. The following statements may be helpful for eliciting feelings of uncertainty with the goal of increasing tolerance in therapy sessions:

- "Yes, I suppose _____ could happen."

- "Actually, I do not know. Anything is possible!"

- "Couldn't it be exciting to not know and be surprised?"

- "Maybe, maybe not."

General Strategies for Challenging Thinking Errors

Once thinking errors have been identified and labeled, it is time to get to work on generating more reasonable or adaptive replacement thoughts. This section includes more general guidelines for supporting clients by systematically challenging maladaptive thought patterns.

FOCUSING ON VALIDITY AND FUNCTIONALITY

An important thing to note is that we are not just challenging the validity of negative thoughts, as often there is a grain of truth to them. We are also questioning the functionality: does the thought help the client move forward and adapt or does it make him feel stuck and upset? If the latter is true, then it is time to pull out your detective hat and find a replacement thought.

SOCRATIC QUESTIONING IN SESSION

Socratic questioning is a form of therapeutic dialogue that supports the child in using logic to challenge negative assumptions. The goal is to use specific questions to facilitate a positive discussion that allows for thoughtful exploration of thoughts and feelings. During Socratic questioning, the therapist takes on the role of guide and collaborator, rather than expert, and works to demonstrate a stance of curiosity while avoiding an interrogative or argumentative style. Additionally, reflection can be a powerful tool in helping the client feel understood and examine her own words. Throughout the process, it is important to continually monitor the child's level of frustration, work to remain empathetic, and support her in tying together thoughts and feelings.

Here is an example of Socratic questioning:

Therapist:	I know we've talked a little about the possibility of summer camp, but I was wondering if you could help me understand why you do not want to go?
Client:	Well, I went last summer and it was the *worst* thing ever! I'm never going back!
Therapist:	Wow, it sounds like it was a difficult experience for you. Can you tell me what made it the worst?
Client:	Yes. No one wanted to be my partner. I know the other kids did not like me at all.
Therapist:	I can imagine that it was pretty stressful to feel like no one wanted to be your partner and that the other kids did not like you. (*Client nods.*) So let's explore what happened and see if we can make sense of the situation, okay?
Client:	Okay.

Therapist:	Let's start at the beginning. When you think back to the first day of camp, can you recall how it started?
Client:	Well, I remember Mom dropped me off a few minutes late, so when I walked in, everyone was sitting in a circle. They were sharing their names and someone moved over so I could sit down. But only the counselor said hello.
Therapist:	Hmmm, so someone moved over and made space to include you? And the teacher said hello? Those sound like friendly things to do.
Client:	I guess, but they probably felt like they had to. So, then I was really nervous, but I shared my name too. Then I remember that we were supposed to pair up to work on an activity, but no one wanted to be my partner, so the counselor told someone to work with me.
Therapist:	So, just to make sure I'm clear, it sounds like you didn't have a chance to ask anyone to be your partner?
Client:	Well, I didn't ask anyone to be my partner because I was feeling too shy.
Therapist:	So no one said "no" to being your partner?
Client:	No, they just paired up with other people. I think a bunch of them already knew each other from school and the few of us who didn't know anyone got paired up.
Therapist:	So it sounds like there were several people who also didn't have partners. If you had known someone there from your own school, do you think you would have tried to pair up with them?
Client:	Probably.
Therapist:	So is it possible that the other kids paired up with people they already knew because it was the first day and they felt more comfortable asking a familiar person to be partners?
Client:	I guess so.
Therapist:	Okay, so maybe they paired up with people they knew because they were feeling shy too, and *not* because they didn't want to be your partner?
Client:	Yeah, I guess that makes sense. (*Client smiles.*)

Looking for evidence. We recommend that children and teens be provided with a structured approach for challenging their negative thoughts both within and outside of session. To do this, they will need to push back on the negative thoughts and seek out evidence that proves the thoughts incorrect or unhelpful. Based on the new evidence, they can create more reasonable or adaptive thoughts and acknowledge the impact of those new thoughts on their emotions. Below we provide a list of challenge questions that can be used as a guide for the child in challenging his negative thinking. Alternatively, specific challenge questions most relevant to the child's negative thought patterns can be pulled from this list or adapted to create a more tailored guide:

Do you think this sounds like any of the "thinking errors" (or "thinking error" characters) we discussed?

What would you tell a friend who had the same thought?

What are the facts in this situation? Is there any evidence that this thought could be false or not completely true? (Can you list three pieces of evidence that suggest it might be wrong?)

What happened in the past when you worried about this?

What is the worst-case scenario, best-case scenario, and most likely scenario? Can you handle (or survive) each of these?

Are you blaming yourself for something that is not completely under your control? Are there others who have played a role or who have some responsibility?

If you look back on the situation a year later, do you think it will still feel as upsetting?

Redirection. Finally, once more adaptive replacement thoughts have been identified and acknowledged, it is time for the child to move on. Discuss with her how to transition by mentally or physically redirecting her attention toward something positive or enjoyable. For example, she may choose to focus her thoughts on an upcoming play-date or engage in a game of basketball. She may create a list of coping actions to engage in when she wants to self-soothe and relax (for example, pet the dog, draw a picture, or talk to a friend on the phone).

Utilizing a Thought-Challenging Diary

After working to identify thinking errors, it is important to circle back to the thought-feeling connection and help the child or teenager examine the impact of his thoughts on his feelings. On the most basic level, it should be emphasized that negative thoughts tend to lead to negative emotions, just as positive thoughts lead to positive emotions. Although we can certainly tolerate some amount of negative emotion, high levels of negative emotion (such as strong anger, sadness, or anxiety), can lead to unhelpful behaviors (such as avoidance, shutting down, or acting out) that interfere with our ability to function well in daily life. One way to help the client develop awareness of his own thought patterns and the thought-feeling connection is through the use of a thought-challenging diary. A thought-challenging diary is a tracking tool that includes columns to write about a "Situation" and related "Negative Thoughts" and "Feelings" (with ratings of intensity levels) (Beck, 1976). In addition, to guide the child or teen in challenging his negative thoughts, a "Challenge and Reframe" column is included in which he practices challenging the negative thoughts (by, for example, listing evidence for and against the thoughts) and generating more helpful alternative thoughts. A final column is included in which the child re-rates the intensity level of the feelings after taking the "new" adaptive thoughts into consideration. The thought-challenging diary should be introduced and practiced in session, and then the child will begin to use it outside of session to log negative or anxious thoughts. When beginning a thought-challenging diary, there are a few things to keep in mind:

INCLUDE FEELING RATINGS

A thought diary should allow the child or teenager to use rating scales to track the level of intensity of emotions (such as a 1-to-10 scale). This allows her to have comparison points, to see patterns of thoughts that elicit strong emotions, and to realize that shifting her negative thoughts to more helpful alternative thoughts can lower the emotional intensity level.

FOCUS ON THE EMOTION (NOT JUST THE THOUGHTS)

If the child is having difficulty identifying negative thoughts, have him work backwards by identifying moments of negative emotion and discussing the situation that produced the emotion. Younger children may need support to verbalize related negative thoughts.

EXTERNALIZE THE EMOTION IF NECESSARY

If the child or teen is able to identify the thought but has difficulty verbalizing the emotion, externalizing the emotion may be helpful. For example, you could say, "If someone said that to your friend, how might your friend feel?"

INTRODUCE THE THOUGHT DIARY IN SECTIONS

For younger children, it may be helpful to introduce the thought diary in steps over several sessions. This way they have the opportunity to practice each component separately.

This sample thought-challenging diary provides categories and descriptions to support the client tracking the situation, initial feeling and affective intensity, negative thought, challenging of thought, alternative thought, and follow-up feeling rating. This diary is presented as a guide and should be adapted as necessary based on the client's developmental needs. (A downloadable version is available at http://www.newharbinger.com/39225.)

Thought-Challenging Diary

SITUATION	FEELING	NEGATIVE THOUGHT	CHALLENGE	NEW THOUGHT	NEW FEELING
Where were you? What was happening?	Label feeling and rate 1–10	What negative thought popped into your head? (Label the type of thinking error)	What evidence do you have to challenge this thought?	What is a new, more adaptive thought?	Rate from 1 to 10

Teaching Relaxation Skills

Utilizing relaxation techniques as a means of self-regulation is an integral part of anxiety management and a great way to cope with day-to-day stress. These skills can be effective in reducing the physiological symptoms of the body's stress response (such as rapid or shallow breathing, increased heart rate, or sweating), which can lead to a calmer mental state and enable the mind to engage more effectively in the cognitive skills of CBT. Relaxation skills can also be beneficial at times directly prior to exposure tasks to enable youth with strong physiological responses to commit to and initiate these tasks.

Preparing for Relaxation

When introducing relaxation techniques to children and adolescents, it is important to prepare them with realistic expectations. Many of the techniques are easy to learn but require consistent practice to be effective. Just as we all know how to run but would need consistent practice to run a marathon, we can all breathe but need consistent practice to master breathing for relaxation. Additionally, not all relaxation techniques are equally helpful for each child, and therapy provides the space to "try on" relaxation techniques like trying on clothes at a store; sometimes it is a perfect fit, sometimes it does not feel quite right, and sometimes we did not expect something to work for us and are happily surprised when it does.

Relaxation techniques are taught and modeled in session, and then the child should be provided a tracking sheet to monitor relaxation practice at home between sessions. Sometimes, the increased focus on body sensations that accompanies self-monitoring during relaxation can be anxiety provoking in itself at the outset. It is important to normalize these sensations and feelings, while continuing to gradually build tolerance to the sensations through short periods of relaxation practice. Reassure the child that these sensations indicate that her body is healthy and working exactly the way it should, and that the sensations will likely subside over time with practice.

Finally, it is important to clarify that the use of relaxation techniques should generally not be encouraged during exposure practice because it may serve as a means of avoidance and dampen the effectiveness of the exposure work. These relaxation skills are most often suggested for use in management of the nervous anticipation of exposure work. During exposure activities, the goal is for the child to tolerate the discomfort of the anxiety and acclimate to the situation without intervention.

Types of Relaxation

Following psychoeducation about the use of relaxation, specific relaxation exercises can be introduced and practiced in session. This section provides a "how to" guide for teaching diaphragmatic breathing, visualization, guided imagery, progressive muscle relaxation, meditation and mindfulness, and relaxation movement to child and adolescent clients.

DIAPHRAGMATIC BREATHING

When done properly, diaphragmatic breathing, or controlled breathing, can be highly effective in modifying breathing and heart rate. The goal of this type of controlled breathing is to regulate respiration by consciously extending each inhale and exhale of the breath in a way that fills the diaphragm. Diaphragmatic breathing is the building block of relaxation and can be paired with other relaxation techniques. The child should begin by sitting up straight or lying in a comfortable position that allows space for the lungs to fill. If it is helpful, he can place one hand on his upper chest and one hand on his abdomen directly below his rib cage, which allows him to feel how the belly will rise and fall (while the chest moves very little) during calm and controlled breathing. The goal is to breathe into the belly, not from the chest. While breathing, the child can either close his eyes or focus them on an object in the room. Each breath will begin with a slow and controlled inhale through the nose, followed by a 1- to 2-second pause, and then a slow and controlled exhale through pursed lips. The length of each inhale and exhale should begin to the count of 3 and then increase to stretch the breath further as the child becomes more skilled. Some creative ways to teach and practice diaphragmatic breathing with children include:

- Blowing bubbles: The goal is to control the breath to blow one big bubble rather than many small bubbles.

- Blowing a pinwheel: Focus on seeing if the child can increase the amount of time she makes the pinwheel spin with each breath.

- Single nostril breathing: Have the child gently press on the outside of the nose to close one nostril, then breathe in and out of the other nostril.

- Taking a stuffed animal for a ride: Have the child lie on her back and place a small stuffed animal or figurine on her stomach (not chest). With each breath, encourage her to take the animal as high (inhale) and then as low (exhale) as she can.

VISUALIZATION

Visualization is the practice of using your mind to focus on a visual image. In essence, it is a vacation for the mind. By vividly picturing a scene with your imagination, your body responds as though you are actually there. The key to visualization is to focus on descriptive details and sensory information, using all five senses (visual, auditory, olfactory, tactile, and gustatory), including colors, shapes, textures, sounds, smells, tastes, and physical sensations. Guided imagery, a form of visualization that involves being guided through the scene by listening to a vivid verbal description, can be very useful with children, as it may initially be difficult for them to picture a scene on their own. There are many useful recordings and scripts that can be used both inside and outside of therapy sessions, or you can collaboratively create a scene with the child based on a personal memory or photograph. Given that relaxing scenarios vary from person to person, it is important to ask the child where he recalls feeling relaxed in the past, which could include anything from a quiet beach to an amusement park. Begin the visualization exercise by asking him to close his eyes and focus on his breathing with several controlled breaths before creating the visualization scene. For younger children who may have difficulty maintaining concentration during visualization, keep the exercise brief and work to encourage their participation by asking them to describe what they "see" in their scene and probing for details to incorporate. This brief sample dialogue demonstrates the integration of sensory information into a visualization exercise:

Therapist: So we are sitting on the beach together right now. What do you see on your beach?

Client: I see my beach towel.

Therapist: I'm wondering what your beach towel looks like and feels like. Can you describe the color and what it feels like to touch?

Client: It has red and blue stripes and is very soft.

Therapist: Ah, yes! I can imagine it now too. I can see the bright red and blue stripes, and when I run my hand over the towel it feels very soft on my fingertips.

PROGRESSIVE MUSCLE RELAXATION (PMR)

Progressive muscle relaxation (PMR) involves systematically tensing and releasing different muscle groups with the goal of reducing muscle tension and leaving muscles in a fully relaxed state. Additionally, the practice of PMR is useful for developing body awareness in children and adolescents by allowing them to thoughtfully experience the contrast between a tense muscle state and a relaxed muscle state. Similar to other relaxation exercises, the child should begin by lying down on her back or sitting comfortably with both feet on the floor. Typically, PMR exercises progress through the muscle groups in a top-down or bottom-up pattern, such as starting with the feet and ending with the facial muscles. For each muscle group, the child is asked to tighten the muscles and hold the tension for the count of 3 before releasing. When she releases, she should let the muscle tension go and allow her body to rest in a loose, relaxed state for 5 to 10 seconds before progressing to the next muscle group. For younger children, it may be helpful to focus on just one or two muscle groups during a session, and to use scripts or recordings to teach and practice PMR, as these may help maintain their attention. Variations can also include doing a full body tense and release for a quick exercise, or squeezing stress balls or other objects with the hands during these exercises.

Combining visualization with PMR exercises can create engaging experiences for the child or adolescent. The samples below demonstrate language that may be helpful in aiding children and adolescents to engage in PMR while targeting specific areas of the body:

- Hands: *Imagine you are squeezing the juice out of an orange. Hold an orange in each hand and now squeeze as hard as you can to get all of the juice out, 1…2…3. Now release and feel how different it feels to have your hands limp and relaxed.*

- Tummy: *Now imagine that your tummy is stiff and as strong as a board. A karate chop cannot even break it! Hold it tight for 1…2…3, and exhale.*

- Jaw: *Pretend you are crunching down on a giant piece of jawbreaker candy. Hold your jaw tightly for 1…2…3. Now relax and let all of the tension go.*

- Face: *Imagine you are smelling a flower and now have to scrunch up your nose to keep from sneezing. Now hold your face all scrunched up for 1…2…3. Now relax your facial muscles.*

- Whole body: *Imagine you are standing in the ocean and with each wave you have to stand tall and tight with your whole body to keep from letting the wave pull you over. Ready, here comes the wave, and hold tight for 1…2…3. Now completely relax your whole body.*

MEDITATION AND MINDFULNESS

The practice of meditation emphasizes focusing one's attention inward by gently observing thoughts, feelings, and experiences. There is a large range of meditation styles, and for children, techniques that provide some structure can help them maintain focus. For example, children may enjoy engaging in walking meditations, chanting positive mantras, or repeating calming noises through breathing (think *Om* but with animal noises, such as doing long exhales while saying "*Mooooooo*"). Additionally, meditation exercises should be time-limited, with the length geared toward the child's age and level of experience.

Mindfulness is the practice of turning your attention to the present by actively building awareness of your thoughts, feelings, physical sensations, and environment

(Kabat-Zinn, 1994). It also involves an element of acceptance and taking a nonjudgmental stance toward your thoughts and feelings. Mindfulness techniques can be especially helpful with managing anxiety, as many worries are about the past (*Why did I say that stupid thing?*) or the future (*What if I fail my test?*). By focusing on the here and now, children can ground themselves and help diminish their anxious thoughts. Specifically, mindfulness practices include focusing on sensory information and body awareness. Some creative techniques for introducing mindfulness to children include mindful eating, mindful movement, and mindful listening to music.

The excerpt below provides sample verbiage for engaging a client in a mindfulness exercise during a session. As always, it is important to adjust the language so that it is easily understood and age-appropriate for each specific client.

We are going to practice being fully aware and present with our body, our surroundings, and our mind, without judgment. Find a comfortable spot to sit and close your eyes. Let's start with the breath. Without trying to change your breathing in any way, just notice each breath as it comes in and goes out. Focus all of your awareness on the sound of the air in your nostrils as you breathe in through your nose, and the sound of the air as it exits your mouth. Notice your belly rise with each inhale, and fall with each exhale. (Pause)

Now I would like you to focus all of your attention and awareness on the sensation of your body on the chair, couch, or other place where you are sitting. Notice the feeling of the chair as it presses against your back and your legs. Notice the strength and support this object provides as it holds your body up. (Pause)

Now take a minute to notice the temperature of the air around you. Is it cold, cool, warm, hot? What does it feel like on your hands...your cheeks? What is the temperature like as you inhale it through your nose? (Pause)

As you practice being aware in this moment, you may find your mind wandering to other thoughts or feelings. This is normal. When this happens, notice the thought without judgment (in other words, it is neither good nor bad, neither right nor wrong). Gently turn your attention back to your breathing and the sensations of your body in the room. You might imagine putting your thoughts and worries in a bottle, corking the bottle, and sending the bottle down a river. Watch the bottle as it floats into the distance. (Pause)

Continuing to breathe comfortably, with your eyes still closed, turn your attention to the sounds in the room. Notice each individual sound you hear one by one. Is each sound loud or soft? Sharp or dull? Immerse yourself in the sounds of the here and now. (Pause) Now see if you can notice the sounds all together around you as you sit in your spot. (Pause)

Finally, I would like you to turn your attention to the sense of sight. When you are ready, gently open your eyes and begin to notice your surroundings. As you look around the room, notice if there is anything that you have never noticed before. Anything that is surprising or unusual. Take note of the details and colors. (Pause) See if you can focus your attention on all that is right here and now, your surroundings, your body, and your overall experience in this moment.

RELAXATION THROUGH MOVEMENT

Finally, controlled movement, such as yoga or tai chi, is another form of relaxation that can be very beneficial for children and adolescents. The active format can increase engagement for children who may have difficulty sitting still and is helpful in creating body awareness. Consider introducing techniques in the session and encouraging the child to practice at home with a video or in a group context by joining a class.

Conclusion

In preparing the child or adolescent for subsequent exposure work, it is critical that they have a strong understanding of the adaptive nature of the fear response. Youth learn that fear is a normal human experience and that fearful sensations cannot hurt them. They learn to identify false alarms or times when this fear response arises when no danger is actually present. A key goal is to increase their awareness of the connection between their individual thoughts, physical sensations, and behaviors. Through understanding how these different systems interact to produce the fear response, they subsequently learn to target their thoughts, actions, and body responses in order to challenge and manage the anxiety. In service of this goal, children and adolescents are guided through the development of strategies to challenge anxious thinking through logical analysis and to calm physical sensations through the use of mindfulness and relaxation skills. This training provides children with tools to manage their feelings and build confidence in their ability to subsequently face their fears.

CHAPTER 5

Structuring and Implementing Exposure Sessions

Just as it takes time to learn to play a musical instrument smoothly and fluidly, exposure therapy sessions require significant clinical skill in managing the structure, pace, content and rhythm of each session. This chapter will be a guide in the step-by-step process for conducting exposure therapy sessions with children, adolescents, and their parents. It will include how to generate a fear hierarchy and use that hierarchy as a guide for successive exposure challenges. We will discuss how to structure sessions to maintain child engagement and motivation; encourage positive and appropriate parent involvement; implement exposures in a variety of settings; utilize effective reinforcement; and help youth cognitively reappraise and emotionally process exposures. Finally, identifying and managing challenges as they arise will help the clinician focus the family and youth on staying the course and persisting in their efforts toward conquering the fear.

Reviewing Key Principles with Clients and Their Parents

Key concepts introduced in beginning CBT sessions should continue to be integrated into each exposure session to make connections between the concepts and real-life examples and to deepen understanding of CBT principles. For most youth, parents play a critical role in the coaching and implementation of exposures. As you can imagine, children vary considerably in their motivation and the skills needed to independently engage in exposures outside of the clinic. We highly recommend that the therapist directly address with the parents the role that you expect them to play in their child's treatment. It is important to set the expectation that parents will be active in assisting their child in recovering from her anxiety disorder.

Share with the parents that their role is to be both coach and cheerleader. They will remind the child of the steps she has agreed to take, encourage her to take the leap, help monitor and track her fear ratings before, during, and after the exposure, and provide praise and encouragement from the sidelines. Therefore, it is paramount that parents are also educated in an understanding of the anxiety cycle, how escape and avoidance increases fear over time, and how approaching the fear gradually will increase self-efficacy and reduce anxiety. This information is integrated throughout the therapy process, as discussed in each section below.

Preparing the Child for Facing Fears

After initial sessions focused on information gathering, psychoeducation, and skills building, the next step is to work with the youth to create a fear hierarchy or ladder prior to the start of exposure work. A fear hierarchy is a specific list of activities related to the feared stimulus that are displayed in order of increasing difficulty or how strongly they generate a fear response (Abramowitz et al., 2011; Barlow, 2002). Creation of a fear hierarchy can often be accomplished within a session or two, although the hierarchy is likely to be modified and adjusted in future sessions as exposure practice unfolds.

Generating Exposure Tasks and Activities

The information that has been collected during the assessment process and initial therapy sessions should be utilized to review with the child which specific activities and situations trigger their anxiety, with the goal of exploring specific steps that might be helpful to work on in challenging the fear. Be prepared with ideas and potential steps for exposure activities specific to the target fear, as many children will not be able to generate these steps themselves. That is, many children have an overall sense of what they are afraid of (for example, being near spiders), but might not be able to identify the steps that will be necessary to extinguish their fear (looking at pictures of spiders, imagining a spider, talking about spiders, watching a video on spiders, going to an insect farm and looking through the glass window, and so on). Older children will likely have more input and ideas for what steps they will consider. When they do have this input, it should be encouraged and ideas prompted.

The more options and steps that can be generated, the better, as this provides greater flexibility and options for the child and therapist in their work together. Flexibility and allowing choices can reduce anticipatory anxiety that may result if the youth feels he is locked into a series of steps he is yet uncertain of his ability to complete. Each proposed activity will also give the therapist useful information on how the fear varies given any number of environmental changes (such as location, others present, physical proximity to the stimulus, and so on). Soliciting information and ideas from parents is important, as they may be more aware or forthcoming regarding the child's fear triggers, maladaptive cognitions, and safety or avoidance behaviors. If the child has multiple fears, the clinician may help the child and parents generate a number of separate hierarchies. For example, there may be a hierarchy of ten items for dealing with separation fears and a hierarchy of seven items for dealing with a spider phobia.

One suggestion for organizing this information is to utilize a visual display of the ideas generated using poster board or a dry-erase board, both for later recall and to track progress over time. The parent, the therapist, or the child can take a snapshot of the board for later use. Children can draw the list in the form of a ladder, with each step on the ladder an exposure item of higher difficulty. Younger children may appreciate decorating the ladder.

Another useful method of organization is to use index cards with one exposure activity written on each card. This allows for flexibility in adjusting the position of items in the hierarchy and adding new items to the list in future sessions. Children can choose an exposure task to practice from the available index cards or add a new exposure task by creating a new card. They can mark a star or put a sticker on each index card as they complete the task. Multiple stars can indicate each repetition of the task and a larger star or smiley face can be added for mastery of the task. For older children and adolescents, a table or checklist developed on the computer can be helpful. Use of a checklist allows them to place a mark next to the activity completed. The list of exposure activities can be increased or adjusted as needed.

Obtaining Fear Ratings for Each Activity

Once a list of activities has been generated, the child is taught how to rate her expected intensity of fear if she were to engage in each of these exposure-related activities. Rating the level of distress is a common practice in exposure work and has been utilized since developed by Wolpe and Lazarus in 1966.

Use of a fear thermometer, with anchor points appropriate for the age and cognitive development of the child, can help her make ratings for each activity. Younger children, who may have difficulty assessing subtle changes in emotion, may do best with a simple scale from 1 to 4. Anchor points on this scale might include: *Calm, A Little Scared, Medium Scared,* and *Very Scared*. They may also benefit from a visual display of facial expressions that increase in physical intensity for each number on the scale. Older children may prefer a scale with 5 to 10 gradations in emotion. The fear thermometer should be tailored so that it can best relate to the emotion being measured (anxiety, discomfort, stress, frustration, and so on). For example, the fear thermometer below assesses anxiety with five possible choices for the child:

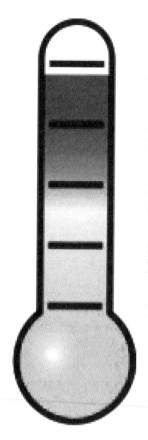

5 = Very Anxious or Scared and I Don't Think I Can Handle It; Panic; Strong Body Feelings

4 = Pretty Scared but I Think I Can Handle It; Moderate Body Feelings

3 = Nervous or Worried, but It Is Not Too Bad and I Know I Can Handle It; Mild Body Feelings

2 = A Little Tense or Worried; Feel Funny or Not Quite Right

1 = Calm and Relaxed

Prior to rating each activity, ensure that the child has an accurate understanding of what each number on the fear thermometer signifies. That is, the physical sensations and thoughts that would be typical at each number on the scale should be reviewed. Have the child provide examples of common activities that he feels would produce that level of emotion. For example, he might endorse lying in bed reading a book as a "1," which represents a calm and relaxed state. When he is thinking about starting his homework, he may feel a "2," or mild tension with some anxious thoughts. A "3" may be working on a particularly difficult homework assignment when he fears inaccuracy.

Once the therapist feels the child has an understanding of the meaning of each anchor point, the next step is to have him rate each potential exposure activity for how scared, stressed, or uncomfortable he expects to feel. In other words, he is asked what his predicted fear rating would be if he were to participate in the exposure activity. Young children may enjoy coloring the thermometer up to the number they endorse for each activity. For example, a question might be phrased as:

Bobby, if you were to let Mom take a walk to her car to get something right now, what number would you be on our fear thermometer from 1 to 5?

Some children may struggle to provide these predicted fear ratings. In these cases, a hierarchy can be ordered according to what they would like to try first, second, and so on. Another option is to have parents provide estimated fear ratings for each situation and utilize those ratings to develop the sequence of exposures. Even in situations where the child is able to estimate fear ratings, it is important to maintain flexibility in the exposures assigned each session, taking cues from both parents and children as to what is most relevant and important to accomplish given progress as well as obstacles from the prior week. Finally, it is reinforced with both parent and child that we will be working as a team to slowly help the child face her fears step by step. Therefore, the parent is included in session to give input regarding hierarchy steps, observe the therapist's use of the fear thermometer and taking of fear ratings with the child, and reinforce the child's hard work in session. Below is an example of a fear hierarchy with steps developed for a child with SAD:

Exposure Task	Fear Rating
Play game with parent in the clinic room with child	2
Play game with child while parent is in waiting room	3
Play game with child while parent is outside the building	4
Write a story imagining parent taking a trip to the store	4
Watch parent drive away and wave goodbye with immediate return	5
Play game with child while parent takes 5-minute trip to store	5
Parent takes 15-minute trip and child is allowed one phone call	6
Parent takes 15-minute trip and child does not make phone call	7
Parent makes short trip but does not tell the child length of trip	8

Structuring Exposure Sessions

Exposure therapy sessions with youth require special considerations in terms of their structure. Typically, a CBT-style format is followed in which the beginning of the session (approximately 5 to 10 minutes) is spent gathering information, assessing progress, and setting the agenda for the session. The content of the middle portion of each session (approximately 20 to 30 minutes) will depend on the current stage of treatment. Early therapy sessions focus on information gathering, psychoeducation, and building CBT skills. Once these activities have been accomplished, the middle portion of session becomes focused on implementing exposure tasks, which are undertaken with the goal of considerable repetition within session. Finally, the end of the session (approximately 5 to 15 minutes) is focused on processing the exposure task with the client and assigning homework. In some cases, it may be beneficial to allot a full hour for the treatment session to ensure enough time is given to exposure practice and repetition.

Beginning of Session: Gathering Information, Reviewing Progress, and Setting Goals

As mentioned, the beginning of session is spent gathering information, checking in regarding progress, and setting an agenda. This period is usually brief, approximately 5 to 15 minutes, with the goal of allowing sufficient time for the rest of session to be used for exposure exercises.

GATHERING INFORMATION AND REVIEWING PROGRESS

During information gathering, the parent and child will review exposure activities that were practiced during the week and the outcome of those activities, any obstacles that arose during practice, and other information related to the current emotional functioning of the child. The amount and quality of information elicited from parent and child will depend on the individual case. For example, children with highly developed self-awareness and self-expression, and those with high levels of internal motivation and desire to participate in therapy, will likely share more information that can be utilized in session. For children with less self-expression and motivation, or for those who are younger and less capable of taking on this role, parents will play a more active role in providing useful information at the outset of each session. In addition, young children may benefit from drawing a picture or role-playing with a puppet to describe the times during the week when they felt anxious, completed an exposure, or used their coping skills.

It will be important to place limits on the sharing of general day-to-day stressors or situations that are not relevant to exposure work. Exposure work needs to be the focus in order to be effective. Priorities should be established early on in treatment regarding which issues are paramount versus those that will be addressed at a later time. That being said, there may be times when an important issue will warrant steering time away from current treatment goals. In those cases, the therapist should check in with the child to determine when and how those issues will be addressed.

SETTING THE AGENDA AND DECIDING ON AN EXPOSURE TASK

Next, an agenda for the session will be set with the child. This plan will be based on the review from the week, progress made, obstacles noted, and information gathered from the child and parent. Including the parent in session allows her to observe the process of deciding on an exposure task with the child and learning what questions are relevant to ask. Use the developed hierarchy of fearful activities to negotiate the exposure task. When considering a starting place, it is useful to provide the child with some limited options. Giving specific options can reduce anxiety and make it easier for him to make decisions. One way you might initiate this conversation is:

Last week you gave me some ratings for different activities that we might practice. There were a few activities you said might make you feel a little anxious or tense and that you could probably handle. I think these might be good starting places. Would you prefer to try _____ or _____ first?

The goals established should be appropriate given current progress in therapy and the developmental capacity of the child. Of note, there is considerable debate as to whether it is most effective to start with a higher-difficulty exposure or to build gradually toward the more difficult exposures (Barlow et al., 2002; Clark & Beck, 2010; Ollendick et al., 2009). Most of the research is based on exposure work conducted with adult populations. Clinically, we find that there are many reasons why moving slowly and gradually increasing difficulty level makes intuitive sense when working with children and adolescents. Rapport, trust, and engagement must be considered. These factors are often negatively impacted when clinicians jump into a high-level exposure too quickly (Abramowitz et al., 2011). Many clients prefer to start at a lower level and gradually build their confidence. This allows them to test the waters—that is, slowly dipping their feet in and gradually entering the water, acclimating to the cold temperature one inch at a time. Success builds on success. While jumping in headfirst may be the fastest way to habituate, for many children this may be experienced as aversive. Further, for protective parents, it may be far less palatable to observe their child starting with high-intensity exposures. Alternatively, in some cases, starting with a high-difficulty item may be feasible if both child and parents are highly motivated for change and open to a faster pace.

WHAT TO REVIEW PRIOR TO THE EXPOSURE TASK

Once an initial exposure has been agreed upon with the child or adolescent, it's best not to delay it. Anxious anticipation of the exposure can increase when too much time is allowed between the agreement to engage in an exposure and the actual exposure itself (Abramowitz et al., 2011). The following guidelines are presented as suggestions for how to mentally prepare the child for exposure tasks. It is not always necessary to review all of these points, and clinical judgment should be utilized in determining which statements may be most beneficial to the individual child.

The rationale for exposure. It may be helpful to briefly review the positive benefits of engaging in these exercises, especially when there has been a lag time between psychoeducation and exposure sessions. Here is an example of dialogue that may be helpful in this regard:

> *Each time you try something on your fear ladder, you are likely to feel some anxiety or fear. But if you stick with it, those anxious feelings will get smaller. The more you challenge your fear, the stronger you get and the weaker your fear gets. Remember, anxious feelings in your body do not last forever and cannot hurt you. We will also be testing whether the bad things you expect to happen actually come true. From our conversations, we have some evidence that those bad things are not likely to happen. Facing your fear can prove this to you. It can also show you that you can handle what happens. Facing your fear is the only way to know for sure whether or not you really need to be afraid of (feared stimulus).*

Positive expectations of success. The therapist should provide brief encouragement that reflects her positive belief in the child's abilities to participate in the exposure. For example, you might state:

> *I know it's hard, but you can do this. Let's start small and build from there.*

Rewards for participation and effort. Many children benefit from a cue or reminder of the incentives available to them for making the brave attempt. For example, you might state:

> *For every exposure you try, you will earn a point. Five points equals a trip to the prize box.*

> *For every exposure you try, you will mark a check to show the completion of that task. Once you reach 10 points, you will have earned your trip to the zoo with Mom and Dad.*

Coping thoughts. The child can be asked to read or review his coping thoughts before engaging in exposure tasks as needed to build confidence to participate in the task (but not during the exposure, for reasons that will be further explained later in this chapter). Here are some examples of coping statements that the child may develop and review:

I am stronger than I think. My nervous feelings cannot hurt me. I can ride the wave of my anxiety. I have felt nervous before and I've handled it.

Bees are not interested in people; they like flowers more! They rarely sting, and only if someone is really bothering them. Even if they did sting me, I would survive. I can handle it.

Relaxation skills. Have the child who is visibly anxious take a few slow, deep breaths or use another relaxation strategy to enter a calmer state before the start of the exposure. However, it is important to avoid the use of relaxation skills during the actual exposure itself, for reasons that will be further explained later in this chapter. For example, you might state:

Let's take a moment to take a few calm belly breaths before we start. In for a count of three, out for a count of three.

Middle of Session: Implementing Exposures

As described, the content of the middle portion of each therapy session, approximately 20 to 30 minutes, largely depends on the current stage of treatment. For therapy sessions prior to the start of exposure work (approximately sessions 1 to 2), content will be composed of information gathering, psychoeducation on the nature of anxiety and the rationale for exposure, and activities to build rapport. The client will also create a fear hierarchy for potential exposure-based activities. As sessions progress, CBT skills are introduced and practiced for general anxiety management (approximately sessions 3 through 5). Some researchers recommend a brief approach to teaching cognitive restructuring and coping skills, spending no more than one session on psychoeducation and these skills prior to implementing exposure-focused sessions. Please refer to chapter 4 for a description of these different models.

Sessions then transition to a focus on exposure-based activities. An exposure task is chosen collaboratively and undertaken with the goal of considerable repetition within the session. Ideally, parents are included in many (if not all) of these sessions to observe the therapist coaching the child through exposures, asking for and tracking fear ratings, providing encouragement, and processing the exposure with the child at the end of the task. Over time, therapists can transition to having the parent take on these roles within session. In doing so, the therapist provides effective training to the parent in being a bravery coach for his child and increases the likelihood that exposures will be effective when conducted outside of session.

Throughout the exposure, it is critical for the therapist and the parent to demonstrate calm, confident demeanors. Uncertainty or hesitancy could be interpreted as a sign that there is indeed a reason to be fearful. The coach's job is to walk the child through the exposure by using a calm voice that conveys confidence in the activity and in the child's ability to handle the experience. Modeling the task for the child can also reduce her anticipatory anxiety. If, after encouragement and review of coping thoughts and potential rewards, the child is still resistant to engaging in the task, the therapist may consider having her engage in a part of the task and shaping behavior toward full participation, or choosing a lower-level task on the hierarchy as a starting point.

TRACKING EXPOSURES

A key component of exposure work is the assessment of changes in the fear rating at varying intervals. This information is necessary data for post-exposure processing. We recommend an exposure tracking form be used to collect fear ratings during exposure tasks. (See sample forms below. Visit http://www.newharbinger. com/39225 to download these forms.) A baseline rating should be collected at the beginning of each exposure. That is, the child is asked a question such as, "What is your fear rating as we are about to start this task?" Ratings are collected at fixed intervals of time (for example, every 1 to 3 minutes) for a task that is continuously occurring, or collected before and after each exposure for activities of short duration (Chorpita, 2007). For example, for a child with a fear of touching doorknobs (as in the case of germ phobia), one might take ratings of his fear level every minute during which time his hand remains on a given doorknob. Continue to take fear ratings once a minute until anxiety reduces significantly (for example, from a "5: Very Scared" to a "2: Tense"). A rating at the end of the exposure is also recorded and the activity is repeated with a different doorknob for generalization. As another example, consider the child with social anxiety who is making a phone call to ask about store hours. Ratings may be taken before and after the exposure, but not during, given both the short duration of the exercise and the likelihood that taking a fear rating will interrupt the child's verbal dialogue. However, this exercise will be repeated by making a number of phone calls of this nature. The child can then observe how her anxiety lessens over time with repeated exposures (after exposure ratings are lower on each successive trial).

Exposure Tracking Log: Before and After

Bravery Task: _____		
Duration of Task: _____		
My Goal: I will complete _____ (# of practices) *or* continue until my fear comes down to a _____ .		
Practice #1		
Fear Rating Before		
Fear Rating After		
Practice #2		
Fear Rating Before		
Fear Rating After		
Practice #3		
Fear Rating Before		
Fear Rating After		
Practice #4		
Fear Rating Before		
Fear Rating After		
Practice #5		
Fear Rating Before		
Fear Rating After		

Exposure Log: Continuous Practice

Bravery Task: _____	
Duration of Task: _____	
My Goal: I will complete _____ (# of practices) *or* continue until my fear comes down to a _____ .	
Fear Rating Before	
Fear Rating at _____ Minutes	
Fear Rating at _____ Minutes	
Fear Rating at _____ Minutes	
Fear Rating at _____ Minutes	
Fear Rating at _____ Minutes	
Fear Rating After	
Fear Rating Before	
Fear Rating at _____ Minutes	
Fear Rating at _____ Minutes	
Fear Rating at _____ Minutes	
Fear Rating at _____ Minutes	
Fear Rating at _____ Minutes	
Fear Rating After	

ASSESSING DISTRACTION, RITUALS, AND SAFETY BEHAVIORS

In addition, the careful clinician will also assess the client's use of distraction or mental rituals during the exposure. Mental avoidance of the situation or stimulus during an exposure through use of other strategies is contraindicated, as will be described in more detail later in this chapter. Similarly, the clinician will want to watch out for the use of subtle safety behaviors during the exposure. For example, in one therapy case, a child with fear of heights consistently stood with one foot slightly in front of the other as an attempt to stabilize herself. She felt this protected her. It was important during exposures to extinguish her use of this safety behavior so that she could recognize it was not needed for her safety. In service of this goal, the therapist or parent can ask the child or adolescent the following questions during the exposure:

Do you notice any rituals while you are engaging in (exposure task)?

Are you trying to distract yourself in any way?

Is there anything you are doing to avoid thinking about or paying attention to this task?

HABITUATION AND THE FREQUENCY AND DURATION OF EXPOSURES

Another critical issue to consider in implementing exposure work is how long the exposure activity should last and how often it should be repeated. One goal of exposure is habituation, the decrease of a physiological response due to repeated experience or exposure to a stimulus (Foa & Kozak, 1986). Habituation is considered one mechanism of change in exposure therapy (Lader & Matthews, 1968; Watson et al., 1972). Many researchers recommend a 50% to 60% reduction in anxiety ratings before termination of an exposure exercise (Abramowitz et al., 2011; Clark & Beck, 2010). Further, repeated and prolonged exposures are generally found to be more productive than shorter ones (Hembree, Rauch, & Foa, 2003; Quirk, 2004). That is, considerable time and repetition are critical for promoting positive changes in fear-related cognitions and greater habituation to the stimulus (Bouchard et al., 2004; Clark & Beck, 2010). Therefore, consider starting with frequent, longer exposures and space them out over time once considerable progress has been made; evidence suggests that this approach results in a stronger maintenance of long-term gains (Barlow, 2002).

The time it takes to habituate to a given exposure task will depend on a number of factors, such as the severity of the fear and the level of challenge presented by the task. As such, allowing for flexibility in the length of sessions or scheduling additional time beyond the 45 to 50 minute time block can be extremely helpful, and at times necessary. Some research suggests that disgust tends to habituate more slowly than fear, and therefore, exposures may need to be longer for cases in which disgust is a primary component (Olatunji et al., 2007). This could apply to exposures with vomit, insects, or other stimuli that elicit both fear and disgust. It will also be critical not only to practice these tasks in session but to assign them for homework as well.

In terms of helping to educate families regarding the concept of habituation, it can be helpful to show both parent and child a graph that demonstrates how habituation occurs within and across sessions (Chorpita, 2007). The general idea is that even though some of the fear may have returned at the start of subsequent exposures, the intensity of that fear is generally at a lower level. For example, during an initial exposure the child may have started at a 7 and anxiety reduced to a 4 by the end of the exercise. When this same exposure task is conducted for a second time, the child's anxiety may start lower, for example a 5 or a 6, and reduce to a 3. At the third exposure, anxiety may start even lower and the time needed to habituate shortens. A line can be drawn connecting these data points to show that the overall trend or slope demonstrates change in the positive direction (in other words, lower levels of fear). This rationale can be helpful in encouraging families to engage in practice between therapy sessions.

TERMINATING THE EXPOSURE ACTIVITY

While complete habituation may not always be realistic, it is obviously not beneficial for a child to abruptly terminate an exposure activity due to fear. In this case, she does not learn to disconnect the feared stimulus from her experience of uncomfortable physical sensations. In future encounters, the child may continue to experience anxious arousal at the same intensity. Cognitively, there are also repercussions. When the child ends the exposure abruptly, expectations regarding future exposures are unlikely to change. That is, she does not learn to recognize the activity as something she can tolerate and handle despite experiencing anxiety. She continues to assume the situation is dangerous and she cannot cope. As a result, considerable attempts should be made to help clients stay the course and complete targeted exposures or adjust the difficulty level and complete easier exposures if necessary. We consider it clinically important to end tasks with a success experience, however small the step taken may be. This increases the likelihood the child will experience improved confidence in her ability to cope with and face the fear in the future.

If the child continues to engage in an activity and, despite a prolonged period of time, anxiety remains heightened, a joint decision may be made to end the exposure. If the exposure is ended in this way and not as a means of escape, the child is more likely to experience the exposure as a success (*I handled it; I managed my feelings; I faced my fears*), despite the continued presence of physiological symptoms throughout the exposure. Many in the field recommend at least a full hour participating in the situation, but this will depend on the nature of the challenge. When a decision is made to terminate the exposure, the therapist should explore with the child the success she made in facing the fear, sustaining attention on the stimulus, and tolerating the anxiety. (See section below on facilitating emotional processing after the exposure.)

Another technique for increasing the willingness to attempt exposures and modulate duration is to allow the child a "controlled escape" (Clark & Beck, 2010). That is, the plan is to persist as long as he can before he needs to stop, with the goal to return to the exposure in a few minutes and increase the length of time engaging in the activity. With this technique, the child is building his tolerance for the exposure through a shaping procedure in which progressive goals help him increase the length of time experiencing the stimulus (for example, spinning in the chair for 30 seconds, 45 seconds, and so on). This technique also prevents termination of the exposure exercise from being viewed negatively or as an indication of a failure.

EXPOSURES TO PROMOTE GENERALIZATION

Exposure work is most powerful when significant repetition occurs in multiple real-life settings in order to generalize skills and mastery (Bouchard et al., 2004; Kendall et al., 2005; Tiwari et al., 2013). While some repetition may be possible within a clinic session, considerable practice will need to occur outside of session. There also may be exposures that are generally hard to approximate within the clinic.

It is therefore recommended that, whenever possible, the therapist hold sessions outside of the clinic and in the relevant exposure environment (for example, at a playground, grocery store, mall, bus, or zoo) Such real-world exposures are critical for generalizing skills and success. Initiating these higher-level exposures will be challenging for both parent and child to navigate and even more so if the expectation is that they take this leap on their own, without initial support. Use of telehealth through secure videoconferencing is an excellent option for maintaining support during exposure tasks and allowing the clinician greater flexibility in conducting a session at the desired location. For example, the therapist might request that an adolescent with a fear of crowds videoconference with her at the mall multiple times during the course of a week. For a child afraid of storms, the therapist might suggest holding an impromptu session via videoconference the next time a storm is approaching. This can help the child take the necessary steps to practice exposures when not in the clinic.

It can also be beneficial to capitalize on opportunities that occur spontaneously within the clinician's office (Abramowitz et al., 2011). For example, the therapist might help the child or adolescent with a fear of vomiting sit near others in the waiting room who appear sick, or might bring it up when she herself is feeling unwell. For a child with a storm phobia, the therapist could head outside with the child when the weather is windy or rainy. For a child with a fear of loud noises, she might process with the child any unexpected noises that occur during session. For a child with an insect fear, the therapist could point out any insects noticed within the office.

End of Session: Facilitate Processing and Assign Homework

The end of the session, approximately 5 to 15 minutes, is focused on processing the exposure task with clients and assigning relevant homework. During this portion of the session, you will review what the child has accomplished, praise his efforts in facing his fear, provide instructions to both parents and youth regarding the implementation of exposure tasks during the upcoming week, and discuss any perceived obstacles.

COGNITIVE REPROCESSING AND SELF-EFFICACY

Despite the historical emphasis on habituation in exposure-based therapy, the fact remains that it is not always possible to achieve a 50% to 60% reduction in fear ratings before an exposure activity is terminated. Recent research suggests that habituation may not be essential for the effectiveness of exposure work (Craske et al., 2008). That is, we cannot assume that the client will experience no fear (or even minimal fear) in the future when exposed to the feared stimulus (although repeated exposures do frequently lead to habituation, as noted above). Instead, the most primary goal may be to increase the individual's self-efficacy and mastery in the face of the feared object or situation, thereby providing corrective information and altering belief systems. That is, the individual no longer predicts the occurrence of aversive experiences in connection to the feared object or situation (Craske et al., 2008; Foa & Kozak, 1986; Hamm, 2009). While habituation is considered temporary and reversible, the cognitive changes associated with self-efficacy and expectations for future encounters offer more long-term, sustained change (Tryon, 2005). Therefore, the important mechanism here is a change in maladaptive beliefs as the client adjusts the way she emotionally processes the fearful experience (Craske et al., 2008; Hamm, 2009). In service of this goal, it will be important to process the exposure with the client so that she interprets her experiences in a more adaptive way and acknowledges her success and achievement in facing the fear.

FACILITATING EMOTIONAL PROCESSING AFTER THE EXPOSURE

Once the exposure has ended, it is important to help the child process and learn from the experience. Praise and encouragement should be provided for engaging in the activity. (For example, "I am proud of you for facing this. You really stuck with it.") You may also wish to have the child describe his success to the parent or repeat the exposure in front of the parent if the parent was not present to observe the exposure task.

In order to facilitate processing, we strongly recommend asking the child a number of questions that encourage a cognitive reappraisal of the fearful stimulus. In addition, these questions might uncover any number of problematic beliefs that interfere with the goal of habituation and greater tolerance of the fear. We present the following questions as a guide in this process, although each therapist should use her own clinical judgment in tailoring questions and processing of the experience in ways that are relevant to each client.

Did fear ratings lessen? Help the child track improvement in his physical sensations during the course of the exposure. Increase recognition that facing your fear becomes easier with practice. The following initial questions may be helpful in this regard:

What happened to your physical sensations during the exposure?

Did the feelings lessen, increase, or stay the same?

How did the feelings change over time?

Reductions in fear ratings during the course of the exposure should be reviewed with the child, along with reductions in the initial rating across exposures. This can demonstrate that habituation is occurring both within and across exposure activities. Younger children may appreciate returning to their body map to record (through coloring or marking on the map) where they noticed physical sensations before, during, and after the exposure activity.

If there was no change in fear ratings, hypotheses can be generated with the child. For example, she may not have had enough time to habituate. She may have engaged in mental rituals or distraction that prevented habituation. The exposure practice undertaken may have been too challenging and could be broken down into a series of smaller and less difficult exposures in the future. Regardless, the child can be encouraged that she is on the right track by taking on an activity that clearly generates anxiety for her. For example, you might state:

You worked really hard today, and even though your anxiety did not come down, we have learned that you can handle the fear when it arises and stick with it. I am really proud of you.

It's worth noting that some children may unintentionally inflate their fear ratings, and therefore it is always helpful when given a number rating to ask the child what sensations they noticed. If the sensations provided do not match the anchor points on the fear thermometer, help him consider whether his fear was truly as high as he was rating. Further, distinguishing between the internal sensations and what is externally observed can also be beneficial for children who are self-conscious regarding the outward display of their anxious symptoms. They may appreciate knowing that what they felt on the inside was not demonstrated on the outside.

Are expectations realistic? Sometimes, a child's hyper-focus on habituation or "getting rid of the anxiety" leads to negative outcomes and beliefs. That is, the child assumes that if she continues to feel some level of fear when presented with the stimulus that something is wrong, the exposure did not work, and—worse—the therapy is not working. Therefore, it is critical that the child understand that some level of anxiety is normal, and the most important goal of therapy is to learn how to handle the anxiety as it arises. Below is an example of dialogue that may be helpful in explaining this concept:

> *While facing your fears will reduce the fear itself, the bigger picture is that it helps you learn that you can handle the fear when it occurs. The nervous sensations may not completely go away, but this is okay! You are learning that even when the anxiety pops up, you can handle it. There will be many situations in your life where you experience some anxiety. This is unavoidable. The goal here is for you to know and trust that you can deal with these feelings when they occur.*

Did the feared consequences occur? Help the child reappraise the fear and recognize that the stimulus is not associated with the fearful negative consequences that he had previously predicted. In other words, the fearful response can be reinterpreted as a false alarm. A useful question along these lines is:

> *Did (the specific negative outcome or worst-case scenario) occur during the exposure activity?*

In some cases, the child will experience or perceive a negative outcome when there was none. For example, he may state, "The bee was about to sting me." Socratic questioning should be used to correct any cognitive misappraisals of the situation. In other cases, a child may perceive a negative outcome solely based on the experience of physical sensations (such as panic sensations or other uncomfortable feelings). Again, it will be important to help clients adjust any thinking errors and negative attributions. The experience of physical sensations of anxiety should be normalized and coping thoughts related to the child's ability to manage those feelings reviewed, as well as the temporary nature of anxiety. Without addressing cognitive misinterpretations, what appears to be a successful exposure may lead to future resistance or even therapy dropout.

Finally, there will also be situations where questions regarding feared consequences cannot be immediately answered, such as when a child is afraid that she will develop a feared disease if she does not wash her hands right away or stands near people who are coughing. In these cases, an additional goal is to help the child tolerate the uncertainty of the situation and the actual possibility that the fear might come true, even though it's unlikely. In this situation, you might have the child repeat to herself that *it is always possible* that she will get a feared disease. The repetition and externalizing of the possibility of the scary outcome allows for habituation to the thoughts themselves. With repetition, the child is likely to no longer have a strong reaction to the thought about getting a feared disease and become more confident in accepting and tolerating the experience of uncertainty.

Did the child cope? The final aspect of emotional and cognitive reappraisal of the fear is to help the child recognize that, despite the experience of fear, he is strong enough to tolerate the physiological response and can stay in the situation without harm. Commentary or discussion that helps promotes the child's confidence in his capabilities will be of critical importance. A useful question in this regard might be:

> *Were you able to handle or tolerate the exercise/activity? Did you handle it better than you expected?*

Most of the time the answer to this question should be "yes." If the child answers "no" even though he fully engaged in the exposure, it will be important to understand the reasons why he interprets the experience as something he had not in fact managed successfully. Attempts to normalize the experience of anxiety may be needed for children whose definition of success is perfectionistic. It may also be helpful to point out the therapist's own positive observations of the child's coping. For example, you might say:

> *Despite your fear, you did not run or try to escape. You answered me when I asked you questions. I know you mentioned your heart was beating fast. At the same time, I saw you handle this by sticking with me and not giving up.*

HOMEWORK ASSIGNMENTS AND PARENT INVOLVEMENT

The last 5 to 10 minutes of session is used for a review of the progress made, assigning homework, and addressing obstacles the family feels may arise during exposure practice outside of session and how they will handle those. In most cases, it will be important to review with both parent and child together to ensure that both parties have a common understanding of the action plan for the week. For older children and adolescents, therapist and client might make a joint decision as to how much parental involvement will be helpful and in what ways.

At the beginning, homework should closely approximate exercises completed successfully within the office. Parents and children should be provided an exposure log for recording out-of-session exposure practice. As discussed throughout this chapter, we strongly recommend parents participate in therapy sessions to learn how to work with their children on exposures outside of session. Parent observation of in-session exposure tasks allows the therapist to model coaching the child through these tasks without participating in accommodating behaviors. It also provides the child an opportunity to show the parent what she is capable of doing and to receive parental praise. Other methods for helping parents learn how to coach their child might involve role-playing how the exposure activity will be conducted in the home or public setting, or having the parent lead an in-session exposure exercise with thera-pist support. Finally, consider providing the parent with a "cheat sheet" of questions to ask the child as she begins an exposure, during the exposure, and at the end of the exposure to process the experience.

Coping Skills and Therapist Talk During Exposure

Coping skills discussed in beginning sessions are designed to give children and ado-lescents increased confidence in their ability to initiate, persist with, and complete exposures. For example, they learn that their feared outcome is unlikely and that their physiological sensations cannot hurt them. They review the rationale for how facing their fears can makes them stronger and more confident over time. They nego-tiate incentives for their brave behavior. After the exposure, they emotionally and cognitively reprocess the experience to develop more adaptive beliefs. In contrast, during the actual exposure, the use of coping skills and cognitive tools is typically contraindicated for a number of reasons.

Coping Skills During Exposure

One main concern with the use of coping skills or thoughts during exposures is that they often serve as a safety behavior (Barlow, 2002). With repeated use, the client becomes conditioned to rely on those safety behaviors when confronting the fear in the future. In other words, he perceives that the coping techniques are required in order to face the feared stimulus. Over-reliance on these tools can also cause the client to attribute success externally to the use of the safety behaviors, as opposed to increasing his own self-efficacy. He continues to feel that he needs to control and dampen the experience, as opposed to accepting it and recognizing that he can handle it.

A second issue with the reliance on mental rituals or coping skills during expo-sures is that they often serve to distract or prevent the youth from fully sustaining attention on the feared stimuli. This distraction can interfere with habituation and can prevent him from accepting and riding out the current emotional experience. Some research has demonstrated that the use of distraction during exposure predicts worse functioning and treatment outcome (Voort, Svecova, Jacobsen, & Whiteside, 2010). When distraction is used, anxiety may repeatedly fluctuate throughout the exposure. That is, increases in anxiety occur when attention is turned toward the stimulus and decreases occur when attention is turned away. The repeated avoidance of the stimuli prevents the client from fully habituating.

In order to assess whether distraction or rehearsal of coping skills are occurring during an exposure, ask the child what he is (or was) thinking about while attending to the stimulus. Is he involved in a mental ritual (such as counting or repeating safe words or ideas)? Is he thinking about a positive image to distract him from the feared image? Is he focused on the use of relaxation skills or another distracting technique? If he is using a strategy for mentally avoiding the feared stimulus, discuss the importance of fully attending to the fear in order to feel stronger and more comfortable with it. Have him monitor his use of distraction and coach him to turn his attention back to the stimulus when his mind wanders. For example, the therapist might state to the child:

I noticed you looked away from _____. In order to get used to _____, it is important to keep looking at it, even though it is hard. I know you can do this.

Is there anything you were thinking about while we practiced?

When the fear lessened, was there something in particular that made that happen?

Sometimes, the child or adolescent resists initiating the exposure without use of a coping skill. In this case, the therapist can help the child gradually reduce his reliance on those skills over time as he becomes more comfortable and confident in facing the feared stimulus and ready to reduce skill use. Below is some language that might be used to help children understand the need to phase out their use of coping skills during exposure work:

Now when we first got started I know that (use of coping skill) made it feel easier for you to (exposure activity). But now that you have had some practice, I would like you to try just observing (feared stimulus) and noticing the feelings in your body, without doing anything to keep your anxiety down. It is important to know that even when we feel anxiety or fear, we can handle those sensations. Just like a spring rain shower, our anxious feelings can come on strongly and quickly. However, they can also slow down and fade away quickly. Accepting the experience and giving it time helps. I want you to know this first hand. I also want you to know that even when the rainstorm is at its peak, you can handle it.

Therapist Talk During Exposure

Careful consideration is also needed regarding whether or not to engage in verbal dialogue during exposure practices. Some researchers recommend little to no discussion during the exposure activity to prevent both the meaning of the stimulus from being altered by the clinician and the client from becoming distracted (Chorpita, 2007). The only conversation that occurs is the therapist requesting fear ratings at varying intervals.

Alternatively, there may be some clinically relevant reasons for engaging in limited dialogue during the exposure. In the initial stages of exposure, verbal encouragement may be critical for motivating the child to continue and sustain the activity. Additionally, talk during the exposure may demonstrate to the child that she is capable of continuing a dialogue even while experiencing physical sensations of anxiety (Abramowitz et al., 2011). In fact, one research study with an adult population found that stimulus-irrelevant conversation during exposure, when it does not impact the ability of the client to fully attend to the stimulus, had no harmful impact and at times was a benefit on the outcome of exposure (Johnstone & Page, 2004).

Therefore, there may be times when limited dialogue during an exposure may have a positive impact. Similar to phasing out the use of coping skills during exposure, therapist talk may be phased out over time. Carefully spaced comments during the exposure can help the child build initial confidence and willingness to participate in exposures. These supportive comments can then be faded over time. The therapist can set the child's expectations for this to occur. Here is an example of a therapist explaining to the child the goal to fade out dialogue during the exposure:

> *You have been doing a great job with (exposure activity). I think you are ready to take the next step and practice without me saying a word. I am going to be very quiet. I will be rooting for you in silence. This gives you the chance to learn that you don't need me here with you to face your fears. That it is you that is handling this.*

Implementing a Reward System

Reward systems have been a standard and integral part of cognitive behavioral therapy and exposure work with children for decades. An individually tailored reward system can substantially facilitate a youth's motivation to work through increasingly challenging exposure tasks. That is, research studies demonstrate that CBT treatment responders are more likely than nonresponders to have been rewarded for their effort (Tiwari et al., 2013). Careful consideration of all aspects of the design and implementation of a reward system will increase the likelihood of its subsequent effectiveness. Families should be provided explicit guidance in developing and utilizing a reward system. The following section will present some key principles and strategies in developing reward systems for use with children and adolescents.

In-Session Reinforcement

The majority of time within each exposure session is devoted to preparing for, practicing, or processing exposure exercises. However, we must also remain cognizant to other needs of the youth that must be addressed, while simultaneously not being pulled too far off course by irrelevant requests or efforts to avoid the hard work of exposure. For example, children with ADHD may need a session with a faster pace or frequent changes in the activity (as long as these changes are not contraindicated when exposure tasks are undertaken). For children with whom developing rapport is difficult or for those who may not be inherently motivated to complete exposure tasks, it can be of benefit to devote a small amount of time at the beginning or end (or both) of the session to a rewarding activity. Young children may also appreciate playing a game with the clinician or choosing from a prize box to acknowledge their hard work. In contrast, children who are older, more introspective, and with greater internal motivation will be capable of engaging in exposure activities for a larger percentage of the therapy session and may not require breaks or rewards during session. However, they may appreciate a limited amount of time to share their interests or to address a current concern.

Bravery Reward Systems

As described above, goals will be negotiated for exposure practices both in and out of session. For out-of-session goals, it will be important to establish with the family what activity will be practiced, at what times of day, in what locations, with what frequency, and who will be present. Goals should be clear and measurable; that is, the child must understand what is expected and what criteria must be met to be successful. Have him record the goal on his exposure tracking log, where ratings can be taken before, during, and after each exposure. Below are some examples of specific and clear exposure goals:

Goal for a child with a fear of being alone in her room:

Avery will practice reading a book in her room for 10 minutes. She will do this once a day, with her parents sitting in a nearby bedroom. She will have the lights on in her room and will practice this after dark.

Goal for a child afraid of something bad happening to her parents when they go out:

Siena will refrain from making a phone call to her mother when her mother leaves on short trips (2 hours or less).

Goal for a child with OCD who is fearful of touching anything dirty:

Noah will practice touching dirty laundry from his hamper three times daily: once in the morning, once after school, and once before bed. This will involve touching and holding items of clothing for at least 3 minutes and until his anxiety ratings reduce by at least 50%, and refraining from hand-washing afterward.

Tracking Goal Achievement

It is helpful to list the goals for the week on a table or on index cards that can provide a visual reminder of the goals accomplished and serve as a tracking tool for the points earned toward designated privileges (see Bravery Goal Chart). The parent should mark a point or tally, or provide a star or sticker, every time a goal is achieved. Goals may be removed or adjusted after repeated and consistent mastery of each one in and out of session.

Some adolescents may benefit from tracking their own goals and checking in with parents to review their progress at a designated time each day. Many families keep the goal chart on a clipboard or hang it on the refrigerator or in the child's room for easy tracking. Younger children often enjoy tangible token systems in which pretend money, stickers, pennies, or marbles serve as tokens for each goal achieved. Tokens can then be "cashed in" for prizes. We strongly recommend that you send the family home with the system written or typed on paper or poster board. In our experience, the level of follow through is dramatically higher when details are not just discussed but also written down.

Providing Positive Feedback

Further, therapists should train parents to provide specific, immediate feedback for goal attainment. Help parents practice the language they need to use to describe the specific positive behaviors they observe as they occur. For example, a parent might state:

You chose something to eat from the menu so quickly. I am so proud of you for making a fast decision. I am marking a point down on your chart!

Teach families to review progress on the goals chart at a designated time each day with a focus on the effort made and positives observed. If the child completed only a portion of a goal, offer positive feedback on progress and express the belief that next time he will take an even greater step forward. For example, the parent or therapist might state:

Matthew, I am so impressed with how you approached that spider today. You watched it climb its web and stood near it for a whole 2 minutes! I know that soon enough you will be able to touch the web and put the spider in your hand. The more you practice, the easier it will get!

Encourage parents to avoid being critical or negative when a child is uncertain or unable to complete a task. Instead, reinforce the need to stay calm and matter-of-fact in tone of voice and demeanor and express confidence in the child's abilities. For example, to encourage practice of brave behavior the parent might say:

I can see you are unsure about going into gymnastics on your own. Let's see if we can come up with a plan to take this step by step. I will stay with you for the first 10 minutes. Then we can practice Mommy leaving the room for short periods of time. How about starting with 5 minutes at a time?

Developing a Reward Menu

Reward systems are generally more successful when rewards are salient and meaningful to the child. They are also generally more effective when they include: a menu with a variety of possible rewards; privileges and activities in addition to tangible items; and immediate rewards in addition to long-term rewards. Finally, rewards should be adjusted as interests change or the child "cashes in" for a specific object. Help the family design a system that feels both reasonable to parents and exciting and motivating to the child.

We recommend exploring a variety of options with the family, including: tangible rewards (such as purchases from a favorite store), privileges (video game time, bike trip, getting nails done), and social rewards (sleepover, special activity with Mom or Dad). The following are some questions that may be helpful in this brainstorming:

How does the child like to spend her time in the evening and on weekends?

What would she like to do more of that is currently limited?

Where would she like to go for a special trip?

What would she like to purchase?

What can parents reasonably provide as privileges in the evening? What time will these be offered? What is within the family budget?

Connecting Goal Achievement with Rewards

The therapist can help parents decide on specific point values to attach to both goals and rewards. They might consider making challenging goals worth more than one point. In terms of rewards, daily ones should be worth a small number of points, while weekly and longer-term rewards should be worth a larger number of points. For goals in which points will be earned at high frequency, consider having the child earn daily privileges, while having enough leftover to save some points each day toward a longer-term reward. It may also be beneficial to help the child understand that she can "cash in" points earned for privileges only at specific, agreed-upon times of the day. Access to privileges and rewards contingent on goal achievement should be restricted at all other times. Brainstorm with parents the environmental variables that should be considered when restricting privileges. How will the child be monitored to ensure reinforcement occurs only at designated times? Finally, it is important to make the rewards achievable. We recommend no point loss for any behavior, as this often quickly reduces the child's feelings of self-efficacy in her ability to earn the rewards.

Here is an example of a goal chart with point values:

Ada's Bravery Goal Chart

	MON	TUES	WED	THUR	FRI
1) Stays in bed all night					
2) Reads book alone in room after dark					
3) Stays with sitter for 1 hour; calls parent on phone no more than 1 time					
4) Walks through grocery store with parent at least 20 feet away					
5) Walks dog with parent walking one block behind					
Points Earned:					
Points Cashed In:					
Points Left Over:					

Addressing Obstacles to Establishing an Effective Reward System

While reward systems serve a vital role in building motivation and momentum within exposure therapy, these systems can backfire when not set up properly and created in a way that takes into account the daily reality and routines of the family. It is therefore of utmost importance to regularly check in and identify any obstacles that arise in the family's implementation of the system. Proactivity in addressing these concerns can mean the difference between developing something feasible and effective versus something the family feels is untenable within their home. Below we present a variety of issues that commonly arise when developing and utilizing reward systems, and some suggestions for addressing each of these issues.

When there is a wealth of noncontingent privileges within the home. If the home is already saturated with noncontingent privileges and items, the child will be less motivated to work for rewards on the designed system. Have a discussion with parents about the benefits of adjusting the household environment so that a greater percentage of privileges are contingent on specific positive behavior, as opposed to free access. Consider that our society rewards effort and hard work with specific positive outcomes (such as income earned at a job, and praise from your boss) and that by implementing a similar system in the home parents are teaching that hard work results in positive outcomes. When children have numerous privileges that are not connected to their behavior, they may develop the expectation that they are entitled to rewards regardless of their behavior (Barkley, 2013). This mindset can inhibit motivation toward achieving goals.

When siblings are jealous of the child who has the reward system. Questions may arise as to how siblings will react to the target child having his own reward system. Parents may want to develop a reward system for the sibling. Create something simple and easy to implement that is focused on a personal goal the sibling wants to work toward.

When the family does not have the time to provide rewards immediately. For families with busy schedules or multiple children in the home, difficulties in tracking goals and providing earned privileges may reduce the effectiveness of the system. Many children cannot tolerate waiting until the weekend for a reward, for example, or will become frustrated if a reward is promised at a certain time and then delayed. Therapists can help families such as these come up with a simplified system, working out in advance how the tasks will be practiced and the rewards administered during the week. Once these have been specified, discuss with parents the necessity of following through consistently when the child earns the rewards, and the risks of not following through (such as the child losing trust or motivation). Role-play and coach the parent during session on how to provide the initial prompt to engage in the exposure, encourage the child during the exposure, record points earned, offer praise, and administer rewards.

When parents put the child in control of tracking points or administering rewards. For most children, this type of plan will not be effective. Many children will be inaccurate or give themselves more points than actually earned, leading to less effort put toward goal achievement. Instead of allowing that level of control, consider having the child be involved by placing the sticker on the chart after the parent reports that she has earned it. Older children may be able to track goal achievement more independently, with parents reviewing their goal sheet and signing off.

When the child's motivation has dwindled. Discuss potential adjustments to the reward system at every session to ensure that it continues to be effective. Are the goals at the appropriate level of difficulty for the child? Do the rewards continue to be salient and of high interest to the child? Is the parent delivering the rewards effectively? Has the child just obtained a large reward and not decided on a new reward to work toward? Brainstorm changes that ensure the child is working toward specific, interesting, and attainable rewards.

When the child loses interest in rewards. It is rare for a child not to have an interest in any reward or privilege. If this concern is reported, ask how the child spends his time in the evenings and on the weekends. What are his hobbies? Consider making some previously noncontingent activities dependent on goal achievement. For example, if the child enjoys drawing, a reward might be a new set of colored pencils, a drawing book, or special time with parents drawing together. For a child who likes to read, extra down time for reading might be provided.

When the child is constantly negotiating or arguing over rewards. Suggest a weekly family meeting time to discuss and negotiate any adjustments to the system with the child's input. Alternatively, you can schedule this time to occur during the therapy session in order to offer guidance and support to the parents. Discuss in advance with the child that no adjustments will be made or negotiated during the week and that the parent alone decides whether a point has been earned. It is also important to coach parents on how to best handle their own frustration levels (including the tone and volume of their voice) and to model appropriate anger management. Parents must be prepared to hold to their limits without giving in when the child negotiates or argues.

Managing Challenges

As previously discussed earlier in this chapter, an attempt to encourage the child's participation in exposure activities should be made through: reviewing the rewards in place, allowing the child input in the exposure activity to be undertaken, starting with low- to moderate-hierarchy items, modeling a calm and confident demeanor, reviewing the child's coping skills, and expressing a positive belief in the child's ability to complete the task. When, despite these actions, the child continues to refuse participation, further problem solving is needed. Below we present some key considerations in this regard.

Adjusting the Initial Exposure

Making adjustments to the initial exposure is warranted for children who repeatedly refuse an exposure task. Adjustments may include the amount, intensity, quality, or other aspects of the exposure. For example, a child with separation anxiety who refuses to consider allowing her parent to leave the therapy office may instead tolerate the parent moving to the far side of the room, then standing in the doorway, then outside the open door, before finally moving outside the treatment room. A child who is unwilling to view a picture or image may instead be willing to talk about the feared image or look at a part of the image. A perfectionistic child who refuses to make a spelling mistake may be willing to spell a word incorrectly after making a spelling mistake is first modeled by the therapist. A child who is anxious about making a phone call may agree to make the call after it is scripted and repeatedly role-played with the therapist.

Assessing the Function of the Behavior

If, after a number of attempts to modify the exposure exercise, resistance continues, the therapist should consider whether the behavior serves another purpose. As a test, suggest an exposure exercise that is not expected to generate anxiety and is unrelated to the fear, in order to determine whether the resistance is associated with the actual fear or whether it is unrelated noncompliance. Children may resist simply because they do not want to participate in therapy, have not built enough rapport or trust with the therapist, do not understand the rationale for exposure exercises, are not motivated by the rewards, have a strong desire for control over their environment, or have a history of noncompliance with adult directives. If further discussion and observation deems one of these issues to be a factor in the resistance, the therapist must first turn his attention to addressing the obstacle. This may involve further rapport building, psychoeducation, parent behavior management training, reward system development, or cognitive work, depending on the nature of the issue.

Maintaining Child Motivation and Engagement

Revisiting the reward system may be necessary to ensure that the potential incentives are salient and highly motivating to the child. A review of cognitive processes involved in the fear may also be warranted. Struggles in this area may signify a need to return to cognitive work, reinforce the rationale for exposure, and review the coping thoughts necessary to build confidence in the child's ability to engage in the exposure tasks. Some questions to be considered include:

When you consider doing (exposure task), what goes through your mind?

What is your biggest worry if you were to try (exposure task)?

In other cases, motivation may be low because the child doesn't recognize the extent or severity of the problem, doesn't feel able to make changes, or is ambivalent about making changes. In these cases, specific questions that are consistent with a motivational interviewing approach (Miller & Rollnick, 2002) may help the child or adolescent increase her desire to work on the given problem and strengthen her belief that the work will likely be fruitful. Below are some questions to explore to increase motivation and engagement, especially when working with older children and adolescents:

When you imagine your life without this fear bothering you, what does it look like? How is it different?

What are the pros and cons of doing exposure work? What are the good things that might happen if you face your fears? What are the bad things you fear might happen? Is it worth the risk? How likely are these bad things to actually occur?

How can I help you get past some of these worries?

What are you likely to achieve if you work on this?

What will happen if we don't work on this?

I've heard or seen you do (note any past successes). How were you able to do that? What worked for you?

Supporting Parents as Exposure Coaches

Despite good intentions, it can sometimes be challenging to engage families in the therapy process. Some parents report that they have difficulty structuring the exposure with their child or finding the time or resources to carry out the exercise. Other parents state that they find themselves unable to withstand their child's resistance to taking part in an exposure or that they feel personally overwhelmed watching their child in distress. They may be unsure what to do when a child complains of feeling physically ill or reports other, plausible excuses for forgoing an exposure exercise. In these cases, it's important to normalize these challenges for the parents and give them tools that they feel they can use in the moment.

First, therapists should discuss the specifics of any planned exposure exercise with the parents in session in order to address any concerns the parents may have or identify complications that the child may not have been aware of. Second, it is essential to stress for the parents that their primary job is to praise any small approximations of success. So if the child's assignment was to go to a birthday party, it is still a success if the child attended the party but sat by himself. Thus, the parent should focus on praising the child for attending (and any other brave behaviors the parent noticed), rather than colluding in the child's frustration at feeling lonely. Third, outlining concrete rules around exposures and managing anxious situations for both the parent and the child can be helpful. For instance, the therapist could help the parent and child identify specific, behavioral indicators of illness that would result in missing an activity or exposure exercise. By setting the rules in the therapy office, the parent may feel empowered to stick firmly to them and avoid negotiating with the child. Fourth, it may be helpful to review with the parent basic anxiety-management skills to help her manage her own anxious reactions to conducting exposures (see chapters 3 and 4). Finally, there may be times in which poor parent-child communication or negative family dynamics serve to reinforce anxiety and impede therapy gains. In those circumstances, it may be best to address these family issues utilizing adjunctive therapies, such as behavioral parent training or cognitive behavioral family therapy.

Conclusion

Implementing exposure therapy for youth requires considerable skill and finesse in developing an effective structure, content, and flow within and across sessions. An important first step is the collaborative generation of a clear and detailed fear hierarchy. This hierarchy is used as an overarching framework or guide for increasing exposure challenges over time that focus on achieving the youth's bravery-related goals. Structuring sessions to maintain child engagement and motivation, encouraging positive parental involvement, utilizing effective in- and out-of-session rewards, and processing the youth's exposure experiences are all important considerations. Helping parents to complete exposure practice outside of session and become effective coaches for their children are also paramount in ensuring success and generalization of treatment gains. Finally, identifying and managing challenges as they arise will help the clinician focus the family and youth on staying the course and persisting in their efforts toward conquering the fear.

CHAPTER 6

Adaptations for Specific Client Populations

More often than not, the real-life clients we work with in our offices are complex and present with co-occurring disorders as opposed to "pure" anxiety disorders. Additionally, children with anxiety disorders who have comorbid diagnoses have historically been found to have higher levels of overall psychological dysfunction (Strauss, Last, Hersen, & Kazdin, 1988). Cognitive behavioral therapy techniques, including exposure work, can be used effectively to treat anxiety disorders in a range of complex cases; however, special considerations and modifications are often needed.

For cases that present with co-occurring conditions, it is important to begin thinking about the prioritization of therapeutic goals at the very beginning of treatment. As part of the assessment process you must consider the severity of each symptom and the impact on the child overall functioning, both in the real world and within the context of the therapy sessions. Additionally, it is important to explore and understand how the disorders may impact or influence one another. Prioritizing treatment goals should be a collaborative process between the therapist, parent, and child. Specifically, symptoms that relate to safety should be addressed first (such as suicidality, self-harm, substance abuse, and aggression), followed by symptoms that create barriers to therapy and exposure work (such as behavioral challenges, extreme anxiety or panic, avoidance of therapy sessions, high parent-child conflict, a poor therapeutic alliance, or high family accommodation).

Related to treatment, there is often a "carryover" effect, in which the CBT skills learned and used for one disorder, such as relaxation and cognitive restructuring, can be retooled and applied to address symptoms stemming from a comorbid disorder. The goal is to support the client with adapting the skills and generalizing them to other challenges, leading to more positive global mental health. There is also the possibility that as the initial targeted symptom diminishes, another symptom may increase or become more acute. In these cases, the therapist must rely on clinical judgment to determine the amount of shift needed in the current therapeutic plan. When possible and safe, it is recommended that the therapist consider splitting sessions to spend a portion of the time addressing the new concern and a portion maintaining focus on the exposure work, rather than abandoning exposures altogether.

This chapter will highlight specific considerations and modifications for a number of the most commonly co-occurring conditions for children with anxiety—including depression, ADHD, oppositional defiant disorder, eating disorders, and developmental disabilities.

Co-occurring Anxiety Disorders

Frequently, clients will experience anxiety symptoms or themes related to two or more anxiety disorders. For example, a child may present with high anxiety related to new places, worries related to being called on in class, and fearfulness and difficulty separating at bedtime. Further, for children and adolescents, co-occurring anxiety disorders are very common, and rates of comorbidity tend to increase with age (Wittchen et al., 2003). For example, it is not uncommon for a younger child to report anxiety related to separation and also identify specific phobias. A teenager may suffer from panic attacks related to school performance and also have a diagnosis of social anxiety or OCD.

When choosing which area of anxiety to tackle first, many times there is no clear-cut answer; there may be considerable symptoms and functional impairment as a result of each domain of anxiety. In these cases, the therapist's role is to support the client and family in evaluating possible starting points and subsequently making a decision as to where to begin. There may be several possible exposure hierarchies to choose from, and we recommend initially focusing on completing one hierarchy before starting another. Once the client has practiced exposure skills with a degree of success on one hierarchy, the therapist can introduce other areas of anxiety to target and work on with the child or adolescent to generalize the skills attained from work on the first hierarchy.

A further complicating factor is that there is often overlap between hierarchies and an exposure may inadvertently target two areas of anxiety at once—such as an exposure with elevators (claustrophobia) being done with strangers present (social anxiety). Acknowledging both factors with the client when creating the hierarchy is important because it may impact the degree of difficulty of the given exposure, initial anxiety ratings of the client, and his willingness to participate in the exposure. With therapist collaboration, the client can then decide where on the hierarchy each exposure task should be placed, and if other exposure tasks should come first in order to facilitate the more difficult one. For example, being physically close to strangers in a non-enclosed space may be a first step to practice before the socially anxious client is able to enter the elevator with strangers, even though the fear being focused on is the elevator phobia.

For other cases of co-occurring anxiety disorders, there is a clear and necessary starting point due to the impact of specific symptoms on the ability to effectively carry out treatment. Specifically, cases in which the client presents with panic attacks or trauma-related symptoms (PTSD) require significant therapeutic work prior to engaging in exposures for other anxiety conditions (such as specific phobia or separation). With comorbid panic disorder, it is quite possible that the child's panic symptoms may occur during exposure exercises and create a significant barrier to success. For this reason, it is highly recommended that the therapist begin by supporting the child in a better understanding of her panic response and developing a higher tolerance for physiological symptoms of panic through interoceptive exposure practice (see chapter 7) prior to engaging in other exposure work. Similarly, a child with anxiety related to trauma will require preliminary trauma-focused intervention to identify specific trauma triggers, better understand his physical reactions to trauma triggers, delineate trauma symptoms from other areas of anxiety, and engage in exposure work designed to help him habituate to distressing memories and the environmental triggers that are connected to these memories. As such, the goal is to address the impairment associated with the trauma and improve overall functioning prior to engaging in exposure work for additional conditions.

Finally, it is important for the therapist and parent to consider the costs and benefits of medication management for anxiety symptoms in the context of therapy. In many cases, anti-anxiety medication may mask anxiety symptoms and therefore make exposure work less effective because the child is not given the opportunity to feel and acclimate to physiological symptoms of anxiety. In other cases, anxiety symptoms are so overwhelming that they impair the child's ability to participate in treatment. In these severe cases, anti-anxiety medication may help to initially alleviate symptoms enough that the child can participate in therapy and begin to learn and practice CBT skills.

Depression

With the exception of co-occurring anxiety disorders, depression is the most common comorbid diagnosis for children and adolescents who present with anxiety. In general, it is estimated that youth with anxiety disorders are approximately eight times more likely to have depression as compared to children without anxiety disorders (Angold, Costello, & Erkanli, 1999; Costello et al., 2005). Additionally, clinical anxiety in children and adolescents, especially if left untreated, is a significant risk factor for the development of comorbid depression (Beesdo et al., 2010; Woodward & Fergusson, 2001). Further, there is considerable overlap in symptoms related to anxiety and depression in children, including negative thinking patterns, irritability and agitation, social withdrawal or avoidance of activity, and challenges with concentration or focus. For this reason, the therapist should be careful to conduct a detailed clinical interview, collect symptom-specific rating scales, and use functional assessment techniques as described in chapter 2 to support the client in understanding the source of observed symptomology (for example, clarifying whether the child is displaying increased irritability in the context of an anxious trigger or, alternatively, negative thoughts and feelings unrelated to anxious triggers) and in prioritizing treatment goals.

When treating a client with both anxiety and depression symptoms, it is especially important to understand the impact of each disorder on the other, and the dual impact of all symptoms on treatment outcomes. For example, in cases where anxiety symptoms began prior to the depressive symptoms (secondary depression), it is likely that untreated anxiety led to high levels of distress, feelings of hopelessness, and negative thinking patterns. These depressive features are likely to remit as the anxiety is targeted through therapeutic intervention and the child begins to feel some relief from the anxiety symptoms, thereby gaining hopefulness and confidence regarding the management of her anxiety. On the other hand, in situations where depressive symptoms pre-date the anxiety, or where the child's predominant emotional state is sadness as opposed to fear, targeting the depressive symptoms first may be necessary. In these situations, it is likely that the level of depression may greatly hinder the child's ability to participate in exposure exercises and complete homework assignments due to a lack of energy, low motivation, or an overly pessimistic frame of mind. Prior to anxiety treatment with exposure work, the client may benefit from CBT targeting depression symptoms, or medication management. For additional information regarding CBT interventions for treating youth with depression, please refer to the *Adolescent Coping with Depression Course* developed by Peter Lewinsohn, or *CBT for Depression in Children and Adolescents: A Guide to Relapse Prevention* by Betsy Kennard, Jennifer Hughes, and Aleksandra Foxwell.

While children with comorbid anxiety and depression can certainly benefit from exposure work, as highlighted above, progress may be slower and some modifications are recommended (Abramowitz & Foa, 2000). Realistically, there will likely be times when depressive symptoms need to be addressed at specific junctures before moving forward with exposure tasks. Although therapeutic gains are expected, it is likely that the rate of change will be slower and therefore treatment will last longer. Due to many of the common symptoms of depression (such as poor concentration, lethargy, and mental confusion), the child or adolescent may also require more repetition and slower therapeutic pacing. Additionally, as described above, there may be a benefit to practicing the application of CBT skills for depressive symptoms prior to targeting anxiety, as these skills may have an impact on anxiety management. For example, using Socratic questioning to challenge negative thinking patterns may help the child build confidence, decrease negative self-talk, and more enthusiastically face his fears during exposure work.

Attention Deficit/Hyperactivity Disorder

Attention Deficit/Hyperactivity Disorder (ADHD) is one of the most common childhood disorders, affecting approximately 5% of the child population (American

Psychiatric Association, 2013). Further, children with anxiety disorders are estimated to be approximately three times more likely to have comorbid ADHD as compared to the general population (Angold et al., 1999; Costello et al., 2005). Attributes inherent to ADHD—including shorter attention span, impulsivity, and difficulty sitting still—can negatively impact treatment outcome for anxiety and the client's capacity to engage in CBT and exposure work (Flannery-Schroeder et al., 2004; Halldorsdottir & Ollendick, 2014; Halldorsdottir et al., 2014). Adaptations are therefore required in order to achieve therapeutic success.

In general, children and adolescents with ADHD thrive in highly structured environments that provide consistency and appropriate boundaries (Barkley, 2013). To achieve this therapeutically, the therapist must work to establish appropriate behavioral expectations from the onset of treatment, including guidelines for participation and general behavior within the office. As with any child, recognizing hard work by providing frequent praise for effort is important for keeping the child engaged and positive.

When considering session structure, follow a consistent routine for each session—such as a check-in followed by homework review and then an exposure exercise to help the client stay focused and anticipate the next task. Additionally, children and adolescents with ADHD often benefit from frequent breaks and repetition, which may lead to slower therapeutic pacing and less material being covered per therapy session. For children with significant inattention, this could include alternating 10 minutes of work time with 3-minute breaks that allow for motor movement and a change of mental focus. Increasing sensory stimulation, such as using a fidget toy, sitting on a yoga ball or disco seat, or changing the environment (by using another office, for example), may also increase focus and decrease fidgeting. Finally, children and adolescents with ADHD typically respond well to very dynamic interactions, opportunities for frequent verbal participation, and high-energy engagement, so look for opportunities to have fun with role-plays and creative exposures.

For children and adolescents with ADHD, challenges with personal insight may also impact therapy. Research suggests that children with ADHD frequently have a "positive illusory bias," a tendency to overestimate their personal competence and level of functioning compared to external estimates from parents and teachers (Owens et al., 2007; Hoza et al., 2002). For example, on self-report measures, they tend to rate themselves as having fewer challenges compared to collateral data gathered from parent and teacher rating forms. Clinically, an underestimation of challenges may impact the client's motivation to work on goals, if she doesn't see the symptoms as a problem, or perceives them as a smaller problem than do others in her life. Additionally, related to exposures, the child may give lower ratings and underestimate the difficulty of exposure tasks on her hierarchy, which can lead to unsuccessful exposure attempts. For this reason, it is recommended that the therapist work with the client to help her understand the personal benefits of treatment and support her with ratings by providing external observations and reminding her of previous experiences for comparison points.

When being introduced to relaxation skills, children with high energy may find it difficult to settle their bodies. Additionally, inattention can make it difficult for the child or adolescent to focus attention inward and develop body awareness related to physical anxiety cues, such as muscle tension or rapid breathing. For this reason, children with ADHD may find it easier to initially engage in more active forms of relaxation, such as progressive muscle relaxation with visualization (for example, squeezing oranges), stretching or yoga poses, or using props for deep breathing (for example, putting a block on the belly to observe the belly rise and fall). Building body awareness can also be supported by fun analogies, such as practicing being as stiff as uncooked spaghetti or as limp as cooked spaghetti (or if it is around Halloween time, moving like Frankenstein and then The Blob).

Regarding therapy homework, children and adolescents with ADHD will likely need greater amounts of support and structure at home in order to manage assignments. It is helpful for parents to have the child complete homework around the same time each day so that it becomes part of his daily schedule. Keeping the assignment posted in a visible place and providing prompts or reminders when necessary may also increase homework compliance at home. As the therapist, it is important to appropriately gauge the amount of homework that the child can complete successfully, and to provide follow-up and rewards for completed assignments.

Finally, for cases in which symptoms related to ADHD are significantly impacting daily functioning, including the child's ability to learn needed CBT skills or participate in therapy, it may be appropriate for the family to consider medication management of ADHD symptoms in conjunction with therapy. When scheduling clients with ADHD, it is best to meet at times of day when the child is not exhausted and when medication is still active, so that he is better able to engage and benefit from therapy sessions.

Oppositional Defiant Disorder

Comorbidity between anxiety disorders and oppositional defiant disorder (ODD) in children is also a fairly frequent occurrence, with comorbid prevalence rates approximately three times higher than in children without anxiety disorders (Angold et al., 1999; Costello et al., 2005). Children and adolescents with ODD often present with behavioral challenges that serve as barriers to effective anxiety treatment—including engaging in power struggles, being overly argumentative, and demonstrating significant anger or irritability (Barkley & Benton, 2013). Additionally, there are often higher levels of parent-child conflict that may impact the ability of the parent to support the child with exposure work at home. If these behaviors are not addressed in the beginning of therapy, they may interfere with the building of a trusting therapeutic working alliance, which is necessary for collaborative exposure work.

Therapeutically, it is important to target significant disruptive and oppositional behaviors before moving forward with exposure-based therapy. Specifically, prior to anxiety treatment, it is recommended that the therapist support the family in developing and implementing a consistent behavioral management plan to address general noncompliance and disruptive behavior in the home and other key settings. Prior to exposure work, a moderate level of collaboration between child and parent should be achieved, with the child complying with a majority of parental instructions and the parent providing consistent positive feedback and rewards for good behavior. For adolescents, while many may be capable of a greater independence with exposure tasks if internally motivated, in other cases, improving the problem-solving and communication skills between parent and adolescent will be critical, especially when the parent is expected to play a key role in treatment. Refer to works by Alan Kazdin, PhD (*The Kazdin Method*), Russell Barkley, PhD (*Defiant Child and Defiant Adolescent Programs*), and Sheila Eyberg, PhD (*Parent Child Interaction Therapy*), for additional evidence-based ideas related to behavioral management, parenting skills, and building collaboration.

Once the family is ready to move forward with anxiety treatment, it is important to continue the focus on structure and collaboration. Similar to children with other comorbid externalizing disorders such as ADHD, children with ODD tend to thrive within environments that are well organized and consistent. Therapeutically, this translates into meeting consistently for appointments, following a consistent structure during therapy sessions, and setting appropriate behavioral expectations and boundaries. Use of a concrete behavioral plan with consistent reinforcement by the therapist creates predictability for the client and allows her to make better behavioral choices in therapy sessions. Immediate reinforcement for positive behaviors (such as verbal feedback or points) is also especially powerful in increasing positive engagement.

Since a central theme of ODD is power and control, it can also be helpful to allow the child opportunities to exercise power appropriately in sessions through collaboration (Barkley & Benton, 2013). Providing her with choices is one way to achieve this sense of control. For example, she could choose between several different exposure exercises or suggest creative ways to complete homework assignments. This sort of compromise allows the therapist to model flexibility and encourages the child to take ownership of her therapy work. Additionally, the therapist can work with the child to reframe anxiety as an opportunity to be powerful by "taking charge" and facing her fears. Finally, as a reward, the child may also enjoy having an opportunity to "play therapist" and direct the therapist through an exposure exercise. Once again, this allows the therapist to model as the child has fun practicing CBT skills.

Eating Disorders

In general, clients diagnosed with patterns of disordered eating—including anorexia nervosa, bulimia nervosa, and binge eating disorder—experience high rates of comorbid mental health issues, including anxiety-related disorders (Hudson, Hiripi, Pope, & Kessler, 2007). Additionally, for clients with co-occurring eating disorders and anxiety disorders, there is often an overlap of symptoms, and the greatest areas of anxiety may relate to food or body image themes. For example, an adolescent female with comorbid anorexia and social anxiety may report that eating in public places is extremely anxiety provoking. Although the target of your exposure work may be social anxiety, there will be times when your exposures also impact eating-related fears. In comorbid eating disorder cases, exposure work can be beneficial as part of a larger CBT-oriented treatment protocol. In fact, an inherent part of therapeutic intervention for eating disorders includes exposure to anxiety-provoking, food-related stimuli to reduce "food avoidance" (Fairburn, 2008). However, it is highly recommended that exposure work be done in collaboration with other professionals, including nutritionists and physicians. Therapeutic work specifically related to the eating disorder should be addressed by an eating disorder specialist while broader anxiety-related symptoms can be addressed through adjunctive anxiety-focused treatment. A team approach to treatment allows for continual monitoring of eating disorder symptoms by the eating disorder specialist and creates a safe environment for exposure work to take place.

Developmental Disorders

For children with developmental disorders, comorbid anxiety disorders are fairly frequent. In fact, certain attributes common in developmental disorders—such as mental rigidity, poor social skills and communication, and sensory sensitivity—can lead to increased daily stress and anxiety levels. For example, a child with autism may experience sensory sensitivity related to loud noises and therefore become anxious and reactive when he observes a fire alarm at school. With treatment modifications, children with developmental disorders can benefit from CBT and exposure work to reduce anxiety-related symptoms (Dagnan & Jahoda, 2006; Newhouse-Oisten, Kestner, & Frieder, 2016; Davis, Kurtz, Gardner, & Carman, 2007).

The first thing to keep in mind when working with this population is that assessment is key to understanding the relationship between the anxiety and the behavior. Since there is a wide range of variance in level of functioning and presentation of anxiety within this population, it is important to take an individualized approach to each case and work to meet the child where she is developmentally. Use of a thorough behavioral assessment is necessary to effectively understand patterns of anxiety, including triggers, the function of each behavior, and the child's attempts to cope. Oftentimes, children with developmental disabilities are referred for therapy due to the disruptive nature of anxiety-related behaviors, such as emotional reactivity or extreme avoidance. It is therefore essential to understand the function of these behaviors, as the child may not be able to fully communicate her fears. Based on the data from the assessment, environmental modifications should also be considered. For example, limiting triggers in the environment, such as by reducing transitions or removing a child before fire drills, may be more effective and timely than behavior modification.

When beginning the treatment phase with children who have developmental disabilities, it is important to consider creative ways to make the CBT model accessible to the child and family. Depending on the child or adolescent's level of personal insight and cognitive ability, CBT skills such as self-monitoring and restructuring of negative thoughts may be very difficult. Additionally, rigid thinking patterns and perseveration on negative thoughts can add an additional layer of difficulty in utilizing cognitive-based skills. In these cases, basic cognitive skills may be taught through repetition of scripted "push back," or challenge thoughts. For example, a child who is fearful of dogs may find it helpful to practice repeating, *They just bark to say a friendly hello.*

Overall, behavioral CBT skills, such as relaxation and exposure exercises, may have the greatest therapeutic impact. These skills should be taught in a concrete and tangible way to help the child learn and remember the new skills. For example, practicing deep breathing with a toy on the child's tummy allows him to see "full lungs" versus "empty lungs" with each deep breath. Similarly, when introducing rating scales, it may be difficult for some children to extrapolate from feelings to number ratings; using a rating scale with pictures or facial expressions as visual cues may be more concrete and effective.

When working therapeutically with children who have developmental disabilities, progress may be more gradual and fears may shift from one stimulus to another more frequently than with other clients. The child may require more repetition and practice of skills during sessions and consistent positive reinforcement for small gains will be especially important for maintaining the child's motivation. As the therapist, you may find it helpful to consider meeting for shorter periods of time, but on a more frequent basis.

For children with sensory challenges, it will also be important to consider the impact of sensory sensitivity on exposure work. Specifically, the child or adolescent may have a lower threshold for engaging in sensory-rich exposures. In these cases, it may be helpful to explore the function of the feared stimulus and sensory aspects, such as helping the child to understand that the "buzzing" noise of a bee is due to the way its wings move when it flies. The child can reframe her worry thought by saying to herself, *The bee is buzzing when it flies to make me some honey.*

Finally, for children with developmental challenges, collaboration with parents and other supporting adults is key to successful treatment. Generally, it is recommended that a portion of the session be spent coaching the caregiver on how to model calmness, provide encouragement and positive reinforcement for facing fears, and generally support the child with exposure exercises. This can be accomplished by having the parent observe portions of each session. The therapist then meets periodically with the parent individually to discuss progress, provide instruction, and give feedback. Additionally, working with teachers or other supportive adults will help the child to practice his skills in other settings and generalize what he learns. For additional information on working therapeutically with clients who have autism spectrum disorder, consider referring to works by Tony Attwood, PhD (*The Complete Guide to Asperger's Syndrome*), and Angela Scarpa, PhD (*CBT for Children and Adolescents with High Functioning Autism Spectrum Disorders*). Furthermore, *Psychiatry of Intellectual Disability* by Julie Gentile, MD, provides additional ideas regarding therapy modifications specific to clients with intellectual disabilities.

Conclusion

Overall, CBT and exposure work can be successful in complex clinical cases; however, it is essential to understand the impact of comorbid symptomology on the child and utilize this data to inform subsequent treatment. In general, as the therapist, it is important to remain flexible in treatment, work collaboratively with the family to prioritize treatment goals, address symptoms that are barriers to treatment, and consult with or refer to other professionals when necessary. Additionally, each comorbid disorder comes with its own unique set of challenges and considerations. Co-occurring anxiety disorders are very common and require in-depth assessment to prioritize which areas to address first. When treating comorbid depression, it is crucial to consider the impact of the depressive symptoms on the child's ability to successfully complete exposure exercises. Externalizing disorders, including ADHD and ODD, will necessitate behavioral management strategies, increased structure, and a focus on building a cooperative therapeutic relationship. Anxiety with comorbid eating disorders requires collaboration with an eating disorder specialist and an understanding of the relationship between food-related stimuli and anxiety. Finally, CBT and exposure work to address anxiety symptoms in children with developmental disabilities requires modifications that make the material concrete and accessible.

CHAPTER 7

Exposure for Panic Disorder

In this chapter, you will find information related to exposure treatment with children and adolescents who have panic disorder. The chapter provides an overview of treatment considerations for this population related to CBT and exposure work, as well as a comprehensive list of exposure ideas and exercises. The information included is intended to support clinicians in creating and implementing an exposure hierarchy that is tailored to an individual child or adolescent client who experiences panic symptomatology and associated impairment, including agoraphobia.

Clinical Presentation and Causal Factors

Children and adolescents with panic disorder (PD) experience unexpected, abrupt, and repeated periods of intense fear or discomfort that peak within a few minutes (American Psychiatric Association, 2013). These anxiety episodes, also known as panic attacks, occur in the absence of real danger. Panic attacks can interfere with a child's home, school, and social life, resulting in the avoidance of situations she fears will lead to a panic attack or where she perceives help may be unavailable. This pattern of avoiding certain places is called agoraphobia. The most intensely avoided situations tend to involve public settings with unfamiliar people and groups (such as restaurants, parks, stores, and crowds; Kearney et al., 1997). When youth with PD are placed in these situations, they often endure them with intense anxiety and need to have a companion or support figure present (Biederman et al., 1997).

Children and adolescents describe physiological symptoms during panic attacks similar to those described by adults with PD (Kearney et al., 1997; Masi, Favilla, Mucci, & Millepiedi, 2000), including dizziness, heart pounding, sweating, shaking, shortness of breath, faintness, and chest pain. Although the physiological symptoms are more prevalent than cognitive symptoms in youth with PD, children and adolescents with PD do report cognitive misinterpretations similar to adults with PD, including a fear of going crazy, losing control, or dying. Furthermore, youth with PD report worry about the implications of a panic attack, have persistent concern about having another attack, and experience a significant change in behavior (such as avoidance of certain activities) related to the attacks (Doerfler, Connor, Volungis, & Toscano, 2007).

Panic disorder has a base rate of approximately 1% to 5% in the community (e.g., Essau, Conradt & Petermann, 1999; Lewinsohn et al., 1993) and around 5% to 15% within clinic referred and hospitalized populations of children and adolescents (Doerfler et al., 2007; Masi et al., 2000). Moreover, nonclinical panic attacks and related symptoms occur at particularly high rates among adolescents in community samples (36% to 63%) (King, Gullone, Tonge, & Ollendick, 1993; King et al., 1997). Panic disorder is most common in girls and adolescents 14 years of age and older, with mid-adolescence considered the median age of onset (Birmaher & Ollendick, 2004). There is also a high frequency of co-occurring internalizing and externalizing disorders in children with PD, with more than 90% diagnosed with another mood or anxiety disorder (Birmaher & Ollendick, 2004). Research suggests that separation anxiety and generalized anxiety are the most common comorbid conditions (Doerfler et al., 2007). In terms of causal factors, there are a multitude of variables that make particular children and adolescents more vulnerable than others to the development and maintenance of panic attacks. Anxiety sensitivity, negative affectivity, stress reactivity, behavioral inhibition, presence of major depression, and early history of abuse or stressful life experiences (in which the child felt a lack of control or predictability), all play a role in predisposing a child to the development of panic (Ollendick & March, 2004).

Exposure Therapy for PD

It is particularly important to uncover and employ effective treatment approaches for youth with panic disorder (PD) as this illness can lead to devastating outcomes. Panic symptoms in adolescence increase the risk of suicidal thoughts and attempts in late adolescence and early adulthood (Boden, Fergusson, & Horwood, 2007). Children with PD experience a high rate of comorbid conditions, particularly mood and other anxiety disorders (Birmaher & Ollendick, 2004). Delays in treatment for children and adolescents with PD result in increased functional impairment and the entrenchment of avoidant behaviors over time (Weissman, Klerman, Markowitz, & Quellette, 1989). Despite these concerns, for children and adolescents with PD, research on effective treatments has been limited in comparison to the breadth of research for adults with the disorder.

Panic Control Treatment (PCT), an exposure-based cognitive behavioral therapy treatment protocol for adults with PD, has a large body of research supporting its efficacy (Craske & Barlow, 2006). This treatment is important to highlight given that the theoretical model has been applied and the treatment adapted for youth with PD (Pincus, Ehrenreich, & Mattis, 2008). The model underlying this approach suggests that the development and maintenance of panic result from faulty connections established between physical cues in the body and panic attacks (Barlow, Gorman, Shear, & Woods, 2000; Clark, 1996). That is, individuals at risk for PD misinterpret and "catastrophize" the experience of normal body sensations (such as dizziness, high heart rate, stomach upset, and muscle tension). For example, an individual might perceive his heart pounding as a sign that he is about to have a heart attack or die. These catastrophic thoughts trigger the body to "sound an alarm" as a result of the perception of danger. The body responds with the "fight-or-flight" response, including an adrenaline rush, as described in detail in chapter 4. Over time, faulty connections are established in which the repeated pairing of subtle physical sensations with subsequent panic attacks leads to the conditioning of panic attacks to these body sensations, even without the occurrence of intervening thoughts. The individual becomes highly sensitized to slight changes in his body cues or sensations, anxiously anticipates panic attacks as a result of these body changes, and starts avoiding any activities or situations that might lead to changes in body cues or that have been associated with panic in the past.

The disconnection of this association between anxious physical sensations and their perceived consequences (panic reactions, cognitive misinterpretations of the physical sensations, and other perceived negative outcomes) is the specific mechanism of action believed to underlie exposure-based treatment of panic disorder. This involves systematic exposure to the feared physical sensations, also known as interoceptive exposure and described in detail later in this chapter; systematic exposure to avoided situations and events that are perceived to be associated with panic attacks; and correction of cognitive misappraisals and faulty predictions of panic attack likelihood and aversive outcomes in these situations. Through repeated exposure to the feared physical sensations and situations without escape or avoidance (and without the occurrence of the feared outcome), clients learn that they can cope with these sensations and situations and that they are not dangerous.

While research on the treatment of children and adolescents with PD has lagged behind that of adults, it is slowly burgeoning. A number of single case studies demonstrate positive findings for CBT approaches in treating the panic symptoms of adolescents with PD (Ollendick, 1995; Hoffman & Mattis, 2000). In particular, a developmental adaptation of PCT, Panic Control Treatment for Adolescents (PCT-A), modifies the PCT protocol by making it more understandable for adolescents (Hoffman & Mattis, 2000). Language is simplified and verbal and visual examples relevant to youth are used to illustrate therapy concepts. Pincus et al. (2010) conducted the first controlled trial of PCT-A. In their randomized study of 13 adolescents, those who received 11 sessions of PCT-A treatment showed significant reductions in panic symptoms, anxiety, depression, and anxiety sensitivity, in comparison to control group participants. Clinical severity of panic continued to improve from post-treatment to three-month follow up and remained stable at six months. No alternative approach exists that offers the research support that exposure-based CBT does for youth with PD.

Clinically Relevant Factors

Ongoing clinical assessment must focus on a clear and detailed understanding of the specific nature of panic-related symptoms and impairment in preparation for exposure therapy. As discussed in chapter 2, the environmental context within which the symptoms present, and the specific nature of the child's cognitions and behavioral responses, are critical considerations in the subsequent engineering of effective exposure exercises. Below we present typical fear triggers or cues, feared consequences, and avoidance and safety behaviors commonly occurring in youth with PD.

Fear Cues

Fear cues or triggers are specific environmental factors or variables that typically elicit the child's anxiety. These are the situations that activate the fear response due to the presence of specific stimuli that are perceived as dangerous or harmful in some way. The following fear cues commonly trigger anxiety in children with PD:

Visiting certain locations where panic is anticipated, panic has been experienced in the past, or fearful cues are present (for example, at the doctor's office, or in a crowded location such as the mall or an elevator)

Any activities in which panic is anticipated, panic has been experienced in the past, or fearful cues are present (for example, at a school performance or athletic competition)

Thinking about, talking about, or hearing others talk about a feared situation or object

Experiencing subtle body sensations that result from hunger, fatigue, or physical exertion (such as dizziness, lack of concentration, shaking, rapid heartbeat, or shortness of breath)

Experiencing physical sensations that result from a specific activity (for example, the experience of pain during a blood draw, feelings of faintness during a medical procedure, nausea on a plane or car ride, or dizziness and butterflies in the stomach when at the top of a tall building)

Being with people or around objects that were present when panic sensations were experienced in the past

Intrusive and ruminative fearful thoughts about the likelihood of panic sensations; the likelihood of danger, harm, or death; or other feared consequences

Feared Consequences

Feared consequences are those environmental conditions and outcomes that the child expects will result from exposure to the feared stimuli. That is, the child's fear is initiated and maintained through her experience, or her belief that these negative outcomes will occur. The following are common feared consequences in children with PD:

Inability to escape, or claustrophobic fears of suffocation (for example, when in an enclosed space such as an elevator or airplane)

Anticipation of aversive physical sensations (such as heart racing, sweating, shaking, throat tightness or choking feeling, dizziness, depersonalization, fainting, or shortness of breath)

Medical emergency or death (for example, fainting and not receiving aid, or having a heart attack)

Loss of control due to inability to stop or manage the panic sensations

Danger or death due to the actual perceived catastrophe or other dangerous situation (such as fear the plane will crash, or fear of losing parents in the store)

Embarrassment from physical sensations (shaking voice, blushing, stuttering, or sweating) being observed by others

Inability to complete an activity or goal (for example, inability to concentrate or fully perform on a test or in an athletic competition)

Avoidance

Children with anxiety commonly avoid the environmental stimuli and situations that trigger their anxiety because they perceive a high likelihood of their feared consequences occurring. The following are common avoidant behaviors observed in children with PD:

Restricting, or refusing to participate in, activities that the child fears will lead to panic sensations or have led to panic sensations in the past (for example, sports or physical exercise, amusement park rides, crowded places, certain forms of transportation, or performance-based situations such as giving a presentation)

Refusal to participate in important activities necessary for maintaining health because the child anticipates it will lead to panic sensations (for example, avoiding injections or blood draws, refusing to eat food on his plate, or avoiding going outside or to crowded places)

Refusal to look at or approach stimuli the child anticipates will lead to panic sensations or have led to panic sensations in the past (for example, looking away while blood is drawn, closing eyes during certain parts of a scary movie, staying in the basement during a storm, or avoiding visual images of the feared stimuli)

Refusal to participate in activities the child has perceived to be dangerous despite low likelihood of actual danger (for example, avoiding various forms of transportation)

Safety Behaviors

Similar to avoidant behavior, children with anxiety often rely on specific objects, individuals, or actions that they believe will protect them from the feared stimuli or feared outcome. Safety behaviors are any action on the part of the child or adolescent that is performed in an attempt to feel safe. The following are common safety behaviors displayed by children with PD:

Staying close to a "safe" person (often Mom, Dad, or a caregiver with whom the child has a close relationship), or refusing to engage in specific feared activities unless that "safe" person is present

Seeking excessive reassurance from parents or other adults to confirm that a situation is safe and the child doesn't have to worry (for example, asking a parent repeatedly if the plane is safe, if the mall will be crowded, if she will generally be okay, if she will experience panic sensations, if she will throw up, and so on)

Refusing to share important information with caregivers in an attempt to avoid the fear (for example, not informing parents about the upcoming field trip to the zoo in an attempt to avoid having to go, or not revealing a physical ailment due to fear of the doctor's office)

Engaging in frequent or excessive checking or information gathering regarding physical sensations or body cues (for example, repeatedly searching the Internet for possible diseases that might be a cause of his physical sensations, or asking his parents to determine whether he is flushed or looks like he's becoming sick, or whether other physical sensations are noticeable)

Engaging in—or demanding that parents engage in—the use of safety behaviors or objects that are perceived as protecting the child from harm (for example, planning an escape route, looking for exits when a feared stimulus is present, carrying a water bottle wherever she goes because she fears a dry throat and choking sensations during panic, or preferring the elevator over stairs because of a fear of dizziness)

Using distraction in an attempt to cope with a feared situation, object, or physical sensation (for example, averting one's gaze from the feared stimuli, listening to music or playing an electronic game, or using relaxation skills such as belly breathing)

Tailoring Exposure Therapy for Panic Disorder

This section is designed to serve as a primer for the implementation of exposure therapy specifically for children and adolescents with panic disorder. It builds on the guidance presented in earlier chapters by offering the therapist specific strategies and modifications for implementing exposure-based work with this group.

Treatment for panic in youth requires particular emphasis on educating the client about the nature of the fight-or-flight response and how panic develops and is maintained over time through conditioned reactions and catastrophic thought processes (in other words, false alarms). Significant time will be spent understanding and exploring the panic cycle for each individual child to uncover situational, cognitive, and physiological triggers and the connection between those triggers. Thereafter, coping thoughts will be developed and practiced to normalize subtle physical sensations and specific triggering situations. Exposures will focus on approaching situations that are avoided due to fear of panic, as well as engaging in activities that generate physical sensations similar to panic and promote tolerance to feared physical sensations. Finally, for some clients, general patterns of over-breathing that contribute to uncomfortable physical sensations will be targeted.

Understanding the Panic Cycle

As panic typically involves feeling a loss of control, and is usually perceived as scary and aversive, it is critical to educate the child on the basics of the fear response as described in detail in chapter 4. That is, panic sensations are a normal and natural response to the presence of real danger; these physical sensations are temporary and harmless; and "false alarms" in our body can occur when we perceive danger in situations that are not dangerous, or when we start to connect certain physical sensations in our bodies with panic (Barlow, 2002).

In order to help their clients better understand how their panic develops and escalates, clinicians are highly encouraged to help them map out a recent panic episode from start to finish. The goals of this exercise are to help the client uncover maladaptive thought patterns, in which danger is mistakenly perceived or predicted, and catastrophic interpretations of physical cues in the body that contribute to the escalation and maintenance of panic. We highly recommend writing down each thought, action, or physical sensation (on a sheet of paper or dry-erase board) in the order that they were perceived to occur, so that the client can see the causal chain of events. Below are some sample questions that can help focus the conversation on understanding the factors that precipitated and maintained the panic.

Where were you when you experienced the panic attack/fearful feelings/anxiety? What were you doing?

What thoughts first popped into your head when you entered this situation?

What feeling in your body did you notice first?

As you noticed this thought or feeling, what happened next? Did it lead to another thought or physical feeling?

What did you do? What did you feel? What did you think?

What other sensations did you start to notice?

Did you have thoughts about those sensations or what they meant?

Below is a sample dialogue that demonstrates how the therapist can use Socratic questioning with her adolescent client to slowly uncover the panic cycle:

Therapist:	You told me that you had a full panic attack on the soccer field yesterday. I'm sorry to hear that. I'd like to better understand how this panic cycle got started. Is it okay if we walk through what happened right before the attack?
Client:	Yeah, I guess, if you think it will help.
Therapist:	Great. Well I'm wondering if you can tell me how you were feeling and what you were thinking when you were approaching the soccer field in your parents' car?
Client:	I don't know…I was okay, I think. Well, maybe I was a little worried about not making any goals. I haven't made a goal yet this season and most of the other kids have.
Therapist:	I see. So you were worried about whether you would make a goal. And did you notice any feelings in your body?
Client:	Not a lot…maybe my stomach felt a bit funny, but that's it.

Therapist: Okay, so from what I understand so far, you had some worry about not making any goals and some mild feelings in your belly, correct?

Client: Yup, that's right.

Therapist: Now, when your stomach felt funny, did any thoughts pop into your head at that time?

Client: Yeah, I hate when my stomach hurts. Last time I had a really bad stomachache and I got scared. But this time wasn't so bad, so I don't get why I would panic. Maybe I should forget about soccer altogether. It's not worth the stress.

Therapist: It's been really hard for you. I get it. Thanks for taking the risk to share with me. I really believe we can work together to help you feel better. These details will give us some valuable clues as to how your panic builds. So, I think what you are telling me is that when you notice stomach sensations, it reminds you of the time you panicked. Is that correct?

Client: Yeah, I guess you could say that's true.

Therapist: And when you think about the previous time you panicked, do you notice any other sensations in your body?

Client: Thinking about it makes me nervous. I mean, it was real bad, you know. My heart probably beats faster, I'm sure.

Therapist: And tell me about when you walked onto the field—what thoughts and feelings did you notice then?

Client: Well, by that time I had been thinking about my stomach for a while because the feelings kept getting worse. I was starting to think, *Here we go again—I bet it's going to happen.* I just knew I was going to panic. I would have to stop playing in the middle of the game and everyone would wonder what's wrong with me. That's so embarrassing. It would be terrible. I would rather quit. And the panic itself, that's bad, too. I breathe so fast that it feels like I'm choking.

Therapist: So let me see if I can put these events in the order they occurred. (*Writing on the board the sequence of events with arrows connecting each one.*) First, you worried you might not make a goal, then noticed some funny feelings in your belly. This led to thoughts about how bad your last attack was and how the panic last time also started with your stomach hurting. Thinking about this made you more nervous and your heart started beating faster. You kept thinking about your stomach sensations and they started increasing. You then predicted that panic was coming because of the sensations in your belly and perhaps your heart. You also predicted that bad things were about to happen: you would not be able to handle the sensations, so you would run off the field. It would be awful, and you would feel embarrassed. The nervous sensations increased until you did panic, at which point you started to fear that you might choke.

It is the clinician's job to help the child or adolescent connect the dots; that is, to understand how his fearful thoughts contribute to, or trigger, increased physical sensations and the development of panic in his body. These thoughts can also influence subsequent actions, which may lead to avoidance or attempts to control the environment, thus reinforcing the fear (as in *I was only safe because I didn't go to that tennis match*). Helping him gain awareness of the power of his thoughts in influencing body reactions and behaviors provides the foundation for understanding the need to actively challenge these unhelpful and catastrophic ways of thinking. The goal is to learn to accept and tolerate uncertainty and ambiguity as part of life and as not inherently "bad." Finally, it is important to highlight with youth that while they may experience short-term relief when they avoid specific situations, in the long run their avoidance prevents them from learning the following key ideas: the situation and physical sensations they are experiencing are not actually dangerous; the negative consequences they perceive are not likely to occur; and they will be able to handle such consequences if they do arise.

Development of the Fear Hierarchy

There are two main categories of exposure that are most relevant to treating a client with panic disorder: 1) exposures to treat the fear of the specific physical sensations that occur as a result of the panic, and 2) exposures to treat the avoidance of specific places, situations, or other environmental cues that have become associated with panic. Both of these pieces are critical to achieve remission of panic symptomatology.

With regard to the latter category, children vary in their areas of behavioral avoidance. For example, a particular child may have had a panic attack when attending her first soccer team practice. As a result, she may associate soccer practice with panic attacks and start to resist future attendance. Another child may feel panic arise when in crowded places such as the mall. Others may feel panic in performance-based situations, such as during tests or presentations. Exposures for each child must be individualized and target the specific area of behavioral avoidance. In addition, the careful clinician will look out for environmental cues that necessitate targeted exposure work. For example, panic may have presented when a child was jumping rope or while an adolescent was at a party with a strobe light. False connections may have been made between environmental cues and the negative event (panic). Therefore, exposures must work to incorporate those specific environmental cues along with the physical locations of avoidance. Finally, exposure work must consider ways to eliminate use of safety objects (such as keeping a water bottle or medication handy during the exposure, or needing parent present) as quickly as possible. If a child resists, you can incorporate gradual elimination as he builds confidence with in vivo exposure work.

Some clinicians may be concerned about the possibility of unintentionally eliciting a panic attack and therefore hesitate to implement exposures that might have that potential. It is important to remember that the treatment model focuses on coping with and managing panic and anxiety, rather than elimination. That is, we strive to "decatastrophize" the experience of panic. Therefore, it can often be a helpful experience for the child to work through the experience of panic during a therapeutic exposure. The therapist can play a critical role here by remaining calm and coaching the client to "roll with" the experience of those sensations without contributing catastrophic thoughts to the experience. The therapist can then process the experience with the youth post-panic to explore a different perspective regarding what transpired, including realistic assessments related to the danger present and the ability to cope. Accordingly, the reduction of panic involves cognitive changes in how we experience panic, not necessarily the complete elimination of panic, and most certainly not the avoidance of panic.

Incorporating Interoceptive Exercises

During exposure work, as always, we want to help the client stay in the situation and "ride out" the emotional experience. In panic disorder, after repeated pairings, strong associations are created between physical cues in the body and the fear response. As the body becomes conditioned to expect panic in response to these minor or subtle internal cues, unexpected panic attacks start to arise in the absence of intervening thoughts and at unexpected times. We call this process interoceptive conditioning.

An important priority for treatment is to weaken these interoceptive connections by decreasing the sensitivity of the youth to these internal cues. In other words, we want the child or adolescent to habituate to the presence of these physical cues in the body and disconnect these cues from the panic response. This means actively facing—in a controlled, systematic, and gradual way—the physical sensations he fears the most. As a result of habituation, cognitions should also adjust: clients realize they are able to tolerate these physiological sensations and that the sensations are not harmful or dangerous. There are a number of important considerations when conducting such interoceptive exposures with youth. First, the child must be able to grasp the rationale and the idea that panic becomes connected to her experience of physical sensations in the body, and that the way to reduce that connection is to help her face those physical sensations step by step. If she cannot understand this line of reasoning, interoceptive exposures may be contraindicated, as they could be experienced as aversive, without particular purpose or meaning.

The most effective interoceptive exercises are those that replicate the specific physical sensations that are associated with the client's fear or distress (Boettcher, Brake, & Barlow, 2016). For example, one child may fear dizziness because he assumes he will faint, while another may be scared of rapid heart pounding and view this as a more aversive experience. Therefore, exercises such as spinning in a chair (to induce dizziness) may be more relevant to the first child, whereas running up stairs (to increase heart rate) may be more relevant to the second child.

It is also considered good practice for the therapist to model the exercise before having the child engage in it. That is, you might spin in a chair for 30 seconds, run up and down stairs, breathe through a straw, or put a heavy sweater on in a warm room. This allows the child to more easily conceptualize the activity and gives her the chance to observe a lack of aversive outcome. We recommend having the client start with brief, 30-second to 1-minute exposures for the full range of interoceptive exercises. As with other exposures, encourage the child or adolescent to stay with the activity for the allotted duration of time and observe any physical sensations that arise. You, as the therapist, should take a fear rating directly before and directly after each activity. This generates useful information regarding which exercises should be actively targeted. For example, a child may have a mild fear response to one exercise, a moderate fear response to another, and a very heightened response to a third. The therapist should then actively tailor subsequent exposures to target the child's specific fears, gradually increase the length of time and repetitions of the exercise, and shorten the lag time between each exercise. For example, a therapist may target jogging up stairs with a client with a starting goal of three flights of stairs, gradually building to five flights of stairs. At the onset, the therapist may wait for the child's heart rate to go back to baseline before starting the next climb. After several repetitions, lag time between climbs will be reduced, such that the child will start each new climb before his heart rate has fully slowed. As with other anxiety disorders, we always suggest structuring exposure activities through the use of an exposure log (see chapter 5). This tracking form highlights the youth's goals for the week, including the specific interoceptive exercises to be practiced and the expected duration and repetition for each. In addition, the form provides a place to record fear ratings before and after each exercise.

With each repetition, look for overall reductions in fear ratings, and process cognitions directly after each exercise using the post-exposure processing questions described in chapter 5. Research by Deacon and colleagues (2013) suggests that the greatest improvements in anxiety sensitivity occur when interoceptive exercises are applied repeatedly for a minimum of eight consecutive trials, with rest periods only long enough to take fear ratings. Exercises continue until the expectancy of a fearful response reduces. However, it is important to note that this particular finding was in an adult population and replication in pediatric PD populations is warranted.

As the child masters each individual exposure, consider increasing the challenge by combining two interoceptive exercises simultaneously (for example, wearing a heavy sweater while jumping up and down) or combining an interoceptive and an in vivo exposure (for example, jumping up and down before entering the mall, or breathing through a straw while riding the elevator). The goal of varying the exposure stimuli is to maximize the effectiveness of these exposures through habituation to a wide variety of situations and experiences, and to generalize positive cognitive changes (Craske et al., 2014).

Considering the Safety of Exposure Tasks

As with any exposure, you need to assess whether there exists any actual danger or safety issues with the proposed tasks. Adjustment may be needed to maintain safety. For example, if an adolescent develops panic symptoms anytime she is walking outside alone in the dark, you will have to consider what actual situational exposures will be appropriate and safe in this regard. Walking down a quiet and dimly lit street in a safe part of town or in the adolescent's neighborhood may be appropriate, while walking alone in an unsafe or unfamiliar area will probably not be. The therapist should also consider the developmental appropriateness of each task, as young children would not typically ride transportation on their own, go into stores by themselves, or have a drink such as coffee that might induce jittery feelings. Finally, and perhaps most importantly, you'll need to consider any medical issues that might make interoceptive tasks contraindicated. Any participant with known cardiovascular or respiratory problems may require adjustments, such as the use of certain medically necessary supports (an inhaler for a child with asthma, for example). Children with medical problems may need clearance from their doctors before engaging in specific exposures that could put them at risk.

Frequency, Duration, and Length of Sessions

As mentioned previously, exposures should be undertaken with considerable repetition and duration as to promote habituation and changes in the cognitive processing of the event. The clinician should assess for a 50% to 60% reduction in fear ratings, and positive changes in the cognitive experience of the event, as indices to guide the frequency and duration of exposures.

Overall treatment length and course will depend on the severity of the symptoms as well as the presence of other interacting anxiety disorders and associated behavioral avoidance. For straightforward cases, treatment is usually short term. For example, the PCT-A model is administered in approximately 11 weekly, 50- to 60-minute sessions. Pincus and colleagues also offers an intensive eight-day treatment model as an alternative approach (2008). For many children with complex presentations that encompass a broad range of behavioral avoidance, overall treatment may be considerably longer. For example, a child fearful of vomiting who experiences panic attacks related to many vomit-related stimuli will require specific targeting of each situation that provokes a panic response and leads to behavioral avoidance.

Cognitive Considerations

As with other anxiety disorders, probability overestimation and catastrophizing play a large role in the development and maintenance of panic. Of particular concern is the misinterpretation of physical cues in the body (as described above). This catastrophizing of normal or subtle body sensations can lead to a cascade of physical symptoms (the panic response). In many cases, the focus of the fear is turned inward as there is no noticeable external danger. Therefore, the child's specific fears and perceived negative effects and consequences of these internal sensations must be explored and challenged to break the panic cycle. Similarly, overestimations of the likelihood of these perceived negative consequences must be addressed. For example, if the child is fearful that his heart will stop beating, coping thoughts are collaboratively developed to combat these fears (such as, *I have been anxious many times before and my heart has not stopped beating; panic alone cannot make someone's heart stop beating*). If the child is fearful that her panic will lead to feeling out of control, coping thoughts are developed that focus on this specific fear (such as, *Last time I panicked I could still do many things I thought I wouldn't be able to do; feeling out of control may be uncomfortable but I don't have evidence that it will hurt me*).

Panic disordered clients also need considerable cognitive challenging of their fears and misattributions related to particular events, places, and objects. Children may believe that their participation in, or presence at, an event or location will automatically trigger a panic attack and they will be unable to cope. A situation which is generally safe, such as riding an elevator, may be viewed as unsafe and lead to panic as a result of the thoughts present (for example, *That elevator is too small, and what if it is not working properly? When I ride that elevator, I know I will panic.*). In these cases, help is needed to separate their panic from the event itself and recognize that it is their thoughts about the event that produce the panic.

Family Education and Support

It is important to ensure that parents understand the nature of the panic cycle and how catastrophizing physical cues escalates the panic response. It is equally important that parents recognize interoceptive and situational exposure work as safe and critical to treatment success. They need to understand their role in helping their child approach fearful situations and challenge anxious thoughts related to his body and the perceived danger of real-life situations. Parents must actively coach their child to participate in events and situations he might have otherwise avoided. We recommend parents participate in parts of the therapy session so they can observe and practice coaching their child in exposure exercises with the therapist present as a guide.

Other Considerations

Breathing retraining is a technique that can benefit clients with PD, with the goal of helping them gain greater awareness of breathing patterns and learn how to reduce over-breathing and shallow breathing. Over-breathing and shallow breathing occur when we breathe from the upper body or chest, as opposed to the diaphragm. These can occur more acutely during times of stress or anxiety or on a subtle level as a general pattern of breathing too heavily from the upper chest. Over-breathing, or hyperventilation, leads to a rapid expulsion of carbon dioxide with each exhale, which can generate increased heartbeat, dizziness, tingling, or disorientation as the balance of oxygen to carbon dioxide in the body is temporarily disrupted. While these sensations aren't harmful, they can be very uncomfortable. For children, we recommend using developmentally appropriate language to explain these physiological effects.

To demonstrate over-breathing, have the client complete an exercise in which she either: 1) takes five deep breaths in and exhales strongly each time, or 2) breathes fast and deep for 60 seconds. Inquire about the sensations she noticed while completing this activity and how similar those sensations were to those she experiences during a panic attack. This exercise is typically an exposure as well as an observational activity, as the child will notice some uncomfortable physical sensations increase and decrease. Parents can also participate in this activity, to enhance their awareness of the experience of their child.

In addition to underscoring with clients that over-breathing is temporary and cannot harm them, it is also important to help them learn how to practice calm breathing techniques to regulate their breathing more effectively. Once the child has a fundamental understanding of these techniques, discuss the goals of becoming more aware of his breathing pattern and learning calm breathing skills that allow the breath to descend to the belly and maintain the right balance of oxygen and carbon dioxide. Teach diaphragmatic breathing as described in chapter 4. Have the client practice 5-minute diaphragmatic breathing regularly during the week, usually starting with practice during calm times and increasing to more stressful occasions thereafter. It is important to note that these techniques are useful as general regulatory strategies *but are not recommended for use during exposure work as a means of anxiety reduction, control, or fear avoidance.*

Exposure Tasks and Activities Guide

As follows, we present a wide list of activities and ideas as a guide for clinicians' use in generating useful and creative tasks for a client's exposure hierarchy. These ideas are not organized in a sequence. Rather, the therapist should always use clinical judgment, as well as parent and child input, in determining the most effective next steps in any series of exposures, and should strive to tailor tasks to the individual needs of each child. Also, please note that while an attempt was made to categorize interoceptive exposures according to the physiological symptom they elicit, most interoceptive exercises elicit multiple physiological experiences. Therefore, exercises within one category may be useful for work within another category as well. Many interoceptive and in vivo exercises were adapted from the following sources: Abramowitz et al., 2011; Sisemore, 2012; and Pincus et al., 2008.

INTEROCEPTIVE EXPOSURES

Suffocation

Sit in a very hot room or location.

Use a space heater or turn the heat on high in the car (outside, not in garage) with windows closed.

Sit outside in the sun on a very hot day.

Sit in a sauna.

Sit in a steam room (or create one with a hot shower if space is enclosed).

Wear a heavy sweater or warm jacket (potentially add a scarf, hat, or mittens) indoors or outside on a warm day.

Ride a crowded bus, metro, or elevator.

Choking/Dry Mouth/Throat Tightness

Create a sensation of tightness around the neck through use of scarf, turtleneck, or other clothing. (Adult presence is advisable, especially for younger children.)

Put a tongue depressor or finger toward the back of the throat to simulate a choking feeling.

Swallow repeatedly and quickly (without drinking liquid).

Hold the swallow in mid action.

Fill mouth with food and pretend to choke.

Eat foods that are difficult to chew (such as steak, peanut butter, or string cheese).

Eat foods that create a dry mouth (such as saltine crackers).

Dizziness

Place head between legs while sitting or standing for 30 seconds to 1 minute, then quickly rise up to standing with head up.

Shake head rapidly from side to side for 30 seconds to 1 minute.

Spin quickly in a chair for 1 minute.

Spin while standing up for 1 minute.

Spin on playground equipment or amusement park ride.

Do 3 to 5 somersaults in a row (then stand up if not already dizzy).

Lay "upside-down" on couch (with back on seat, legs over back cushion, and head upside-down over side of couch) for 30 seconds to 1 minute.

Heart Palpitations/Increased Heart Rate/Sweating

Climb or run up multiple flights of stairs.

Run in place for 1 minute.

Do jumping jacks for 1 minute.

Jog in place while lifting knees high for 1 minute.

Hold the push-up position (or "plank" position) for 1 minute.

Lift a heavy object.

Dance around the room for 1 minute.

Ingest caffeinated food or beverage—such as chocolate, tea, or coffee. (Make sure the item is developmentally appropriate and not prohibited by dietary or family rules.)

Hyperventilation/Shortness of Breath

Breathe through a straw for 1 minute while holding nostrils closed.

Breathe in and out of a paper bag rapidly (1 breath every 2 seconds) for 1 minute.

Hold breath for 30 seconds to 1 minute.

Depersonalization/Derealization

Stare at a specific location (such as a dot on the wall, bright light, or other object) continuously for 1 to 3 minutes.

Sit in a dark room with strobe light.

Sit in a dark room with fluorescent light.

Stare at a moving spiral.

Sit in a dark room with no light and stare into darkness.

Nausea/Stomach Sensations

Read in a moving car.

Eat "heavy" food (such as a rich, cream-based casserole).

Eat until "overly full."

Eat prior to engaging in physical exercise (example: eat a snack and then do 20 jumping jacks).

Tighten stomach muscles for 1 minute.

Eat spicy foods or put hot sauce on food.

Eat certain feared foods.

Cough deeply and repeatedly.

Role-play gagging and pretending to vomit in the toilet. (Pour a can of split pea or minestrone soup into toilet as "vomit.")

(For other nausea-related exposures, please see the section on emetophobia in chapter 10.)

Feeling Embarrassed

Participate in situations likely to generate physical sensations of embarrassment (examples: wear clown hair in public, cough a lot or make other noises, clap hands abruptly).

When in public or other social situations, purposefully demonstrate the following:

- Shaky hands

- Shaky voice

- Stuttering or mumbling

- Heavy breathing

- Fearful facial expression

(For additional embarrassment-related exposures, please see chapter 13.)

SITUATIONAL EXPOSURES

Visual/Auditory Exposure

Draw picture of a feared situation or past panic experience.

Listen to audio clips of sounds related to panic symptoms (such as loud/fast breathing, rapid heartbeat).

Listen to an audio or video clip of someone having a panic attack (for example, from a movie or an audiobook).

Watch stimulating or exciting TV shows or movies.

Watch clip from TV show or movie with a feared or scary scene.

Watch clip of person in the feared location (examples: walking through a crowded mall, giving a presentation in front of a large group, participating in a sports game, riding a bus or train).

Imaginal Exposure

Create a script with all of the details of a previous episode of panic or a situation where panic is expected; imagine being in the situation while therapist reads the script multiple times. Therapist audio-records the youth reading the script and has him listen to the audio clip multiple times.

In Vivo Exposure

Transportation

Stand at the bus, metro, or train stop; watch vehicles arrive and depart.

Enter and exit the vehicle (bus, metro, train) without taking a ride.

Ride transportation for short (5-minute) ride or one stop.

Get on and off transportation frequently (example: take train one stop, get off train and wait for next train, then take that one another stop; repeat this process).

Stand while holding handrail on vehicle.

Give money or swipe card to ride the transportation.

Ride transportation for longer periods of time or multiple stops in a row.

Ride transportation through tunnels.

Ride transportation with various different family members or friends.

Attending and participating in events

Approach the location and sit in car with familiar adult (parent, therapist, caregiver).

Stand outside location with a familiar adult for a period of time.

Say hello and talk to fellow attendee who is also outside.

Enter the party or event for 1 to 5 minutes before returning outside.

Enter the party or event for increasingly longer periods of time.

Sit at table or location that is not next to a familiar adult for 1 to 5 minutes.

Sit apart from familiar adult for increasingly longer periods of time.

Allow familiar adult to use the restroom or leave location for 5 minutes at a time.

Allow familiar adult to use the restroom or leave location for longer periods of time.

Follow the above procedure for attendance at athletic, academic, musical, theater, or other social events.

For event performance, stand with the rest of the group during performance or sit on the bench with rest of team, even if not participating or ready to perform.

Start to participate in small increments or steps (examples: play an instrument or in a sports game for only a few minutes at a time, use gestures but do not yet sing at a group music performance).

(Please refer to chapter 8 and chapter 13 for additional exposures related to separation and performance anxiety.)

Crowded locations

Approach the store, mall, or restaurant at a time when it will not be crowded.

Stand outside and move gradually closer to the door.

Walk in and out of the door multiple times.

Walk into the location and stand near the door.

Walk further into the feared location.

Ask an employee a question about store hours or for help finding a particular item.

Make a purchase or order food.

Approach more crowded areas of the location or go at a time of day when it will be crowded.

Reducing Safety Behaviors

Avoid carrying or taking medication to reduce experience of any physical sensation.

Refrain from using relaxation, meditation, electronics, or other forms of distraction to dampen or avoid experience of physical sensations.

Refrain from carrying safety objects such as a water bottle, cough drops, paper bag, and so on.

Have parent refrain from providing repeated reassurance or answering related questions (such as "Will I panic?" or "Do you think I'm having a heart attack?"). Have client take responsibility for using thought challenging as needed. See chapter 3 for a detailed discussion on ways to mitigate parent accommodation behaviors, including appropriate parent responses.

Reduce frequency of looking up physical symptoms/sensations on the Internet or using other resources to assess conditions.

Case Example

A 17-year-old girl presented with frequent panic attacks which were initiated and maintained by both interoceptive conditioning and a number of core situational fears. In addition to panic disorder, this adolescent presented with a specific phobia of nausea and vomiting, which was intimately connected to her panic. Her fear of vomiting and associated panic led to significant food restriction, rigid food preferences, fear of feeling full or bloated after meals, and sensations of nausea before, during, and after eating.

Initial sessions were focused on educating the client about the connection between her catastrophic thoughts about her physical sensations and the escalation of panic. Of note, this client had memories of numerous episodes of vomiting that she experienced as traumatic. She believed that vomiting again would be "terrible," that subtle feelings of nausea were highly likely to lead to both panic attacks and vomiting, and that the panic and nausea would never end. After considerable education on the panic cycle and thought challenging (cognitive restructuring) to counter these maladaptive beliefs, an exposure hierarchy was developed with activities that targeted all triggers of panic (food intake, exercise, physical sensations including dizziness and nausea, transportation, and other activities she feared would lead to nausea).

Imaginal exposures were conducted using scripts of her previous memories of vomiting. After a number of sessions focused on repeated imaginal exposures, the client reported feeling less consumed by those memories and less fearful when recalling episodes of vomiting. Exposures also focused on looking at pictures and videos of vomit, smelling and looking at fake vomit, and pretending to gag and vomit into the toilet. Obstacles to participation in home exposures were addressed, including difficulty looking at the pictures and videos outside of the clinic. Videoconferencing with the therapist was initially used to support the client in initiating these exposures in the home setting.

Exposure work transitioned to interoceptive exercises, with the goal of building confidence in managing and "decatastrophizing" subtle body cues. This client initially struggled with activities such as spinning in a chair and climbing stairs, as feelings of dizziness led to sensations of both panic and nausea. However, repetitions of these exposures resulted in mastery of these activities and reduced anxiety levels. She was able to start incorporating exercise regimens back into her lifestyle, something she had avoided previously.

Exposure work also included goals of increasing her food intake, expanding the variety of foods she consumed, and establishing a healthy meal plan. These goals were the most difficult for this adolescent. Food was brought into session to practice increasing food intake and tolerating the physical sensations that resulted from this increased intake. Parental involvement was encouraged to reinforce and plan interoceptive and situational exposures at home. In addition, the family was referred to a nutritionist to collaborate on ensuring healthy meal plans and the maintenance of adequate weight. Safety behaviors were reduced, such as carrying her water bottle and eating food while listening to music as a distraction. This client also practiced eating meals directly prior to other activities, such as working out, walking, or attending an event—something she had previously avoided due to her concern that this would increase the likelihood of panic and vomiting.

At termination, this client was eating consistently, experiencing fewer and less intense panic attacks, using her coping skills effectively to challenge catastrophic thinking and manage physical sensations, and engaging in less avoidance as related to all of the situations described above. Given the complexity of this case and the multiple areas targeted within treatment, therapy continued over the course of one year.

Conclusion

Children with PD experience unexpected, abrupt, and repeated episodes of panic that peak within a few minutes. These anxiety episodes occur in the absence of real danger. The repeated experience of panic attacks and fearful anticipation of future attacks interfere with their home, school, and social life, resulting in the avoidance of situations in which they fear a panic attack may occur or help may be unavailable. Delays in treatment for children and adolescents with PD result in increases in functional impairment and the entrenchment of avoidant behaviors over time. Fortunately, research into the treatment of youth with this disorder is burgeoning, and recent studies demonstrate positive effects of exposure-based CBT. This chapter reviewed diagnostic information, key treatment considerations, and implementation of exposure-based CBT for children and adolescents experiencing panic disorder. Samples of specific exposure tasks were provided for consideration in creating individualized exposure hierarchies with clients. Finally, a case example was used to illustrate the clinician's role in implementing CBT skills and exposure tasks with a specific case of PD in an adolescent.

CHAPTER 8

Exposure for Separation Anxiety

In this chapter, you will find information related to exposure treatment with children and adolescents who have separation anxiety disorder (SAD). The chapter provides an overview of treatment considerations for this population related to CBT and exposure, as well as a list of possible exposure tasks. The information included is intended to support clinicians in creating and implementing an exposure hierarchy that is tailored for individual clients who experience SAD symptoms and associated impairment in a variety of contexts.

Clinical Presentation and Causal Factors

The clinical manifestation of SAD in children and adolescents involves a "persistent and developmentally inappropriate fear when separated from home or individuals with whom the youth is attached" (American Psychiatric Association, 2013). SAD is diagnosed in patients under 18 when they display excessive fear during separation events for at least four weeks. Children with SAD experience distress when alone, separated from, or anticipating separation from, an attachment figure. They often demonstrate reluctance to engage in activities without their attachment figure, worry about accidental separation or harm to the attachment figure, worry and reluctance to sleep away from the attachment figure, repeated nightmares, and somatic symptoms when anticipating or experiencing separation from an attachment figure (American Psychiatric Association, 2013). The distress these children experience at separation commonly leads to a number of behavioral manifestations including emotional outbursts, begging, whining, demanding the attachment figure stay, physical clinging, aggressive behavior toward the attachment figure, and excessive attempts to seek reassurance from the attachment figure regarding their own safety or the safety of the attachment figure.

As it is developmentally appropriate for young children to have a strong attachment to their parents, it is important to distinguish between developmentally appropriate worry and that which is disproportionate for the age and situation. Whereas infants and toddlers display an anxious reaction when separated from attachment figures, most young children learn that their parents will return. In contrast, children with SAD often display extreme reactions when anticipating a parent leaving them with a babysitter or attending a playdate or sleepover at a friend's home without their parents. Similarly, it is developmentally typical for children to be nervous before attending a new activity or separating from parents for long periods of time (such as a week at an overnight summer camp), yet most children soon adjust. When the anxiety interferes with the child's ability to attend such activities because he is too distressed in anticipation of or during the activity, or is resistant or refusing to attend activities or be away from the attachment figure, the diagnostic label is applied. As separation fears are more developmentally appropriate at a young age, a specifier of early onset SAD is provided to children under age 6 whose anxiety and distress is excessive for their young age.

Lifetime prevalence rates for childhood SAD are estimated at 4.1% according to data from a nationally representative survey of US households known as the National Comorbidity Survey Replication (Shear et al., 2006). Approximately one-third (36.1%) of cases in childhood persist to adulthood when left untreated (Shear et al., 2006). Twelve-month prevalence of SAD is .9%, the lowest of the anxiety disorders (Kessler, Chiu, Demler, & Walters, 2005). SAD is significantly more common among girls than boys, and most (86.1%) children with SAD have at least one other comorbid condition (Shear et al., 2006).

SAD develops through an interaction of biological and environmental factors. Environmental contributors to SAD include parental temperament and parenting style, which interact with a child's more fearful temperament (Ginsberg, Siqueland, Masia-Warner, & Hedtke, 2004; McLeod, Wood, & Weisz, 2007). Parenting styles that limit the child's sense of autonomy and control by being overly intrusive, (for example, by taking over a task that a child could do independently), are associated with higher levels of anxiety, and in particular, SAD (Chorpita & Barlow, 1998; Wood, 2006; McLeod, Wood, & Weisz, 2007). An insecure or anxious attachment style is also moderately associated with SAD (Eisen & Schaefer, 2005).

Exposure Therapy for SAD

There is significant evidence for the benefit of CBT involving exposure therapy to reduce symptoms of SAD (Ehrenreich, Santucci, & Weiner, 2008). Numerous randomized trials have compared CBT for child anxiety to a waitlist control group and have found significant improvements (Barrett, Dadds, & Rapee, 1996; Kendall, 1994; Kendall et al., 1997). While most studies of CBT include a range of childhood anxiety disorders, children with SAD compose a substantial percentage (17–23%) within trials that include a variety of primary anxiety disorders (Kendall, 1994; Kendall et al., 1997). The Coping Cat program (Kendall, 1994; Kendall & Hedtke, 2006) is the original CBT program developed for child anxiety. It is administered in an individual format. Alternative CBT programs are administered in different modalities. The FRIENDS program, for example, is administered in a group format with increased family involvement (Barrett, Lowry-Webster, & Turner, 2000). A randomized trial comparing individual and family-based modalities of CBT found equivalent results for child-reported anxiety, yet found that family-based Coping Cat was more effective when both parents had an anxiety diagnosis (Kendall et al., 2008). A preliminary study found evidence that training parents in cognitive behavioral therapy, without their child present, was also effective in reducing SAD (Eisen, Raleigh, & Neuhoff, 2008). Most cognitive behavioral therapy programs have been developed for, and evaluated in, children over 7, given the cognitive demands involved in challenging maladaptive thought patterns. To meet this gap, parent-child interaction therapy (PCIT) was adapted for the treatment of SAD in young children aged four to eight. This treatment focuses on parenting skills through teaching child-directed and bravery-directed interactions, in combination with the use of graduated exposure work (Pincus, Santucci, Ehrenrich, & Eyberg, 2008). Consistent with the fact that younger children are less capable of, and benefit less from, cognitive restructuring, this particular CBT component is not a focus of the PCIT for SAD protocol. Initial results from a randomized controlled trial (RCT) demonstrate the effectiveness of this PCIT with exposure for young children with SAD (Carpenter et al., 2014).

Clinically Relevant Factors

Ongoing clinical assessment must focus on a detailed understanding of the specific nature of the child's anxious condition in preparation for exposure therapy. As discussed in detail in chapter 2, the environmental context within which the behavior presents, and the specific nature of the child's cognitions and behavioral responses, are critical considerations in the subsequent engineering of effective exposure exercises. Below we present typical fear triggers or cues, feared consequences, and avoidance and safety behaviors commonly occurring in children with SAD.

Fear Cues

Fear cues or triggers are specific environmental factors or variables that typically elicit the child's anxiety. These are the situations that activate the fear response due to the presence of specific stimuli that are perceived as dangerous or harmful in some way. The following fear cues commonly trigger anxiety in children with SAD:

Attending school or an activity (examples: sports, music lesson, playdate, birthday party, summer camp) without an attachment figure present

Attending events with large crowds where separation is anticipated (concerts, large sporting events, crowded shopping malls)

Anticipation of sleeping away from home without attachment figure present (sleepover, overnight field trip, overnight camp)

Anticipation of an attachment figure departing (leaving for work, leaving after a planned visit to school, leaving the child's bedroom at bedtime)

Waiting for an attachment figure who is late (late for pickup, late returning home from work)

Learning of a parent's plans to leave the child with an alternate caregiver (hiring a babysitter, leaving the child with relatives while away)

Environmental aspects that feel challenging to the child (being in the dark at night, not knowing many peers at a birthday party, not feeling skilled at the required sport or activity)

Feared Consequences

Feared consequences are those environmental conditions and outcomes that the child expects will result from exposure to the feared stimuli. The following are common feared consequences in children with SAD:

Harm befalling the attachment figure (example: parent will get into a car accident)

Harm befalling the child (getting kidnapped, monsters in the house, getting hurt or injured as a result of absence of attachment figure)

Attachment figure will leave and never return

Becoming separated from an attachment figure

Becoming lost in a public or crowded location; not being able to find attachment figure

Feeling worried and not having the comfort of attachment figure

Inability to cope with or tolerate an activity or social experience

Difficulty sleeping or experiencing physical symptoms (vomiting, headache) without comfort of attachment figure

Avoidance

Children with anxiety commonly avoid the environmental stimuli and situations that trigger their anxiety because they perceive a high likelihood of their feared consequences occurring. The following are common avoidant behaviors observed in children with SAD:

Refusal to attend new activities without attachment figure present (playdates, lessons, sports)

Staying in close physical proximity to attachment figure while attending activities (physical clinging to caregiver)

Prolonged and difficult separation when asked to attend an activity without attachment figure

Resistance or refusal to attend school

Resistance or refusal to prepare for the separation event (refusal to eat breakfast or get dressed in preparation for school)

Resistance or refusal to sleep alone (falling asleep only with attachment figure present, frequent visits to attachment figure's room, sleeping in attachment figure's room)

Resistance or refusal to attend crowded events where separation is possible

Refusal to sleep outside of the home without attachment figure present

Resistance or refusal to be in parts of the home alone (the basement, upstairs without attachment figure present)

Resistance to being cared for by alternative caregivers (babysitters, relatives)

Refusing to eat or engage in other behaviors that might elicit nausea or other uncomfortable physical sensations when separated from attachment figure

Safety Behaviors

Children and adolescents with anxiety often rely on specific objects, individuals, or actions that they believe will protect them from the feared stimuli or feared outcome. Safety behaviors are any actions the child performs in an attempt to feel safe. The following are common safety behaviors displayed by children with SAD:

Staying close to attachment figure during an activity (holding hands, clinging)

Excessive reassurance seeking about the well-being or plans of the attachment figure (repeatedly asking what time she will return home, repeatedly confirming plans)

When separated from attachment figure, maintaining frequent contact through texts or phone calls, to be reassured of attachment figure's well-being

Sleeping with or nearby attachment figure

Ritualized routines when separating from attachment figure

Frequently checking the time when awaiting return of attachment figure

Carrying an object belonging to attachment figure

Using safety items or engaging in activities perceived to keep them safe (keeping a light on at bedtime, closing closet doors, sleeping with a blanket over the head, keeping the radio or TV on when alone in the home)

Maintaining proximity to a phone when separated from the attachment figure

At school, making frequent trips to the school nurse with physical complaints or to request calling attachment figure

Tailoring Exposure Therapy for SAD

This section is designed to serve as a primer for the implementation of exposure therapy specifically with the population of children with SAD. It builds on guidance presented in early chapters by offering the therapist specific strategies, modifications, and special considerations for carrying out this work with children with SAD.

Exposure sessions for SAD typically involve the child or adolescent gradually separating from the attachment figure both in terms of physical proximity and salience. Further, as attachment figures play a significant role in the maintenance and treatment of SAD, consistent and considerable involvement of attachment figures is indispensable. We strongly recommend that therapists consider evaluating parental accommodation of the child or adolescent's avoidance and use of safety behaviors. Oftentimes, in an effort to be helpful and reduce children's anxiety, parents allow children to stay near them, avoid difficult situations, and/or be in frequent contact to ensure the child is doing well. Parents may allow and inadvertently reinforce the use of safety behaviors such as carrying something belonging to the attachment figure at all times or being in excessive contact with the attachment figure (for example, carrying around a cell phone at all times of day, including when in school or while sleeping). As avoidance and safety behaviors serve to maintain and reinforce SAD, it is critical to evaluate these factors, teach parents skills for reducing their enabling or accommodation of these behaviors, and incorporate the reduction of such behaviors into the fear hierarchy.

Development of the Fear Hierarchy

Exposure sessions for SAD typically involve the child or adolescent gradually separating from the attachment figure, in terms of both physical proximity and salience. Prior to conducting exposures outside of the therapy office, it is an important initial step to have the child practice separating from his attachment figure within the office. This may mean having the parent sit in the waiting room, take a walk around the building, or drive to a nearby store while the child stays in the therapy office. The degree of difficulty (distance of the attachment figure from the therapy office, or length of time away from the office) should gradually be increased as the child masters each step.

Fortunately, opportunities to separate are plentiful. However, at times they may require extra planning, as they may be deviations from common routines. For example, the parent might drop the child at the front door and then park, instead of entering with the child, or she might plan to purposefully be late or have an alternative caretaker pick up the child from an activity. It is important to collaborate with other individuals with whom the child may interact during separations—such as teachers, coaches, babysitters, school counselors, or school nurses. Adults working with children with SAD should be provided information about the importance of not accommodating avoidance and limiting reassurance.

Exposures and cognitive challenges should be tailored to the needs of the child and based on information gathered from the functional assessment. For example, some children may be comfortable separating from an attachment figure during daylight but afraid of monsters under the bed that appear during darkness. In those cases, exposure tasks would focus on tolerating being in the dark alone. In vivo exposures might involve staying in a dark room alone for increasingly longer periods of time and with the attachment figure gradually increasing physical distance from the child. In contrast, for a child afraid that something bad will happen to his parent and she won't return, the practice could involve the parent arriving later than planned, with the delay of arrival gradually increasing. It is often helpful for the therapist to model for the attachment figure how to respond when the child experiences distress. It is important that the child learns to engage in brave behaviors with reduced therapist involvement over time.

Oftentimes youth fear separation from an attachment figure because they worry that they will become anxious or physically "sick" and will not have their attachment figure nearby for comfort. This is particularly difficult for many children at bedtime or when sleeping away from home. Attachment figures often help soothe children experiencing somatic symptoms of anxiety and therefore children become nervous about coping with such symptoms alone. Similarly, many children who worry about being unable to fall asleep without their attachment figure nearby overestimate the negative effects of delayed sleep or being tired. Interoceptive exercises will be important to incorporate into treatment (as described in chapter 7) when the child experiences a fear in anticipation of body cues or sensations. For example, practicing being tired and lacking sleep without being near the parent is a useful interoceptive exposure in the example above.

ASSIGNING HOMEWORK

As most separation from attachment figures occurs in real-life settings (school, sleepovers, parents leaving for work, and so on), it is very important for the child to practice exposures regularly outside of session. The child should be assigned separation tasks each week, increasing the length of time of the separation, increasing the physical distance of the separation, or decreasing the use of safety objects and rituals. For example, in the case of a child who struggles to sleep in her own room throughout the night, treatment might involve first setting up a bedtime routine involving starting the night in her own room. The child might then be challenged to stay in her room for gradually increased periods of time each night prior to going to her parents' room. She would receive a reward the following morning after each night in which she successfully met her stated goal. When the child did join parents in their room, they would set limits, such as requiring that she sleep in a sleeping bag on the floor, as opposed to joining them in bed. Parents would also be encouraged not to engage in conversation with her when she entered the room.

Alternatively, if the child is in the beginning stages of therapy and not yet ready for practicing a separation, she could learn to tolerate separation-related distress by engaging in imaginal exposures (for example, imagining the attachment figure is leaving), uncertainty training (for example, exposing herself to thoughts of the uncertainty of the attachment figure's safe return through auditory or written rehearsal of the feared event), or decreasing the amount of reassurance provided by the attachment figure. Many children with anxiety disorders have difficulty tolerating uncertainty (Comer et al., 2009). For children with SAD, this often may mean it is difficult for them to not know when a caregiver will return. Repeated exposure to thoughts that are uncertain can lessen the emotional arousal associated with such worries. Please refer to chapter 4 for additional information on uncertainty training.

USE OF TELEHEALTH

Telehealth can be an invaluable tool in treating SAD, given the importance of conducting separation exposures outside of the session during real-life moments of separation. For example, a therapist can schedule a telehealth session in anticipation of the child going on a playdate. The therapist can coach the child to remember his coping thoughts and relaxation skills in anticipation of the separation, review the plan for brave coping, and stay on the videoconferencing call as the child says goodbye to his attachment figure. If the child becomes distressed during the separation, the therapist can model for the parents how to stay calm without providing reassurance or reinforcement for negative behaviors. Similarly, videoconference sessions can be scheduled for times at home when the attachment figure may be leaving the house— for example, to walk the dog or run a brief errand. Many children with SAD have difficulty staying home when the attachment figure leaves the house, and some may even become distressed when parents are on different floors of the home or in the yard while the child is inside. The therapist can stay on a videoconferencing call with the child as the parent leaves to walk the dog or go into the yard, coaching the child to use his coping skills to stay calm and providing reinforcement for progress.

Considering the Safety of Exposure Tasks

Exposures tasks for SAD often involve encouraging the child to complete a task independently from an adult. When prompting a child to be away from an attachment figure or alone, it is crucial to first ensure that the task is safe and to clarify any risks with the family. If a child is planning to stay home alone while her caregiver walks the dog or completes a brief errand, it is important to assess the child's chronological age and developmental readiness to be alone. Certain states have laws stating the minimum age a child can be left home alone, ranging from as young as 8 (Maryland) to as high as 14 (Illinois).

Similarly, it is often helpful in the treatment of their anxiety for a child to practice separating from adults in public or crowded places. This may include being dropped off at an activity and walking in alone, completing a scavenger hunt in a public place such as an office or grocery store, or navigating a building such as a school or stadium on his own. Prior to the exposure task it is important to assess the child's developmental readiness for the task. Review with the child steps he can take if he becomes lost—including how to read signs, identifying which adults are safe to approach (employees of the store, for example), and selecting a meeting point. If a child will need to use an elevator to navigate the building, it is helpful to assess the child's familiarity with elevators and, if necessary, review with him how to use it.

Cognitive Considerations

Children with SAD tend to hold specific beliefs that predispose them to and maintain this condition. These misinterpretations should be addressed through cognitive restructuring work, as described in chapter 4, with the goal of helping the child build confidence in facing her fears and a more adaptive perspective when evaluating separation situations. Core beliefs of children with SAD tend to involve the following: 1) a misinterpretation of ambiguous situations as dangerous, 2) an underestimation of their ability to cope with situations, and 3) a focus on failure and a negative bias (Eisen & Schaefer, 2005). These factors ultimately lead to avoidance as the child perceives failure and catastrophe likely and views herself as unable to cope. This makes her less likely to enter new situations or persist in the face of difficulty. Children should be reminded of their coping thoughts and skills directly prior to and after exposure tasks.

Family Education and Support

Exposures for SAD by design involve not only the child with anxiety but also the attachment figure or figures. Oftentimes parents of children with anxiety have their own worries about dangerous things that may happen or about their child's ability to cope successfully without their support. For some caregivers, separating can be just as—if not more—difficult for the parent as it is for the child. It is important to provide psychoeducation to parents on the goals of exposure therapy, highlighting the likelihood of increases in anxiety in the short term during exposures in order to achieve an overall reduction in anxiety and ability to cope with such anxiety. It is useful to validate the caregivers' reactions to their child's distress, which may include both the urge to soothe, reassure, and accommodate the child and frustration with the child's behavior. Helping parents recognize that these reactions are normal is helpful in decreasing their own stress and their ability to serve as coping models for their child. Attachment figures should be encouraged to recognize their own anxiety about potential separation and practice coping thoughts and relaxation techniques to stay calm during exposure tasks.

Parents should be assured that they are not "bad" for their natural attempts to soothe and protect their child. At the same time, helping their child learn to soothe himself and cope with such anxiety is an important part of parenting. Parents should be warned about the likelihood of "extinction bursts"—that is, rises in anxiety symptoms and negative behaviors in children when no longer receiving accommodation or reinforcement during their anxiety. Attachment figures should be encouraged to continue to adhere to their exposure plan and ignore such behaviors. Further, it is important to prompt attachment figures prior to the exposure to identify ways they can soothe themselves and tolerate their own distress while watching their child be upset. It is important for the therapist to model for the parents how they should act during the exposure and to provide frequent praise and reinforcement for staying calm while witnessing the child's distress.

Oftentimes children with SAD will stay with a parent during an activity (such as a birthday party or basketball lesson) or accompany the parent on errands to avoid separation. Parents often accommodate such avoidance in an effort to reduce their child's distress or prevent disruption to the family. Instead, families should be encouraged to use such moments as natural opportunities to practice their skills and limit avoidance. Sometimes such opportunities need to be created. For children who have difficulty sleeping away from home, for example, parents can plan sleepovers at relatives' and friends' houses, varying in degree of familiarity and length of time away from home.

ADDRESSING REASSURANCE SEEKING

Children with anxiety often seek repeated reassurance from their attachment figures. For example, questions such as "Are you coming back? What time? Where will you be?" are common, even when the child knows the answers. Parents often attempt to soothe and comfort their child by answering such questions, often repeatedly, and assuring the child that nothing bad will happen. However, continually answering such reassurance questions can maintain the child's anxiety and his reliance on the attachment figure to cope. He is likely to feel comforted for a short time, but then become nervous again and feel an urge to repeat the question to be calmed. Attachment figures can use these questions as a natural opportunity to practice encouraging the child to answer his own questions as a way of coping. In other words, rather than answering the question, the attachment figure can note it is a "reassurance" question and encourage the child to answer it himself, develop his own coping thought, or tolerate the uncertainty of not knowing. Many times children ask such questions an excessive number of times per day. Attachment figures can begin to reduce the frequency by providing a limited number of index cards with the title "Reassurance question," or other symbolic tokens that the child must turn in in order to have a reassurance question answered. The child makes the choice to either use his question card or answer it on his own. When the limit for the number of questions allowed per day has been reached, the attachment figure refuses to answer such questions. The child should also receive a reward for each reassurance question card not used.

Exposure Tasks and Activities Guide

Following, we present a list of activities and ideas as a guide for clinicians' use in generating useful and creative tasks for a client's exposure hierarchy. While some sections may be loosely organized according to an increasing level of difficulty, they are not meant to be utilized in sequence. Rather, the therapist should always use clinical judgment and parent and child input in determining the most effective next steps in any series of exposures, and should strive to tailor tasks to the individual needs of each child. Many of the ideas below are based on the Coping Cat treatment (Kendall & Hedtke, 2006).

FEAR OF ENGAGING IN ACTIVITIES ALONE OR WITHOUT ATTACHMENT FIGURE

Visual/Auditory Exposure

View images of places the child may be avoiding (examples: school, sleepaway camp).

Read the website or brochure of activities the child may be anxiously anticipating. Many summer camps have videos that show what a typical day at camp is like. Schools may have a calendar of activities or sample schedule.

View images of crowded places where the child may be inadvertently separated from the caregiver (examples: festivals, amusement parks, concerts, sporting events).

Read stories about children attending a new school (example: *The Night Before Kindergarten*, by Natasha Wing).

Watch developmentally appropriate video clips on YouTube or other online sites, showing children successfully navigating the particular anxiety-provoking situations (examples: a kindergarten classroom, a gymnastics class, a crowded mall).

Videoconference with a staff member who can give the child a video tour of the feared location.

Imaginal/Role-Play Exposure

Role-play saying goodbye without a lengthy hug or ritual. Have the child practice calm statements such as, "Bye, Mom. See you at pickup!"

Role-play entering an activity according to the expected routines (example: hanging up her jacket and putting her backpack in a cubby).

Role-play being at an activity with parents and walking away to engage with peers (examples: sports practice, playdates, birthday parties, neighborhood block parties).

Imagine various scenarios (attending playdates, birthday parties, or camp without the attachment figure) and address the thoughts and feelings that come up. Repeat the script while gradually working in coping thoughts and responses.

If the child is nervous about what may happen while the parent is away, encourage him to make a "worry recording" starting with the phrase, "It's always possible that…" (Example: for a child worried about being left with a babysitter, the recording may include worries that the babysitter will be mean, the child won't have fun, or the parents won't return.) The goal of the worry recording is for the child to externalize worries and habituate to hearing these uncertainty statements, in order to reduce their overall impact on the child.

In Vivo Exposure

Practice gradual separation from the attachment figure in the therapy office (example: starting with the parent directly outside the door with the door open). It may be helpful for the attachment figure to give the child an initial reason for leaving, such as having to make a phone call or complete paperwork in the waiting room.

Gradually increase the number of minutes the child will stay in the therapy room without her parent.

Ask the attachment figure to leave the office for extended periods of time and extended distances while the child stays in the therapy room. (Example: the attachment figure can first walk to the door of the building and return, then walk to his car and return, then take increasingly longer walks around the building.) This plan may take place across many sessions. If the child remains nervous after the initial challenge, repeat that challenge prior to increasing the distance from the child or time away from the child.

Ask the attachment figure to drive off the premises of the office and return (example: drive to a nearby traffic light).

Ask the attachment figure to drive to a nearby store and pick out a fun reward for the child and then return.

Take a walk with the child away from the office without the parent present. Gradually increase the distance or length of time before returning.

Practice the parent "dropping off" the child and separating from her. Begin by joining parent and child at the door to the building and entering the office with the child, with the parent staying at the door. Gradually work toward the child being dropped off at the front door and entering the office as the parent parks the car.

Arrange with parents to drop off the child and have the child enter another place or activity alone (examples: a friend's house, school, sports lesson) while the parent parks.

Have child enter a part of the home where he fears being alone (examples: basement or upstairs while family is on main floor) for increasing periods of time.

Gradually increase the distance and duration of separation from attachment figures at home during activities the child fears doing alone (examples: showering, sleeping).

Ask attachment figure to go outside (example: into the yard) while child stays inside.

Ask attachment figure to take a walk in the neighborhood of increasing duration/distance while child stays home (with a sibling or other adult, if child is too young to be left home alone).

Have child play in yard while attachment figure stays inside home.

Have child take a walk in the neighborhood without attachment figure. (If too young to walk alone, can walk with a sibling or friend.)

Have child gradually increase physical distance from parents at an activity (examples: baseball practice, playdate).

Have child attend activity without parents present (examples: school, sports lessons).

Have child attend a playdate or birthday party without attachment figure present. Gradually increase the difficulty of doing so by planning activities with less familiar peers.

Have child stay home with a substitute caregiver (examples: relative, babysitter) while parents leave the home for gradually increased periods of time.

Reducing Safety Behaviors and Avoidance

Have parents set limits on the number of reassurance-seeking questions (examples: "What time are you coming back?" "Will you be here?") that their child can ask about an activity involving being away from their parents.

Encourage parents to frame appropriate reassurance as factual statements such as, "I plan to pick you up at 4 p.m.," rather than statements such as, "I will always come back."

Limit ritualized goodbyes (example: a set number of hugs or kisses).

Reduce safety behaviors such as turning all the lights on for the child or searching empty rooms for monsters.

Discourage carrying safety objects, such as a mother's bracelet, to an activity away from the attachment figure.

Limit the frequency of contact (texts or phone calls) between child and attachment figure when they are separated. Graduate to the child completing the activity without any contact with the attachment figure.

Encourage attachment figure to complete errands (examples: walking dog, grocery shopping) without bringing child along.

Encourage attachment figure to leave child for a period of time without phone or with phone turned off.

Encourage use of alternative caregivers such as babysitters or relatives.

WORRY ABOUT HARM TO OR LOSS OF ATTACHMENT FIGURE

Visual/Auditory Exposure

Read an age-appropriate book about the topic of death.

Read news stories about car accidents or natural disasters.

Watch an age appropriate TV show or movie in which a caregiver dies.

Create and listen to a worry loop tape with statements such as "My parents might get into a car accident and die" to learn to externalize and tolerate uncertainty worries.

Imaginal/Role-Play Exposure

Imagine a parent is late to pick up the child from school or another activity. Encourage the child to imagine who is there, what they are doing, what they are thinking, and so on.

Conduct a "What would happen if…" role-play. For a child who fears that her mother will have a car accident and not return, the child and therapist would act out everything that would happen from beginning to end in this situation, including how she would feel, what she would be told when she receives the news, the changes that would occur in her and the family's daily routine, who would care for her, and so on.

In Vivo Exposure

Ask the attachment figure to pick the child up a few minutes late from a therapy session.

Ask the attachment figure to pick the child up late from an activity.

Practice other in vivo exposures listed above under "Fear of Engaging in Activities Alone or Without Attachment Figure," as they are relevant and related to fear of harm to or loss of attachment figure.

Reducing Safety Behaviors and Avoidance

Limit reassurance that the parent will definitely be safe.

Limit telling the child a specific time that he will be picked up.

Vary which adult picks the child up from an activity.

WORRY ABOUT GETTING LOST

Visual/Auditory Exposure

View images of crowded places (examples: sporting events, concerts, festivals).

Read news stories about children getting separated from their parents.

Read statistics about child kidnapping and encourage child to calculate likely risk.

Imaginal/Role-Play Exposure

Create a recording in which the child imagines being inadvertently separated from her attachment figure. Record the child describing the event, how she feels, what she thinks, how she responds. Listen to the recording repeatedly.

Conduct a "What would happen if…" role-play in which the child role-plays being accidentally separated from his attachment figure. The child can practice identifying fears, using strategies to stay calm, and thinking up actions to take to safely reunite with an adult.

In Vivo Exposure

Travel throughout the office building separately from the child. (Example: the child and adult agree to take different stairways and meet on the second floor, or one takes an elevator while the other takes the stairs.)

Engage in a scavenger hunt created by the therapist in the therapy office building. The child can navigate the building independently to find rewards or clues leading to a reward.

Engage in a scavenger hunt in a store. Ask the child to separate from the attachment figure (or therapist), locate products on her own, and meet at a designated location. (Example: the child can be given a shopping list instructing her to find shampoo, rice, and a favorite candy bar, and meet at the front of the store. The child and adult can then return the items to the shelf and purchase the candy bar as a reward. This can be repeated with various levels of difficulty from a small, familiar store to a larger grocery store, and then a large warehouse store or department store.)

Attend crowded events such as large concerts, sporting events, or festivals.

Challenge the child to visit a restroom or a concession stand independently.

Visit unfamiliar places where the child may feel increased worry about getting lost.

Reducing Safety Behaviors and Avoidance

When developmentally old enough, limit use of hand holding or tugging of parent's clothing.

WORRY ABOUT SLEEPING ALONE OR AWAY FROM HOME

Visual/Auditory Exposure

View images of feared creatures. These may include ghosts, monsters, characters from books or movies (example: Chuckie), or Internet memes (example: Slenderman), depending on the child's fear.

View clips on television or YouTube videos of feared scenes or characters (examples: Dr. Who, Zombies in Minecraft).

Read books that include images or characters that the child is nervous about.

Read about anticipated experiences that may involve sleeping away from home (examples: overnight school field trips, overnight camp) on brochures and websites.

View photos of past experiences at overnight field trips or summer camp.

View videos on overnight camp's website, or other videos of children engaging in and coping with the activity or situation.

Imaginal/Role-Play Exposure

During daytime, role-play bedtime rituals (examples: putting on pajamas, brushing teeth, reading stories), complete with the attachment figure leaving the room.

During daytime, role-play the child having difficulty falling or staying asleep and seeking the attachment figure's support. The attachment figure can practice calmly redirecting the child back to his bedroom and ignoring his repeated requests for comfort.

Role-play the child separating calmly from the attachment figure at a bus stop for school or camp. Visit the bus stop and have the child practice calmly saying goodbye as the attachment figure walks away (or, if developmentally appropriate and in a safe location, parent can drive away briefly).

Interoceptive Exposure

Spin around in a chair to experience headache and nausea.

Plan a very busy day to induce feeling tired and engaging in activities anyway.

Plan for the child to intentionally stay up later than normal to induce feeling tired. Process her ability to cope and the temporary nature of the fatigue.

In Vivo Exposure

Gradually decrease the amount of time the attachment figure spends in the child's bedroom at night.

Gradually decrease the number of check-ins the attachment figure participates in as the child is falling asleep (example: from every 5 minutes to every 10 minutes, and so on).

Gradually increase the distance from the attachment figure to the child's bedroom at night (example: beginning with the parent at child's bedside, then in a chair or on the floor in child's room, then directly outside the bedroom with door open, then directly outside the bedroom with door closed, then in another room on same floor, then on another floor of home).

If child is currently sleeping regularly in attachment figure's bedroom, gradually increase the amount of time the child must stay in his own bedroom before switching rooms.

If child is sleeping in attachment figure's bed nightly, gradually shift where she sleeps to a chair or the floor in bedroom, then (if needed) to the hall outside bedroom, then to child's bedroom.

Have child practice nighttime routine (example: changing into pajamas, brushing teeth, getting tucked into bed) at a close relative or friend's home, and then taken home before falling asleep. Repeat as needed, gradually increasing the time spent away from home.

Have child stay overnight at a close relative or friend's home.

Have child stay overnight at a less familiar relative or friend's home.

Have child stay overnight for multiple nights at a relative or friend's home.

Have child attend single night of overnight field trip with attachment figure as chaperone sleeping separately.

Have child attend multiple nights of overnight field trip with attachment figure as chaperone sleeping separately.

Have child attend overnight field trip without attachment figure for single night, increasing to multiple nights.

Have child attend a brief overnight camp.

Have child attend a longer overnight camp.

Reducing Safety Behaviors and Avoidance

Avoid setting up a comfortable place for the child to sleep in the attachment figure's bedroom.

Avoid having attachment figure fall asleep in child's bedroom.

Limit visits to the child's bedroom to check on the child.

Limit comfort and reassurance provided during visits from child to attachment figure.

If there are multiple bathrooms in the home, encourage child to use child's bathroom rather than attachment figure's bathroom when needed during middle of the night.

Provide a "bedroom pass" that the child must exchange in order to enter attachment figure's bedroom. Define brief length of visits (example: no more than 10 minutes). Start with three passes and gradually decrease the number allowed. For each pass not turned in, allow the pass to be exchanged for a specified reward.

When child is sleeping away from home, limit the number of phone calls or texts to the attachment figure.

Encourage attachment figure to ignore texts or phone calls after reaching agreed-upon maximum number.

Prohibit the use of phone/texting completely during sleepovers.

Lengthen response time between texts.

Discourage child from bringing cell phone during overnight field trips or summer camps.

When child is sleeping away from home and does have the option to call, discourage attachment figure from helping him count down to the next phone call or visiting day. Rather, encourage them to focus on the present and fully engaging in activities without attachment figure.

When saying goodbye to a child leaving for a long period of time, attachment figures may consider refraining from expressing how sad they are to say goodbye to the child.

When writing letters to children who are sleeping away from home, attachment figures may consider refraining from describing events the child is missing at home, sharing sadness, or expressing very strongly how much they miss their child.

Case Example

An 11-year old boy presented to the clinic due to difficulty separating in the morning to go to the school bus, refusal to attend playdates, and anxiety about upcoming plans to attend an outdoor education trip with his middle school. Treatment began by establishing rapport and helping the client to feel comfortable in the therapy office. He was very nervous and tearful when separating and sought repeated reassurance from his father in the waiting room that he wasn't going to leave. His father initially provided significant reassurance and repeatedly responded by saying, "I'll be right here."

When presented with the option of starting with a game of his choice the child was eventually willing to go back to the therapy office as long as the door remained open. After a few minutes of being engaged in the therapy room, he was willing to close the door. After several weeks, he easily came back into the therapy office on his own. However, some weeks his father requested that he join the session at the beginning to check in. During sessions when he and his father began session together, the child had significantly more difficulty separating. After speaking privately with his parents, we agreed that they would communicate a message by a note or join at the end of session, rather than join him in the beginning.

The client began by practicing separation challenges within the office. First, his father was asked to take a walk outside of the office. The child was nervous and watched from the window. His father then took a longer walk around the perimeter of the office building. During the next session, the client practiced being "dropped off" at the front door. Together with his therapist, the client and his father walked to the front door of the building. His father stayed outside as the child entered the building with the therapist. He was nervous and asked repeatedly for reassurance. He then repeated the challenge with the therapist walking in behind him. He expressed fear that the receptionist would yell at him, yet he successfully entered anyway. At the next session, he repeated those challenges and also practiced having his father drop him off at the front door and entering the office independently while his father parked the car.

Each week he also worked with his parents and therapist to plan a weekly separation challenge outside of the office. He began by being rewarded for boarding the school bus calmly. He then scheduled a playdate at the home of a close friend with whom he felt comfortable. Next, he practiced staying home alone while his father walked the dog. Lastly, he prepared for his outdoor education field trip. He began asking his older brother about his outdoor education experience, viewed photos of previous trips, and started packing. He practiced by attending a sleepover at a close friend's house. He also role-played saying goodbye calmly at the site of the school bus stop. On the day of the field trip he was nervous and fearful, initially crying in the car ride, yet he was willing to get on the school bus and ended up enjoying his field trip.

Conclusion

Children with SAD experience distress when alone, separated from, or anticipating separation from an attachment figure. They often demonstrate reluctance to engage in activities without their attachment figure, worry about accidental separation or harm to the attachment figure, or have repeated nightmares or somatic symptoms when anticipating or experiencing separation from an attachment figure. Given the significant toll this anxiety can take on the child and family, addressing these concerns is of paramount importance. There is significant evidence for the benefit of CBT involving exposure therapy to reduce symptoms of SAD. This chapter reviewed diagnostic information, key treatment considerations, and implementation of exposure-based CBT for children and adolescents experiencing SAD. Samples of specific exposure tasks were provided for consideration in creating individualized exposure hierarchies with clients. Finally, case examples were used to illustrate the clinician's role in implementation of general CBT skills and exposure tasks with real clients experiencing SAD.

CHAPTER 9

Exposure for School Phobia

In this chapter, you will find information related to exposure treatment with children and adolescents who have school phobia. School phobia treatment can be complex and requires a high degree of collaboration with parents and schools, which can create challenges for clinicians. The information included in this chapter is intended to support clinicians in creating and implementing an exposure hierarchy that is tailored to each individual client. Ideas for exposure tasks and activities are provided for consideration in creating individualized hierarchies. Finally, case examples are used to illustrate the clinician's role in implementation of CBT skills and exposure tasks with real clients who experience school-related anxiety.

Clinical Presentation and Causal Factors

School phobia, also frequently incorporated under the broader clinical terms of "school avoidance" or "school refusal," occurs when a child or adolescent refuses to go to school or experiences significant distress around the idea of attending school. There are a wide range of behaviors that fall under the umbrella of school avoidance behavior: missed classes or periods of the school day, a span of nonattendance, frequent tardiness, disruptive morning routines, attending school but with somatic complaints or verbalized fear or dread, and excessive pleas or attempts to avoid school. A school phobia often begins with an overall apprehension or nervousness around school. The child may talk about not wanting to go to school or about school feeling bad for an undefined reason. The feelings may evolve into tantrums, especially during the morning routine, or crying at school or during drop-off. An adolescent's resistance may present as stubbornness; the teen may refuse to get out of bed in the morning, deliberately not complete homework, or refuse to get out of the car during drop-off. For all ages, physical symptoms often co-occur with the emotional upset (Egger, Costello, & Angold, 2003; Honjo et al., 2001). The most common of these include upset stomach, vomiting, diarrhea, headache, dizziness, shortness of breath, rapid heartbeat, and an overall "off" feeling.

The *DSM-5* does not designate school phobia as a distinct disorder; however, it is often a symptom of other disorders, most commonly generalized anxiety disorder, depression, separation anxiety disorder, social phobia, or oppositional defiant disorder (Egger et al., 2003; Kearney & Albano, 2004; McShane, Walter, & Rey, 2001). At any given time, researchers estimate that about 2% to 5% of school age children experience issues with school refusal (King & Bernstein, 2001; Suveg, Aschenbrand, & Kendall, 2005). School phobia presents equally among boys and girls and across different ethnicities and races. Refusal can occur at any point during a child's educational career, though some studies have found anxiety-based school refusal to be more prominent at transition points, between ages 5 and 6 or between ages 10 and 13 (Fremont, 2003; King & Bernstein, 2001; Pellegrini, 2007).

School phobia stresses and disrupts a family considerably. Parents often find themselves exasperated with their child as they try to coax, prod, demand, or yell in an attempt to convince the child to attend school. Many parents become anxious and overwhelmed as they realize that their child will not attend school and they need to find emergency childcare, cancel work meetings, or rework their plans for the day. With increasing noncompliance, a sense of urgency develops and parents may feel desperate to change the child's behavior.

There are a host of factors that may contribute to school-based anxiety. Consider the following contributing variables: stressful family dynamics, such as a parent who is ill or the death of a family member; recent child illness; returning after long breaks such as school vacations; adolescent power struggles; changing schools; social concerns, such as being bullied or teased; academic stress and perfectionism; learning disabilities; and sensory sensitivities that impact the child in the school setting (Kearney & Albano, 2007).

Exposure Therapy for School Phobia

Unlike truancy, in which case the child or adolescent is believed to be missing school solely to enjoy rewards outside of school, and which is often accompanied by an anti-school attitude, school phobia is hallmarked by significant underlying anxiety and a pattern of school absences related to avoidance of this anxiety (Kearney, 2008; Berg, 1997; Berg, Nichols, & Pritchard, 1969). It is important that the assessment process focus on differentiating between cases of anxiety-based school refusal and cases in which the child or teen refuses school solely to gain rewards outside of school (such as being with friends, or staying home and playing video games), in which case exposure therapy would not be indicated. School phobia leads to higher amounts of school absenteeism, which in turn increases family stress, impacts academic progress, limits social exposure, and increases the likelihood of school dropout (Kearney, 2008; Lamdin, 1996; Rumberger, 1995). Additionally, each day that a child is out of school can make it more difficult for her to return due to the increased stress of compounding missed instruction, makeup work to be completed, and family resources used. Impairment is significant and effective treatment is critical for this population.

The practical skills-based approach of CBT, including exposure treatment, is a great tool for providing effective and timely symptom reduction and increasing school attendance. Current research comparing psychosocial interventions for school refusal indicates that the behavioral and cognitive strategies of CBT are superior in providing a decrease in anxiety-related symptoms and long-term improvement of school attendance (Pina, Zerr, Gonzales, & Ortiz, 2009; Kearney & Silverman, 1999; King et al., 1998; Last, Hansen, & Franco, 1998). Specific exposure work—including graduated exposures, systematic desensitization, in vivo exposures, and role-plays—was found to be a key component in successful school phobia treatment models (Moffitt, Chorpita, & Fernandez, 2003; Hargett, 1996; Hagopian & Slifer, 1993; Houlihan & Jones, 1989; Kolko, Ayllon, & Torrence, 1987).

Exposure-based CBT for school phobia differs from many other areas of anxiety treatment, as it requires significant collaboration with the school. Additionally, the timeline is critical to creating momentum and success. Due to pressure for the child or adolescent to return to school as quickly as possible, exposures tend to move more quickly and may include brief, daily therapeutic follow-up to make necessary adjustments and modifications of the exposure plan. The goal is to collaborate closely with the child, family, and school to create an exposure plan that appropriately challenges the child to make continual progress without overwhelming him. Additionally, prior to beginning exposure work for school phobia, a significant amount of preliminary work must be done to prepare the parent or caregiver, child, and school. The CBT model for school phobia and school refusal emphasizes parent training, contingency management, reduction of reinforcement in the home setting, and cognitive restructuring and coping strategies (relaxation) in addition to exposure tasks. In-depth information related to these strategies is provided in chapters 3 through 5.

Clinically Relevant Factors

Ongoing clinical assessment must focus on a clear and detailed understanding of the specific nature of the child's anxious condition in preparation for exposure therapy. As discussed in chapter 2, the environmental context within which the symptoms present, and the specific nature of the child's cognitions and behavioral responses, are critical considerations in the subsequent engineering of effective exposure exercises. As follows, we present typical fear triggers or cues, feared consequences, and avoidance and safety behaviors commonly occurring in children with school phobia:

Fear Cues

Fear cues or triggers are specific environmental factors or variables that typically elicit the child's anxiety. These are the situations that activate the fear response due to the presence of specific stimuli that are perceived as dangerous or harmful in some way. The following fear cues commonly trigger anxiety in children with school phobia:

Psychological symptoms (examples: heart racing, nausea, stomachache, rapid breathing) related to anticipation about going to school or possible experiences at school

Thoughts or mental replaying and imagery of previous negative school experiences

Physically separating from the parent or caregiver at the beginning of school

Having the school bus arrive for pickup to go to school

Situations, such as working on homework, that might elicit worries about making mistakes (perfectionist thinking)

Situations that require performance (examples: giving a presentation, reading aloud, playing a game in gym class)

High-sensory situations (examples: fire drills, noisy lunch rooms, unstructured time at recess)

Receiving corrective feedback from teachers or perceiving social judgment from peers

Witnessing or experiencing negative or aggressive peer interactions (teasing, bullying)

Engaging in competition (academic or other) at school

Feared Consequences

Feared consequences are those environmental conditions and outcomes that the child expects will result from exposure to the feared stimuli. That is, the child's fear is initiated and maintained through her belief that these negative outcomes will occur. The following are common feared consequences in children with school phobia:

Overwhelming emotionality following separation from parent/caregiver

Abandonment by parent/caregiver

Harm to, or death of, parent/caregiver while away

Social judgment or rejection by peers

Panic in anxiety-provoking school situations

Unbearable embarrassment related to negative performance or corrective feedback

Catastrophic consequences of making a mistake

Unavoidable danger or physical harm in high-sensory or unpredictable environments

Avoidance

Children with anxiety commonly avoid the environmental stimuli and situations that trigger their anxiety because they perceive a high likelihood of their feared consequences occurring. The following are common avoidant behaviors observed in children with school phobia:

Engaging in acting-out behaviors, such as temper tantrums, to avoid separation or going to school

Refusing to get out of bed on school days, or engaging in excessive stalling during morning routine

Citing physical symptoms as reasons for not being able to attend school

Avoidance of school-related conversation, such as discussion about grades

Refusing to work on schoolwork

Going to the guidance counselor or nurse's office frequently during class time

Skipping classes or leaving school without permission

Avoiding other school-related activities (extracurricular opportunities, sporting events, clubs)

Safety Behaviors

Children with anxiety often rely on specific objects, individuals, or actions that they believe will protect them from the feared stimuli or feared outcome. Safety behaviors are any action on the part of the child or adolescent that is performed in an attempt to feel safe. The following are common safety behaviors displayed by children with school phobia:

Seeking reassurance from parent/caregiver by asking repetitive questions related to school attendance (examples: "Do I have to go to school tomorrow?" "What if I get sick at school?")

Frequently calling or texting parent while at school

Wanting parent/caregiver to come into the school building or classroom

Becoming rigid with school routine, such as only sitting next to certain peers or only attending certain classes

Engaging in distractions, such as playing a video game on the way to school, to tolerate anticipatory anxiety

Tailoring Exposure Therapy for School Phobia

This section is designed to serve as a primer for the implementation of exposure therapy specifically for children and adolescents with school phobia. It builds on guidance presented in earlier chapters by offering the therapist specific suggestions for what must be uniquely considered when carrying out this work with youth with school phobia. That is, additional strategies and modifications to the treatment approach will be discussed that are of paramount importance to implementing exposure-based work with this group.

School refusal cases are intense; a family often presents for treatment after parents have tried multiple strategies without success, and they often feel desperate for their child to return to school. Due to this urgency, it is important to act as quickly and effectively as possible. As with other anxiety-based avoidant behaviors, continued avoidance of the feared stimulus (school) increases the anxiety and fear response to the stimulus. For school refusal cases, each successive day a child misses school makes it harder for him to return.

Development of the Fear Hierarchy

As with any good fear hierarchy, exposures for school phobia should be tailored specifically to the child or adolescent. The functional analysis will guide the clinician in creating an individual hierarchy based on the specific feared stimuli. A child who avoids school due to a teacher she has perceived as mean will work through a hierarchy that is fundamentally different from that of a child who avoids school due to his fear of the school fire alarm. In both cases, though, the child needs help learning how to reenter the school building and reengage in a classroom setting. Further, it is common for children with school avoidance issues to develop somatic concerns (such as stomach pains, headaches, or dizziness) before or during the school day. When children develop fear in anticipation of these somatic complaints, it becomes important to incorporate interoceptive exposures into treatment. These exercises, as described in chapter 7, serve to reduce the anxiety associated with, and increase tolerance of, uncomfortable physiological sensations.

In almost all school phobia cases, collaboration with the school team is essential. School administrators and teachers often need a clinician's help to understand underlying psychiatric concerns that may be leading to the avoidance, rather than assuming the refusal is due to belligerence or opposition. School staff are crucial collaborators as the exposure steps are carried out. It is best to inform parents of the necessity for collaboration at the intake appointment and to obtain a release from parents allowing direct communication with the school. It frequently takes time to establish contact with the school and determine the best person with whom to communicate. Additionally, some school staff accept feedback and suggestions willingly, while others are frustrated by requests to give a student extra attention or accommodations. Working to validate teachers' concerns and brainstorm together about changes that are least disruptive to the class can help to build rapport. In addition to teachers, administrative staff and other school personnel are often helpful in the reintegration process. For example, a school secretary may be helpful in meeting a child at the school door to walk her to her teacher, or a child may consider the school nurse or guidance counselor his "safe" person at school—someone he can seek out in times of increased anxiety (Nuttall & Woods, 2013). It is also imperative that parents know immediately if their child is not in class. For older kids, this may require extra staff checking to see if the student is in each class.

The family and school also need to work out an attendance plan. Goals should be realistic and attainable. Alternative schedules often need to be arranged with school administrators, and the guidance counselor may need to adjust a child's schedule if full school days are too intense for the student to handle initially. For example, a student may feel comfortable attending her elective classes but not core classes. In this case, the student could begin reentry by attending his electives and only one core class, adding additional core classes every three days. For those classes a student is missing, the teachers may need specific guidance on preparing makeup work and the rationale for doing so. Communicating with teachers directly may be helpful, although it can become cumbersome with middle school and high school students who have a host of teachers. For older kids and adolescents, the guidance counselor may be most effective with teacher coaching. You may choose to communicate directly with the counselor, and the counselor can help the teachers manage the work dissemination. Some students are able to complete the missed work easily while others may become overwhelmed and anxious with the amount of outstanding work. In the latter case, arranging modified or reduced workloads can alleviate some of this stress.

It is best when parents and school can be flexible in both managing the reentry schedule and completing makeup work. As the clinician, you should be in close contact with designated school staff to ensure that the hierarchy remains appropriate and realistic. You should set up a specific schedule for the parents and school regarding the details of ongoing exposures (where, when, for how long, and with what frequency). If appropriate, parents should also get permission to access school grounds (car loops, playgrounds, fields) when school is not in session. Exposures in these environments can be done while children are in school clothes, with backpack on, and after a typical morning routine, to create realistic exposure opportunities outside of school hours. A behavior chart may be necessary to capture daily progress, or a daily email update from a staff member may be helpful.

The school team will undoubtedly be recording the number of absences and late arrivals, but it may also be helpful for parents and children to keep a home record of this data; children and adolescents are often unaware of how quickly the missed days accumulate. Older children—adolescents in particular—may feel motivated to change when they visually see the absences accumulating, equating to failing of a class or repeating of a grade.

Children and adolescents are often motivated by external rewards. Positive reinforcement can accompany successful completion of a hierarchy step. For example, if a 6-year-old completes her morning routine before school with a positive attitude, the parent may add something special to her lunch box. Or, for example, a 12-year-old may earn 10 minutes of video game time for every class he successfully attends. Immediate, positive reinforcement is preferable to negative consequences. Reinforcement should be granted when the student completes a realistic step, not withheld until he is attending all day, every day without issues.

Considering the Safety of Exposure Tasks

It is always important to consider safety while engaging in exposure activities. For school exposures, the school's nurse or health technician may need to be informed of the student's condition. This will help the nurse or technician understand how to address a child who may complain consistently of physiological symptoms related to the exposure that are rooted in anxiety. For example, if a school avoidant student experiences rapid heartbeat and fast breathing related to exposures, the health staff should be informed so that they can encourage use of distress tolerance skills rather than immediate attempts to alleviate symptoms through avoidance. For children working on exposures related to school drop-off, it is important to be mindful of the busy and fast-paced movement of cars and buses during the school drop-off time, because their heightened state of arousal may decrease their judgment regarding safety.

Clinicians and parents also need to be prepared for the possibility of an extreme response that sometimes occurs with preteens or adolescents: a threat to harm themselves. Some teenagers are so afflicted by the anxiety and committed to avoiding it that they threaten to hurt themselves (as in engaging in cutting behavior, threatening to run away, or threatening suicide), thinking that these threats will cause the parent to back down and leave them alone. These threats should always be taken seriously, but without terminating overall exposure work. If a teen threatens extreme behavior, you or the parent should clearly state that safety is a priority, and if the teen cannot guarantee safety, she will be taken to a crisis center or hospital. Clearly state, however, that after safety is reestablished, the exposures will continue. The adolescent needs to understand that threatening harm to oneself is not a successful avoidance tactic, and parents should respond with clear consequences rather than abandoning all requests and therefore enabling such behavior.

Frequency, Duration, and Length of Sessions

Factors such as frequency of exposures, duration of treatment, and length of session vary considerably depending on the nature of the school avoidance. Generally, however, the more frequent the exposure sessions, the faster the progress will be. For example, if a school avoidant child attends one class a day and adds a class to his schedule every two weeks, progress will be very slow. For this reason, it is often helpful to meet with a family several times a week during the most intense phases of the exposure work. You should actively train parents to be effective exposure coaches so that they can help the child engage in exposures outside of session time. In some cases, because of parents' work schedules, it may only be possible to meet once a week. In these cases, the weekly therapy session should be extended in length to allow for both parent coaching and child exposure, and the child should practice imaginal exposures frequently throughout the week.

Due to the intense interplay between parents, school, and child, a single therapist may be unable to support the needs of all three parties. In this case, it might be helpful to refer the case to another therapist who also specializes in school avoidance issues for dealing with one aspect of the treatment, or a larger therapy practice that has the resources for the parents to see one therapist, the child to see another, and a third clinician who can maintain contact with the school as well as act as case manager.

Cognitive Considerations

Initial work on building coping thoughts can encourage the client to begin the exposure process and return to school despite his discomfort. It is important that the therapist validate the child's feelings and demonstrate confidence that he can "handle it." The client can work in session on writing a script for challenging his worries about returning to school. For example, a younger client may find it helpful to practice saying, *My stomach feels upset when I go to school, but I will be okay. And when I practice going to school a little bit at a time, my stomachaches will actually get better!* An adolescent might state, *All I want to do is stay home and play games on my phone because that's when I feel the calmest. The problem is, every day that I do this, it makes it harder to go back to school, and I know deep down that I can't avoid this forever. I can handle going to school even if it is uncomfortable, if I face my fears a little at a time.*

Another challenge you may encounter while working with clients who experience school phobia is anticipatory anxiety that occurs on Sunday evenings or following holiday breaks. Often the child may improve in her functioning during the typical school week, but become stressed and anxious every Sunday when thinking about returning to school. This can lead to a rough Sunday evening and Monday morning for the child and family. Working specifically on challenging thoughts related to anticipatory anxiety, shifting mental focus to more enjoyable activities on Sundays, and engaging in relaxation strategies at bedtime are recommended. Additionally, we recommend coaching parents on reducing their responses to reassurance seeking; planning enjoyable, low-stress activities to engage in; and following a consistent nighttime routine on Sundays. Although Sunday evenings may remain difficult in the short-term, the goal is to use these strategies to make it easier over time and hopefully the client will begin to look forward to her relaxing Sunday routine.

Family Education and Parental Involvement

Following a thorough assessment, preliminary work related to parent education and coaching must be addressed prior to starting exposure tasks. This foundational work should include tools for building cooperation within the parent-child relationship, appropriate boundary setting to regain parental control, behavioral strategies for managing attention-seeking behaviors (clinging, crying, tantrums), enacting a point system for reward of positive behaviors, developing a consistent morning routine, and coaching on how to support and engage with the child during exposure tasks. Along with this comes overt messaging to the child that school attendance is expected and non-negotiable. Many families find it helpful to have a concrete set of "school attendance exceptions," such as a fever of 100 degrees or more, vomiting or diarrhea, bleeding or injury requiring emergency medical intervention, scheduled doctor's appointments, and so on. Additionally, for some children who have sleep challenges that impact their ability to get up for school in the morning, work related to sleep hygiene may also need to occur in conjunction with exposure work.

Finally, parents often unknowingly enable their child's school avoidance behaviors and need support to identify and reduce these barriers in order for exposure tasks to be successful. For example, the parent may have difficulty tolerating his child's distress, and therefore is more likely to let the child stay home when she clings or has a stomachache. Other parents may worry about their child being able to handle teasing, failure, or a stern teacher. Helping parents to identify their own worries about school attendance and reassuring them of their child's ability to handle distress is key. In situations where the parent is struggling significantly with separating from the child, it may be helpful to have the other parent or a familiar adult temporarily do the school drop-offs.

Exposure Tasks and Activities Guide

As follows, we present a wide list of activities and ideas as a guide for clinicians' use in generating useful and creative tasks for a client's exposure hierarchy. While some sections may be loosely organized according to an increasing level of difficulty, these tasks are not designed to be utilized in sequence. Rather, you should always use clinical judgment, as well as parent and child input, in determining the most effective next steps in any series of exposures, and should strive to tailor tasks to the individual needs of each child.

Visual/Auditory Exposure

Read developmentally appropriate books about school and anxiety-provoking school-related experiences, such as bullying or giving presentations.

Look at pictures of the child's school, including images of the external building and drop-off area, classrooms, and people who work there.

Have a younger child draw pictures of his classroom.

Write out the class schedule and discuss the most difficult parts of the day.

Look through a school yearbook and focus on people and places that are the most anxiety-provoking.

Practice exposure to sensory-related stimuli from the school setting (such as listening to recordings of fire alarms, noisy cafeterias, or loud teachers).

Listen to a recording of the school morning announcements.

Work on homework and classwork assignments. If perfectionism is a part of the issue, practice making mistakes while working on classwork.

Listen to a recording of an intimidating teacher or administrator while gradually increasing the volume.

Listen to a recording of a class lecture on a difficult subject.

Listen to a recording of "worry thoughts" the child identifies (such as, *My parents will forget to pick me up, I might be bullied, I might fail a test*, or *What if no one likes me?*).

If the social aspects of school are an area of anxiety, watch movies or television shows that highlight uncomfortable or unkind social dynamics (examples: *Mean Girls, Glee*).

Make a recording of the parent's voice and play it during school to feel connected, rather than calling or texting the parent.

Spend time perusing the school website. Consider creating a "website scavenger hunt," where the child has to search and read the different webpages to find things.

For adolescents, have them join classes via teleconferencing if allowed.

If available, use virtual reality technology or 360-degree video technology to help the child "experience" the school environment.

Imaginal/Role-Play Exposure

Have the child reenact anxiety-provoking school experiences and scenes with puppets or dolls.

Practice steps of the morning routine (waking up, getting ready, packing materials, eating breakfast, getting into the car, traveling to school).

Role-play positive responses to parental requests (example: the parent saying, "Good morning—time to get up!" and the child saying, "Okay. Here I come.").

Practice parent and child separating and saying goodbye. Prior to role-playing with the child, the parent should be coached separately on using a positive and encouraging demeanor and keeping the goodbye brief.

Pretend to go to school, or pretend to be in a class that is challenging or engaged in an anxiety-provoking situation. Take turns playing the role of teacher and student.

Role-play engaging in anxiety-related school tasks (such as entering a room late, raising your hand, giving a presentation).

Take turns pretending to be someone in school who teases or is unkind; practice assertive responses.

Role-play how the child would handle it if the parent were late to pick him up.

Imagine going through the morning routine and tolerating anticipation anxiety.

Imagine riding the school bus, walking into school, attending a difficult class, coming into contact with anxiety-provoking peers, or tolerating distressing physiological sensations.

Imagine separating from the parent and saying goodbye.

Imagine the parent coming late to pickup.

In Vivo Exposure

Engage in interoceptive exposures that mimic the uncomfortable physiological sensations. As a higher-level exposure, engage in these tasks while simultaneously imagining a school-related anxiety-provoking situation.

Stay engaged with peers from class and school; arrange playdates or hangouts, meet peers at the school playground or athletic fields.

Have child participate in running errands or other daily activities, even when she complains of minor physical discomfort (headache, nausea, fatigue).

Get ready for school, including going through the entire morning routine.

Get out of the car or ride the school bus (without necessarily attending school yet).

Walk into the building, greet school staff, and walk to class.

Drop child off for other school-related events (after-school activities, tutoring).

Attend easiest classes first and advance slowly to more difficult ones. Determine mini rewards throughout the day for attending classes (example: lunch with a favorite teacher or in a special room).

Enter the school building but make arrangements for the child to spend portions of the school day with the adults he is most comfortable with (favorite teachers, support staff, or administrators). Ideally this would be a reward for having attended a more difficult part of the day.

Sit outside of a classroom to hear a softer version of an intimidating teacher, or sit in the class with earplugs that have been approved.

Give the child a helping role or job at school to help her feel valued and important (examples: helping set up lunchroom, reading books to students in lower grades).

For particularly hard classes, allow student to start class by coloring, or solving a puzzle. Sometimes a "warm up" and slight distraction can help a student handle the rest of the class.

Arrange for a child's friend or a guidance counselor to meet the child at drop-off or at the child's locker in the morning.

Arrange a carpool so that the child separates from an adult other than parent.

Reducing Safety Behaviors and Avoidance

After gradual reintroduction, give permission for the child to miss school only for predetermined, limited reasons: fever of 100 degrees or higher, vomiting or diarrhea, bleeding or injury requiring emergency medical intervention, scheduled doctor's appointments, and so on.

Coach parents to resist responding to every text or call while the child is at school. Sometimes it is helpful to have scheduled times to call or text the parent, and then work to gradually reduce contact.

Have parents refrain from providing repeated reassurance or answering repeated questions (such as "What if I feel like I'm going to throw up again?"). Teach parents to respond to their child in a way that allows him to learn to reassure himself. (For example, ask him, "How do you think you could handle that?" or "How would you deal with those hard feelings?")

Work with school staff to reduce safety behaviors and avoidance at school. (Example: encouraging child to return to class after a brief check in with the school nurse or counselor, rather than staying out of class for long periods of time.) Having an agreed-upon plan among the child, parents, and school staff makes this much easier.

Encourage the child to interact with a variety of classmates and teachers within the school setting.

Work with parents to be consistent with behavior systems at home that limit positive reinforcers (examples: television, extra attention) on days that the child is home from school.

Case Example

A 12-year-old seventh-grader was referred for therapy following a steady decline of school attendance over several months and a current three-week lapse in school attendance due to migraine headaches. He also had symptoms related to ADHD, social anxiety, and mild depression. He was under the care of a neurologist, and migraine pain was well managed with medication. The client was referred for cognitive behavioral therapy because of the physician's concerns regarding his resistance to returning to school, the impact of the underlying school-based anxiety on the client's migraines and school attendance, and family dynamics enabling the client's school avoidance.

At the time of intake, the client presented as very polite, but generally communicated minimally, often responding with one-word answers or saying "I don't know," and appearing moderately anxious based on nonverbal cues. Interestingly, he denied feeling anxious at the time of intake but reported having a mild headache. His parents expressed concern about his resistance to returning to school and reported that even talking about school or homework often led to conflict. This conflict was creating a pattern wherein the parents would then withdraw due to concern that additional stress might increase their son's headaches. This family dynamic had started out of concern for their son's health, but was now perpetuating a cycle of school avoidance that was impacting the teen's academic success and increasing school anxiety and absences.

This case was particularly challenging due to the complex combination of individual and family factors. Initial treatment began with a blend of individual sessions and separate parent sessions. The individual sessions focused a great deal on psychoeducation about anxiety and CBT, building coping strategies such as relaxation, exploring worry thoughts related to returning to school, and practicing cognitive restructuring to challenge overly negative patterns of thinking related to school. The task of simply discussing school was anxiety provoking in itself, and this difficulty was openly acknowledged. Core areas of school-based anxiety included fear of large amounts of makeup work, failing seventh grade, physically walking into the school, classmates inquiring about the long absence, classes with large amounts of writing, and making it through a full school day. Additionally, since the client reported that a large source of motivation was related to peer engagement, the teen was encouraged to increase social engagement and seek out opportunities to participate in school-related social events.

At the same time, parenting sessions were focused on supporting the parents to reduce enabling behaviors by setting boundaries and appropriately communicating expectations regarding daily school attendance (warm yet firm, non-negotiable stance), reducing reinforcers in the home environment on days when their son refused school (no access to electronics and limited parent interaction), limiting phone contact during school hours (calls accepted only when made by the school nurse), and enacting a reward plan (family contract with items earned for meeting school attendance goals). The largest hurdle for the parents was accepting that their son may experience some pain while at school, but that he was strong enough to cope with the pain. Overall, they were in agreement that school attendance with mild pain had more potential for success than missing school.

Once the family was at a point where school reintegration could begin, collaboration with the school became the focal point. Based on the client's worries about returning to school, the school guidance counselor worked with teachers to arrange appropriate accommodations to make the transition easier. Specifically, the amount of makeup work was greatly reduced, the client's schedule was rearranged to begin the day with a preferred class (gym), the opportunity was given to replace an advanced class with an extra elective, and the client was offered support for writing assignments. The school also reached out to the client and his family to reassure them that they were invested in supporting him and helping him pass seventh grade.

Prior to the first day back, exposure activities included a "walk through" of the school after hours, role-playing how to handle questions from classmates, and jointly emailing teachers to confirm makeup work. Based on client anxiety scale ratings, and in agreement with the parents and the school, the exposure hierarchy for reentry was as follows: enter school and meet with guidance counselor for school tour; enter school and attend gym class; enter school and attend classes up until lunch; attend classes until lunch and meet with a teacher during lunch to discuss status of makeup work; attend school through lunch and then return for final class of day; attend for the full day.

With positive support, parent consistency of expectations and reinforcement, and school collaboration, the client was able to make steady progress and return to school full-time within a few weeks. The teen also joined several school clubs and a sports team, which served as additional reinforcers for consistent school attendance. Once he had reached full-time status, the parents worked to maintain the "non-negotiable" stance on school attendance for all children in the family.

Conclusion

School phobia has been found to lead to a higher incidence of school absenteeism, which in turn increases family stress, impacts academic success, limits social exposure, and increases the likelihood of school dropout. Given the significant impact this anxiety has on the child's educational and social functioning and the family system, addressing these concerns becomes of paramount importance. Current research comparing psychosocial interventions for school phobia indicates that the behavioral and cognitive strategies of CBT are effective in decreasing anxiety-related symptoms and improving long-term school results. This chapter reviewed diagnostic information, key treatment considerations, and implementation of exposure-based CBT for children and adolescents experiencing school phobia. Samples of specific exposure tasks were provided for consideration in creating individualized exposure hierarchies with clients. Finally, case examples were used to illustrate the clinician's role in implementing general CBT skills and exposure tasks with real clients experiencing school phobia.

CHAPTER 10

Exposure for Specific Phobia

In this chapter, we review diagnostic information, key treatment considerations, and the implementation of exposure-based CBT for children and adolescents diagnosed with a specific phobia. The information included in this chapter is intended to support clinicians in creating and implementing an exposure hierarchy that is tailored to each individual client. Ideas for exposure tasks and activities are provided for consideration in creating individualized hierarchies. Finally, case examples are used to illustrate the clinician's role in implementation of CBT skills and exposure tasks with real clients diagnosed with specific phobia.

Clinical Presentation and Causal Factors

The clinical presentation of specific phobia in children and adolescents involves a persistent and pervasive fear of a specific object or situation that is endured with severe distress and active avoidance (American Psychiatric Association, 2013). Being in the presence of the feared object or situation often results in behavioral reactions such as crying, clinging to parents, refusing to participate in activities, attempting escape, and, sometimes, aggressive behavior in an effort to avoid the fear. The fear is considered out of proportion to the actual danger posed by the specific object or situation. Physiologically, children experience a variety of reactions in response to the feared stimulus, which can range from mild stress and tension to severe panic attacks. There is typically a significant impact on the family as a result.

Phobias are extremely common among children and adolescents, presenting in approximately 3% to 9% of children (Kim et al., 2010; Ollendick, King & Muris, 2002) and approximately 15% of 13- to 18-year-olds (Merikangas et al., 2010). Estimates of the median age of onset for specific phobias range from 7 to 11 years, with many children reporting their first symptoms as early as age 5 (Kessler, Berglund, et al., 2005; Stinson et al., 2007). Phobias of animals, the dark, insects, and blood-injury have been found to arise earlier in childhood (Lipsitz et al., 2002; Ollendick & March, 2004), whereas situational phobias such as fear of flying, heights, and travel often begin in late adolescence or adulthood (Barlow, 2002; Lipsitz et al., 2002). Girls have higher rates of specific phobias as compared to boys (Bener, Ghuloum, & Dafeeah, 2011; Ollendick & King, 1994; Ollendick et al., 1995). Over 60% of children with specific phobias have a comorbid disorder, with 50 to 75% of those comorbid children having another anxiety disorder, separation anxiety being the most common (See Ollendick & March, 2004 for a review).

There are a multitude of causal factors that lead to the development of specific phobias. A genetic vulnerability toward anxiety typically plays a role (Eley et al., 2008). In addition, children often develop phobias subsequent to a negative or aversive experience with the specific object or stimuli (Hamm, 2009; Menzies & Clarke, 1995; Ollendick et al., 2002). They draw faulty conclusions regarding the future likelihood of occurrence of these negative scenarios and may harbor doubt regarding their own coping abilities. Further, many children experience panic sensations when faced with scary circumstances, with some children interpreting these sensations as scary and potentially harmful. Finally, children may feel more vulnerable to external threats due to their reliance on adults to care for them. Phobias can be inadvertently reinforced by well-intentioned caregivers, who model anxiety due to their own specific fears, or allow the child to avoid her fears so as to prevent discomfort, anxiety, or tantrums.

Catastrophic and inaccurate beliefs regarding the fear are common contributors to both the development and maintenance of specific phobias. Children can overestimate the danger in a variety of situations, such as getting struck by lightning, a burglar breaking into the home, or being in a plane crash. They may have an inaccurate understanding of the reality and facts in a number of real-life situations as well as imaginative thinking, which may increase fears. Young children especially have a hard time distinguishing between what is real and what is pretend. They may develop fears of monsters under the bed, or specific movie characters. Media can exacerbate children's fears. News reports of storms and other natural disasters are often fearmongering, presenting the worst possible scenarios as likely to occur.

Exposure Therapy for Specific Phobia

The specific mechanism of action in the exposure-based treatment of specific phobia is the disconnection of the association between the specific feared behavior, object, or situation and its consequences (such as anxious physical sensations, perceived or actual negative outcomes, and maladaptive cognitive beliefs). Exposure seeks to minimize the negative reinforcement that results when avoidance of the stimuli leads to positive outcomes, such as relief of, or a reduction in, anxiety and increased perception of safety. For children and adolescents, exposure-based CBT is considered the most efficacious and promising treatment for specific phobia, with some studies reporting response rates between 80% and 90% (Silverman et al., 1999; Öst, Svensson, Hellstrom, & Lindwall, 2001; Pina et al., 2003). Treatment components typically include a series of graduated exposures (for example, imaginal, interoceptive, and in vivo), as well as participant modeling, cognitive restructuring, and contingency management. A number of clinical trials have demonstrated that youth treated with exposure demonstrate better outcomes at post treatment when compared to treatments without an exposure component, such as psychoeducation (Silverman et al., 1999; Ollendick et al., 2009). Further, in these studies, treatment gains in exposure conditions showed maintenance at 6- and 12-month follow-up.

Evidence is also accumulating to suggest that some specific phobias may be treated in as little as one or two prolonged exposure sessions. That is, there have been a number of research studies demonstrating clinical improvement of symptoms in children with specific phobias after one exposure session that lasts from 2 to 3 hours (Ollendick et al., 2009; e.g., Öst et al., 2001). Generally, scheduling longer treatment sessions or conducting multiple sessions per week may be beneficial in promoting habituation and between-session maintenance of treatment gains (Öst, 2012).

An interesting spin on exposure practice involves the use of advanced computer technology to create a virtual environment that simulates a feared stimulus or situation. Several studies are demonstrating efficacy of the use of exposure via virtual reality (VR) in the treatment of specific phobias in children (See Bouchard, 2011 and Ollendick & Thompson, 2013 for reviews). Many companies offer software that can be purchased online. For clinicians with access to virtual reality equipment, this technology may allow for additional exposure opportunities, is engaging to youth, and may be particularly helpful when addressing a feared stimulus that is hard to access. For those without access, some video games now offer headsets with three-dimensional (3-D) viewing glasses, and IMAX movies in 3-D offer realistic experiences as well (Peterman, Read, Wei, & Kendall, 2015).

Clinically Relevant Factors

Ongoing clinical assessment must focus on a detailed understanding of the specific nature of phobia-related behaviors and impairment in preparation for exposure therapy. As discussed in detail in chapter 2, the environmental context within which the behavior presents, and the specific nature of the child's cognitions and behavioral responses, are critical considerations in the subsequent engineering of effective exposure exercises. As follows, we present typical fear triggers or cues, feared consequences, and avoidance and safety behaviors commonly occurring in children with specific phobias:

Fear Cues

Fear cues or triggers are specific environmental factors or variables that typically elicit the child's anxiety. These are the situations that activate the fear response due to the presence of specific stimuli that are perceived as dangerous or harmful in some way. The following fear cues commonly trigger anxiety in children with specific phobias:

Visiting certain locations where harm is anticipated and fearful cues are present (examples: dentist office, grassy park, airplane, elevator, bodies of water)

Observing, interacting with, or participating in a procedure related to feared stimuli (examples: watching a dog off-leash in the park, riding an elevator, receiving or watching an injection)

Thinking about, talking about, or hearing others talk about the feared situation or object

Physical sensations (examples: experience of pain during blood draw, feelings of faintness during a medical procedure, nausea on a plane or car ride, dizziness or butterflies in stomach when at the top of a tall building)

Fear of having a panic attack or losing control when exposed to fear cues

Feared Consequences

Feared consequences are those environmental conditions and outcomes that the child expects will result from exposure to the feared stimuli. That is, the child's fear is initiated and maintained through his experience, or his belief that these negative outcomes will occur. The following are common feared consequences for children with specific phobias:

Suffocation or inability to escape (example: when in an enclosed space such as an elevator or airplane)

Physical pain (examples: prick of needle, shark or snake bite, bee sting)

Death of self or loved ones (example: falling from a high place)

Loss of control (example: in enclosed places)

Damage or destruction (example: home destroyed in a fire)

Contamination (as in blood draw or injection phobia)

Fainting (as in blood or injection phobia)

Embarrassment if peers or others observe the fear reaction

Disgust (example: with blood) (Olatunji et al., 2007)

Avoidance

Children with anxiety commonly avoid the environmental stimuli and situations that trigger their anxiety because they perceive a high likelihood of their feared consequences occurring. The following are common avoidant behaviors observed in children with specific phobias:

Restriction of, or refusal to participate in, activities that might lead to exposure to feared stimuli (for example, won't attend a soccer game on a windy day, won't attend school when a fire drill is anticipated, won't go to restaurants or other crowded places, won't go to a park where dogs are often present)

Refusal to participate in important activities that are necessary for maintaining health (examples: receiving an injection or blood draw, eating certain foods, going outside)

Refusal to look at or approach stimuli (examples: looking away while blood is drawn, closing eyes during certain parts of a movie, staying in basement during a storm, avoiding visual images of the feared stimuli)

Safety Behaviors

Children with anxiety often rely on specific objects, individuals, or actions that they believe will protect them from the feared stimuli or feared outcome. A safety behavior is any action on the part of the child or adolescent that is performed in an attempt to feel safe. The following are common safety behaviors displayed by children with specific phobias:

Staying close to their "safe" person (often a caregiver with whom the child has a close relationship) or refusing to engage in specific feared activities unless that "safe" person is present

Seeking excessive reassurance from parents or other adults to confirm that a situation is safe and that they do not have to worry (example: asking a parent repeatedly if there will be a dog at a friend's home they are visiting, if there are any sharks in the lake, or if a dental procedure is safe)

Refusing to share important information with caregivers in an attempt to avoid the fear (examples: not sharing about the upcoming field trip to the zoo, or the presence of a physical ailment due to fear of the doctor's office)

Frequent or excessive checking or information gathering (For example, a child with a fear of storms may repeatedly check news and weather reports. A child afraid of a fire in the home may read exhaustively from informational websites and pamphlets regarding ways to protect herself and her home from fires. Alternatively, children may enlist adults to engage in checking behavior for them. They may want an adult to look in the closet for monsters or check the grass for insects.)

Demanding that parents engage in the use of safety behaviors that are perceived as protecting them from harm (for example, a child may insist that a smoke alarm be installed in every room of the house, that the family retreat to the basement when the forecast predicts a storm, or that the stairs be taken instead of the elevator).

Distraction (example: averting one's gaze from the feared stimuli, listening to music or playing an electronic game, or using relaxation skills such as belly breathing)

Tailoring Exposure Therapy for Specific Phobia

This section is designed to serve as a primer for the implementation of exposure therapy specifically for youth with specific phobia. It builds on guidance for conducting exposure therapy presented in earlier chapters by offering the therapist specific suggestions for what must be uniquely considered when carrying out this work with youth with specific phobia. That is, additional strategies and modifications to the treatment approach will be discussed that are of paramount importance to implementing exposure-based work with this group.

Treatment for specific phobia is consistent with the broad principles of implementing exposure therapy as described in chapter 5. The child, therapist, and parent work together to collaboratively develop a fear hierarchy, or a number of small fear hierarchies, depending on the number and breadth of the concerns. The child is taught to provide fear ratings for his expectations of the level of fear when engaging in each possible scenario. He is also taught cognitive challenging and relaxation skills to increase his confidence in initiating exposure tasks and for post processing of exposure experiences in new, more adaptive ways. Prior to exposure work, a task is chosen and an exposure tracking form generated for recording fear ratings before, during, and after the task. Concrete data from fear ratings during the exposure is collected with the goals of the child learning that approaching the fear reduced its intensity over time, anticipation of the event was not as bad as the actual event itself, and understanding that he was able to cope with the experience. Finally, reward systems are used to increase motivation and engagement in exposure tasks.

Development of the Fear Hierarchy

Exposures, as well as cognitive challenges, should be tailored to the needs of the child and based on information gathered from assessment. For example, some children may be comfortable swimming in lakes but have a fear of oceans because of the waves. In such cases, exposure tasks would focus on tolerating the sensory aspects of ocean waves. In vivo exposures might involve a trip to the ocean or a water park with a wave pool. In contrast, other children may have a fear of being in crowds at the beach and will require exposures directed toward this specific fear, which may include video exposures to crowded locations, imaginal exposures using detailed imagery of being in a crowded location, and slowly entering public locations with varying crowd sizes.

In some cases, assessment will indicate that the child is fearful of having a panic attack or other intense physical sensations as a result of exposure to the feared stimuli. In these cases, incorporation of interoceptive exercises to teach the child to cope with and habituate to her physiological sensations will become an important component of exposure work. (See chapter 7 for a discussion on interoceptive exposures.) For example, an adolescent who has a panic attack on a plane during a particularly turbulent plane ride may subsequently fear that if he takes a plane ride again, he will experience another panic attack. The focus of his fear then becomes the experience of aversive physical sensations on the plane. He also worries about embarrassment if others observe his panic attack, and being stuck on the plane without an opportunity for escape when panic occurs. Therefore, the fear of the physical sensations and negative outcomes as a result of these sensations are a primary component of his plane phobia and must be a direct target of treatment.

If you're not able to confront the actual object or situation of the phobia (for example, a tornado, shark, or bear) or if it's a fear of something rare or difficult to control (such as taking a plane ride, or a severe storm), focus should be placed on incorporating imaginal exposures, reducing avoidance of places where the object or situation may be more likely (such as the beach, forest, or airport), and reducing the use of safety behaviors in these locations (such as refusal to put feet in the water at the beach because of shark phobia, or checking weather reports for storm phobia) (Abramowitz et al., 2011).

SHAPING APPROXIMATIONS OF THE BEHAVIOR

In many phobia cases, small, concrete steps are needed to encourage the child to initiate tasks and build confidence. For example, in one clinic situation we had a child who was afraid of putting his head under water. Swim staff at his local pool had been unable to make progress with him on this behavior and as a result, he could not participate in his swimming lessons. In our clinic session, the therapist brought in a large, transparent tray with about one foot of water and played games in which the client earned points for approximations of the desired behavior (putting his head under water). Exposure work began with dabbing our eyes and ears with water and then putting one ear under water. We gave the child time to get used to the sensations and talk about each sensation he noticed. As he became comfortable with this, the therapist modeled putting her mouth and nose (but not eyes) under water and blowing bubbles. The therapist made silly faces and played games such as having him guess her emotion as she made facial expressions with her mouth in the water and he watched underneath the transparent container. The therapist talked about the physical sensations she noticed when putting her face in the water. After about 15 minutes, he was ready to try. He put both mouth and nose in the water and blew bubbles.

VARYING PHYSICAL PROXIMITY TO THE PHOBIC STIMULUS

In many cases, the physical distance or proximity of the child to the phobic stimuli is a key variable that will be slowly modified during exposure tasks. For example, we worked with a middle school student with a fear of smoke alarms. At home, she had significant anxiety in anticipation of the noise the smoke alarm would make if it were triggered. After implementing both imaginal and audio/video exposures, this youth agreed to stand at the far side of a parking lot while we set off the smoke alarm. She initially required a distance of 200 feet away from the alarm. While the alarm was not audible at this distance, agreeing to her terms reduced her resistance and allowed her to initiate the exposure. She was then willing to slowly move closer to the alarm. Within 45 minutes she was standing next to the alarm as it went off, with minimal anxiety.

MODELING THE DESIRED BEHAVIOR

It is often helpful for the therapist to serve initially as a model for the desired behavior or interaction (Ollendick & March, 2004). For example, with a child with a dog phobia, the therapist may lie down and allow the dog to sniff him prior to requesting that the child engage in this behavior. Modeling should be faded out over time as the child learns to engage in brave behaviors with reduced therapist involvement.

COLLECTING MATERIALS FOR EXPOSURES

In many cases, the therapist will need to locate materials for the planned exposure tasks prior to the session. For a child with an insect phobia, dead or live insects may be collected from various locations in advance. The therapist may search the Internet and the library for pictures and video clips of insects. She also might collect objects such as feathers or leaves that create a sensory experience similar to an insect's touch. For exposure sessions outside the clinic, the therapist might plan and schedule a visit to the local museum, nature center, or zoo.

For the child with a needle phobia, a needle kit including an alcohol swab, needle/syringe, tourniquet, and local anesthetic cream should be obtained. For other medical fears, additional equipment such as stethoscopes, blood pressure cuffs, dental tools or drill, reflex hammers, and so on, may be applicable. The therapist might search the Internet and library for medical images, using search terms such as *needles*, *injections*, *doctors*, *dentists*, and so on. She may obtain clips from TV shows that show medical scenes appropriate for the child's age. Coordination with a doctor's office also may be necessary to gain access to patient rooms and collaborate with medical professions for opportunities to view blood draws or role-play medical procedures with office personnel.

A specific phobia of dogs requires advance planning to locate appropriate and friendly animals to utilize for exposure tasks. Clinicians should consider contacting owners of certified pet therapy dogs or local dog trainers. Trainers can often be hired to bring dogs of various breeds and sizes to multiple exposure sessions.

Considering the Safety of Exposure Tasks

While in most cases danger is minimal, safety is always an important consideration when conducting exposure work. Exposure to the elements may present actual dangers at times. When heading outside with a child with a storm phobia, consider whether there is active lightning, severe winds, or other reasons it is recommended to stay indoors. For children with a fear of a specific animal or insect, use research to make informed decisions regarding the extent to which you can expose the child to the stimulus in question. For example, there are animals and insects that can be approached from a distance but should not be held or touched. Children with medical problems may need clearance from their pediatrician to engage in exposures during which fainting may occur.

Frequency, Duration, and Length of Sessions

There are many considerations to be taken into account in determining the frequency, length, and duration of treatment. Initial severity of the phobia, child motivation, and parent capabilities are just a few variables that will impact treatment. Some children and families may be amenable to and successful with massed practice. This will involve longer or more frequent meeting times and may be better suited for youth with a high motivation for change. Other families may prefer weekly sessions, with homework assignments in between, as these may feel more manageable and less overwhelming. When possible, it can be beneficial to utilize session observations (regarding the child's progress, willingness to continue, habituation to items on the hierarchy, and signs of fatigue or declining coping capacity, for example) as a guide to determine the optimal timing for a session break. It is helpful to end each session on a positive note and with an experience of success.

Family Education and Support

Parental accommodation can be particularly striking in specific phobia cases. For example, the parent may experience a similar phobia and may inadvertently model the feared behavior and cognitions, or not trust the child's ability to face his own fear. A detailed assessment should determine the specifics of any accommodating behaviors and steps should be taken to address these within and outside of therapy sessions. For example, in a particular case of a child with an intense fear of dogs, we found that the child often handled in-session exposures well, but a pattern of not completing exposures outside of session quickly developed. In discussing the concern with the family, it became evident that the mother was having a great deal of difficulty supporting the child with the assignments because of her own fear of dogs. Although the mother was verbally supporting her son with assignments, her nonverbal cues (facial expressions, physical hesitation, and so on) often increased his anxiety about approaching dogs. The mother agreed to work separately on her own fear of dogs, and the child began completing homework assignments with other trusted adults in his life. At the conclusion of treatment, both mother and son had made great progress in reducing avoidance and were encouraging each other to continue to face their fears. Please refer to chapter 3 for a more in-depth discussion on addressing parent accommodation and promoting positive parent involvement.

Exposure Tasks and Activities Guide

As follows, we present a wide list of activities and ideas as a guide for clinicians' use in generating useful and creative tasks for a client's exposure hierarchy. While some sections may be loosely organized according to an increasing level of difficulty, these tasks are not designed to be implemented in sequence. Rather, the therapist should always use clinical judgment, as well as parent and child input, in determining the most effective next steps in any series of exposures, and should strive to tailor tasks to the individual needs of each child. Some of the following ideas have been adapted from Sisemore (2012) and Abramowitz et al. (2011).

CHOKING

Visual/Auditory Exposures

Use the word "choking" and draw a picture of a person choking. You can start with a drawing of a stick figure with its mouth open and work up to more realistic pictures.

Look at pictures of people choking.

Watch video clips from the Internet or movies where people are choking or gagging (examples: *Super Size Me* and *Mrs. Doubtfire*). Choose clips that do not involve death or harm.

Imaginal/Role-Play Exposures

Watch others pretend to gag or choke. Make pretend gagging and choking noises and gestures.

Recall a previous incident when choking sensations occurred.

Imagine all aspects of choking (food getting lodged in throat, not being able to inhale, and so on).

In Vivo Exposure

Fill mouth completely with food and pretend to gag or choke.

Reducing Safety Behaviors and Avoidance

Eat foods that are avoided. Start with foods that provoke mild anxiety and move to eating food that child endorses as more difficult (for example, foods that are difficult to chew—such as steak—or sticky or gooey ones, such as gum, peanut butter, or string cheese).

Refrain from carrying perceived safety objects or keeping them nearby (examples: water bottle, cough drops).

Have parent refrain from providing repeated reassurance or answering repeated questions (example: "Will I choke if I eat this food?"). Teach parents to say to the child, "What do you think?" when asked for reassurance, so the child can learn to answer for herself.

DOGS

Visual/Auditory Exposures

Say and repeat the word *dog* and name specific types of dogs (examples: golden retriever, collie, poodle). Add other dog-related vocabulary (examples: *barking, wagging, panting, licking, growling*). The therapist can use word games such as crossword puzzles, spelling bee challenges, hang man, word scrambles, or rapid naming to make this activity engaging for the child.

Read stories about fictional dogs (examples: *Clifford, Scooby-Doo, 101 Dalmatians*).

Look at and describe pictures of fictional dogs.

Look at and describe pictures of real dogs. Depending on the child, you may need to start with the portion of the dog that is least anxiety provoking (examples: ear or paw) and then move toward looking at the whole dog. Additionally, the therapist should move from looking at pictures of friendly-looking, smaller dogs and progress toward larger, more aggressive-looking dogs.

Listen to audio recordings of dogs. Again, the exposures should begin with less threatening sounds (whimpering, whining, panting, friendly barking) and progress toward more aggressive sounds (loud barking, growling).

Watch video of friendly dogs, such as a dog show.

Imaginal/Role-Play Exposures

Engage in role-plays that involve mimicking dogs. This can be fun for younger kids and helps them to understand the function of a dog's behavior. (Example: "A dog barks to say 'hello;'" "a dog sniffs you to check you out.")

Imagine interactions with dogs using vivid verbal descriptions.

Have child imagine being in the presence of a dog while incorporating other sensory exposures. Include exposures to address any other sensory concerns or triggers the child may have related to dogs (examples: dog smells, the feel of touching dog fur, the feel of a dog breathing on him, the feel of a dog's wet nose).

In Vivo Exposures

Listen to the sounds of a real dog in a separate, adjoining room with no visual contact. Make sure dog is a well-known family pet or professionally trained dog.

View a real dog that is confined to a crate or behind a fence. The goal is to have the child gradually move closer to the confined dog until she is able to sit directly beside it.

View and then approach a dog on a leash. The child gradually moves closer to the dog until close enough to touch. As a first step, it may be helpful for the therapist to model approaching the dog.

Touch a dog on a leash. The child will start by touching less anxiety-provoking areas (tail, paw, back) and move toward touching more anxiety-provoking areas (nose, mouth, teeth).

View and approach other dogs. Homework assignments should include opportunities to practice the same skills with other safe dogs.

Increase the variety of interactions with dogs (examples: walking a dog on a leash, feeding a dog, giving a dog a command).

Have dog jump up and put paws on lap or chest. Lie down and allow dog to sniff or eat treat that is placed on the belly or forehead. Therapist modeling of these interactions first is often very helpful.

Increase time spent with dogs and spontaneous interactions with dogs. These interactions include playing with dogs off leash and engaging with friendly dogs with less training.

Visit an animal facility, humane society, pet store, or dog park. Interact with dogs as appropriate and dogs that center staff have identified as friendly and not posing a risk.

Reducing Safety Behaviors and Avoidance

Stay on the same side of the street as a leashed dog walks by. Do not move farther away to avoid the dog.

Visit the homes of friends who have dogs.

Go on walks in the neighborhood or other outdoor areas, such as parks.

Reduce use of safety objects or behaviors such as carrying a long stick on walks in the neighborhood, or always using a bicycle.

Have parent refrain from providing repeated reassurance regarding the safety of each animal or answering excessive questions from child. Teach parents to say to the child, "What do you think?" when he asks for reassurance, so he can learn to answer for himself.

ELEVATORS AND ENCLOSED SPACES

Visual/Auditory Exposures

Use and repeat the word *elevator* and elevator-related terms (examples: *doors, floor, buttons, 80th floor, stuck elevator*).

Work with the child to draw pictures of elevators or, with a younger child, engage in play with elevator-related themes.

Look at pictures of elevators. Pictures should include both the exterior of the elevator and the inside, with the doors both open and closed.

Imaginal Exposures

Imagine all steps involved in riding an elevator—walking into the elevator, noticing the interior fixtures, pushing the button, watching the doors close, feeling the elevator rise or fall, feeling it come to a stop, watching the doors open, and stepping out of the elevator.

Imagine riding a glass elevator that goes up one or several floors.

Imagine an elevator getting stuck, pushing the call button, someone coming to aid, and waiting for help.

Interoceptive Exposures

When the fear is associated with panic sensations, incorporate interoceptive exposures to learn to tolerate and habituate to those physical sensations (examples: spinning in a chair, shaking head vigorously, breathing through a straw or paper bag).

In Vivo Exposures

Stand at the elevator and push the call button.

Stand in a familiar elevator with the doors open, first with the therapist and then independently. The amount of time for the exposure can be gradually increased until the child can tolerate the amount of time it would typically take to ride the elevator several floors.

Stand inside a familiar elevator and allow doors to almost close or close briefly, first with the therapist and then independently.

Stand inside a familiar elevator with the door closed for an extended amount of time, first with the therapist and then independently.

Ride a familiar elevator, first with therapist (several times) and then independently. Begin with one floor and then gradually increase. Start with elevator without others present and work toward riding a crowded elevator.

Work to generalize skills by practicing exposures with unfamiliar elevators.

Work to tolerate uncertainty (regarding how long the ride will take or how crowded the elevator will be) by riding elevators with others who choose the floor.

Exposures For Other Enclosed Spaces

For fear of other enclosed spaces, apply the previous steps to another location. Have the child discuss, draw and view pictures of, imagine, and confront in vivo small, enclosed spaces such as closets, small rooms without windows, subway train cars, or the inside of an airplane, as relevant.

Practice activities that create claustrophobic sensations (example: sitting in a small space with the door closed, or with others in the space to create a crowded environment).

Wear tight-fitting clothing or a turtleneck or scarf. Sleep under a heavy blanket or inside a sleeping bag. Increase temperature of the room to make it feel stuffy.

Reducing Safety Behaviors and Avoidance

Reduce use of stairs over time. Take elevator whenever possible. (Depends on step the child is currently working on.)

Sleep in bedroom or use bathroom with the door closed.

Have parents refrain from providing reassurance about the safety of the elevator. Teach parents to say to the child, "What do you think?" when he asks for reassurance, so he can learn to answer for himself.

Have child ride the elevator without parent or other safety person.

Reduce avoidance of certain locations where child feels stuck or enclosed (examples: sitting in a traffic jam, being in a crowded school meeting).

INSECTS

Visual/Auditory Exposures

Use and repeat the word *bug* and other insect vocabulary (examples: *beetle*, *fly*, *tarantula*, *wings*, *insect*, *spider*).

Look at drawings of bugs or have the child create her own.

Play with toy bugs, including figurines, puppets, or stuffed animals.

Look at and describe pictures of real bugs. The therapist should begin with the least anxiety-provoking pictures, or portions of pictures, and move toward more anxiety-provoking pictures. Read descriptions about each bug.

Listen to bug sound recordings (buzzing, chirping, clicking, or hissing) and other sensory exposures that imitate the physical sensations of bugs (example: use a feather to imitate the feeling of a bug crawling on the child's arm).

Watch video clips of insects. Start with audio off and progress to both audio and video.

Imaginal Exposures

Imagine an insect, using a vivid verbal description, and imagine interactions with bugs.

In Vivo Exposures

Look at, approach, and touch real bugs that are not alive (examples: bugs in glass jars or magnifying boxes, locust shells).

Look at, approach, and touch bugs in a cage, plastic bag, or container (Andersson et al., 2009)(examples: ant farm; bee in a bug cage; live bug exhibit at a museum, nature center, or zoo).

Observe bugs outdoors, in their natural environment (Andersson et al., 2009). Look at, describe, touch, pick up, and catch nonpoisonous bugs. Places should include specific locations that the child typically avoids, such as standing near a flowering plant if fearful of bees or playing in the grass if fearful of ants.

Clean spider webs from closets, garage, or other locations. Take down and look at an abandoned wasp nest. Turn over rocks where insects may be hiding. Visit beekeeper and watch bees swarm.

Catch bugs in the home. Look at them and touch them before they are taken outside.

Reducing Safety Behaviors and Avoidance

Reduce and then eliminate checking for bugs in closets, corners of home, or other locations child is concerned about.

Approach spider webs and other locations where bugs are present.

Play in tree house or on the playground. Walk in grass and other outdoor areas that have been avoided.

Have child (instead of parent) take care of and dispose of insects in the home. Reduce parents' role in cleaning cobwebs and removing insects.

Have parent avoid providing repeated reassurance or answering repeated questions such as, "Are there any bugs here?" Teach parents to say to the child, "What do you think?" when he asks for reassurance, so he can learn to answer for himself. Parent should not check areas of the home or outdoor locations for insects at the child's request.

LOUD NOISES

Imaginal Exposures

Imagine scenes with a variety of loud noises, such as standing in a noisy crowd, sitting at a desk at school when the fire alarm sounds, or watching a lightning storm and hearing thunder. Create visual detail using a script, or discuss details to help child create imagery. Make sure to include all five senses (sound, sight, touch, taste, smell).

Visual/Auditory Exposures

Watch video clips of a variety of loud noises (examples: shouting, fire alarm or smoke alarm, fireworks, thunder, infant crying, nails on a chalkboard). Start with noises that create mild anxiety and work toward those that create greater fear. Start with audio off and imagine the sound while watching the video. Proceed to watching the video with audio on low volume and work to a higher volume. Vary sound level as you listen.

Listen to an audio recording of loud noises while closing eyes and imagine being in that location (example: imagine being outside while listening to thunder).

Listen to an audio recording of relaxing music interspersed with loud noises.

In Vivo Exposures

Clang pots and pans together, play and explore sounds on musical instruments, pop balloons, or make various loud vocal noises (examples: squealing, screeching).

Practice listening to loud noises in a variety of public settings (examples: attending a sporting or music event, watching fireworks, going to the movies). Focus especially on those locations that have been previously avoided.

Listen to a loud noise that will be produced within some time interval, but child does not know exactly when (examples: set alarm to ring on phone, clock, or smoke alarm during session).

Have others surprise the child by hiding and then popping out and yelling, "Boo!"

Have family member create a loud noise in the home (examples: sound air horn, set off smoke alarm, turn TV on loud volume) at various intervals.

Reducing Safety Behaviors and Avoidance

Avoid wearing earplugs, covering ears, or moving away from the noise.

Reduce avoidance of activities or use of alternate routes where loud noises are common or likely.

Reduce parental overprotective behaviors such as checking or making adjustments for the child (example: checking battery status of smoke alarm, checking volume on TV or alarm, checking how crowded a room is before child approaches, checking to see if neighbor's dog is outside).

Reduce child information seeking and checking in an effort to avoid loud noises (examples: researching where fireworks will take place and how far away they will be, researching the maintenance of smoke alarms, checking volume on electronic devices).

Have parent refrain from providing reassurance that loud noises will not occur.

FICTIONAL CHARACTERS

(Examples: Maleficent, Voldemort, Chucky, clowns, puppets, monsters)

Visual/Auditory Exposures

Discuss visual and auditory qualities and physical aspects of the feared image or stimulus.

If the fear includes difficulty saying the name of the person, image, or object, practice saying the name repeatedly. (Therapist can first model this, then have the child practice.)

Audiotape the character's name repeated orally by the therapist or child and give assignment to listen to the tape during the week.

Read lyrics or words spoken by the character. Start with lyrics or phrases that are less feared. Use a monotone, calm voice at first. Start with just one sentence or phrase and repeat. Eventually use the typical inflection, melody, and rhythm used by the character and build to reading all of the lyrics or a whole passage from the movie or book.

Draw pictures of the feared character. Draw parts or portions of the feared stimulus. Discuss the pictures.

Make a puzzle by cutting a printed picture of the image into pieces and have the child put the pieces together.

Fold a printed picture of the stimulus into five to ten strips (like an accordion). Show the child one part at a time, with praise and rewards as you add each additional strip.

If a doll or three-dimensional figure of stimulus exists, slowly expose the child to seeing and touching the doll.

Create a mask of the character and take turns wearing the mask and pretending to be the character.

Imaginal Exposures

Create a written script that describes the visual and auditory details of the feared character or incorporates an action of the character. Have child imagine the character as you read the script.

Create a written script that describes a past experience with the feared image that resulted in fear or stress. Have the child imagine being in the situation as you read the script. Repeat script until anxiety reduces.

Visualize speaking to or touching the feared image or character.

Look at pictures of the feared character or performer outside of costume; view "behind the scenes" video clips, including those that show the person applying makeup or costume, or view an interview with the actor who plays the character.

Listen to audio clips of the feared character speaking, or music from the movie. Start with audio on lowest volume and play for a few seconds. Build tolerance to longer exposure and increasing volume. Start with a large physical distance between the child and the speakers as needed.

Watch video clips of the feared character. Play the video for a brief duration with no volume. Allow child to stand at a distance she feels comfortable with to start. Build tolerance to longer exposure, child moving closer to video screen, and adding volume slowly.

In Vivo Exposures

Set goals for being in places and situations where there is a higher likelihood of exposure to the visual or auditory aspects of the feared character.

Attend an activity where specific exposure to the feared image will occur (examples: going to the movie theater, attending a concert, going to a theme park).

Reducing Safety Behaviors and Avoidance

Reduce avoidance of locations and activities where exposure to the visual or auditory image may be likely (examples: refusal to turn on TV, watch certain channels, or go to locations where TV or movie may be on).

Reduce need to rely on alternate routes when anxious (examples: refusing to allow parents to drive in the direction of a billboard that displays the feared character).

Have parent refrain from providing repeated reassurance regarding the absence of the character in a particular location. Teach parents to say to the child, "What do you think?" when he asks for reassurance, so he can learn to answer for himself.

Reduce elaborate rituals or checking behaviors, such as looking under the bed before going to sleep, checking closets in bedroom, and checking locks on doors in the home.

Reduce reliance or need to have safety person nearby.

NAUSEA AND VOMITING

Treatment Considerations

There is a paucity of research on children with emetophobia, despite research suggesting an early onset of the disorder (Lipsitz, Fyer, Paterniti, & Klein, 2001). Adult research suggests that a large proportion of individuals with emetophobia experience unrelated panic attacks and significant gastrointestinal symptoms as part of the panic attacks (Lipsitz et al., 2001). The onset of emetophobia often follows medical illness or an aversive experience with vomiting. Theoretical models suggest that this leads to a hypervigilance of gastrointestinal cues and a tendency to interpret benign cues as threatening (indicating that vomiting is likely) (Boschen, 2007). Given the heightened sensitivity to these cues, interoceptive exercises that induce nausea (for example, through dizziness) and other gastrointestinal symptoms are particularly important in treatment.

Visual/Auditory Exposures

Say and repeat the word "vomit" and other related words. Create a tape with words repeated for child to listen to at varying intervals.

Discuss characteristics of vomit and sensory aspects of vomiting (examples: sensation and taste in throat, sensations in stomach).

Draw pictures of vomit. Draw picture of person with mouth wide open and vomit coming out. Draw and discuss scenes from previous incidents when vomiting was experienced or witnessed.

Look at pictures of real vomit and people vomiting. Start with pictures where vomit appears at a distance and move toward pictures with greater visual detail.

Print pictures for child to take with her and practice viewing at home and in other settings.

Print pictures of people vomiting, as well as pictures of people who are calm and happy. Have child look at shuffled pictures to practice tolerating the uncertainty of when he will view someone vomiting.

Watch video clips of people vomiting. Check video clips in advance of session to ensure they contain no inappropriate language or illegal behavior.

Imaginal/Role-Play Exposures

Create script for, and imagine details of, a traumatic event experienced that involved vomiting. Read script with repetition until anxiety reduces.

Create script and imagine family member or friend vomiting.

Imagine having eaten something rancid. Imagine feeling nausea and vomiting.

Have therapist and then child make gagging and vomiting noises and engage in vomiting motions.

Watch familiar others and family members simulate throwing up (for example, kneeling by the toilet, making gagging and then vomiting noises, and spitting out a concoction of food) (Maack, Deacon, & Zhao, 2013; McFayden & Wyness, 1983).

Interoceptive Exposures

Practice interoceptive exposures that create the experience of nausea such as spinning in a chair or shaking head back and forth for 30 seconds.

In Vivo Exposures

Use tongue depressor or finger to create gag reflex (Forsyth, Fusé, & Acheson, 2008).

Wear belt to create pressure on belly, or drink soda to create bloated feeling.

Eat and then go for a walk or engage in other physical exercise.

Create fake vomit, place it in a container, and have child sit across the room from the open container. Slowly move closer to the container and view and smell the fake vomit.

Note: There are a number of recipes for fake vomit that can be found on the Internet. Most involve using a chunky soup such as split pea or vegetable, combined with ingredients such as crushed cereal or oatmeal, canned tomatoes, vinegar, uncooked eggs, and sour milk or cream to create a rancid odor. Some recipes suggest that you heat the mixture or allow it to sit in a warm temperature for a number of days before using.

Touch fake vomit and smear on clothing. Have child bring an extra shirt so she can change after this exposure.

Expose the child to other foods with strong odors, particularly those that are actively avoided and may elicit nausea (examples: aged cheese, sour milk).

Taste vomit-flavored jelly beans and mix with other jelly beans to create uncertainty.

Eat food or drink water until feeling full.

Reducing Safety Behaviors and Avoidance

Eat foods previously avoided due to vomiting fear. Shellfish and meat are often avoided due to fears that they may not be fresh. Leftover or undercooked food is also commonly avoided.

Eat foods on the plate that have been mixed together or are touching.

Refrain from checking behaviors such as looking at expiration dates on food items, checking ingredient list (unless there is an allergy or other medical reason), or having someone else check the food for the child by taking a bite first.

Go to locations where vomiting or nausea was experienced in the past and which may be currently avoided. Refrain from using alternate routes in order to avoid specific places that are associated with a previous vomiting incident.

Engage in activities that are feared to elicit nausea (examples: boat or train ride, amusement park ride, exercising). Eat before engaging in these activities. Engage in these activities without safety person.

Refrain from carrying or keeping perceived safety objects nearby (examples: water bottle, antacids, garbage pail next to bed).

Offer support to family and friends who are sick or perceived as getting sick (examples: offering to get a tissue, sitting in the same room and talking).

Have parent refrain from providing repeated reassurance or answering repeated questions (examples: "Is that food okay?" "Is it fresh?" "Will I get sick if I eat this?" "Is anyone at Grandma's house sick?" "Do you feel sick?").

Have parent refrain from checking child's forehead to make sure he doesn't have a fever. Teach parents to say to the child, "What do you think?" when he asks for reassurance, so he can learn to answer for himself.

If vomiting is witnessed, do not hold or plug ears, avoid eye contact, or run from the situation.

NEEDLES, BLOOD, AND MEDICAL PROCEDURES

Treatment Considerations

A significant number of individuals with fear of injections report a history of fainting upon exposure to fear cues (Ritz, Meuret, & Alvord, 2014). Blood injury phobia elicits a unique physiological response pattern in which the initial fight-or-flight response is followed by a stage of parasympathetic response in which the heart rate slows and blood pressure falls (Ritz et al., 2014). As a result, patients often experience sensations of sweating, shaking, and faintness, with some losing consciousness. Therefore, blood and injection phobias require unique considerations in their treatment. Some of the safety behaviors that patients utilize (such as averting the eyes during a procedure, distracting with music, lying with legs elevated) may actually reduce the frequency of fainting. A careful functional analysis should be used to assess the extent to which these behaviors have been helpful and have prevented feared consequences. Further, some arousal-reduction strategies actually may increase the probability of fainting by reducing blood pressure further (Abramowitz et al., 2011). It is important to check the child's medical condition to ensure that fainting is not risky in her particular case. Discuss with the family physician to clear treatment with the child's provider prior to starting any exposure work.

Exposure combined with applied muscle tension is considered the "gold standard" treatment for blood injury phobia (Öst & Sterner, 1987). Applied muscle tension involves brief sequences of voluntary contractions of the arm, leg, and chest muscles followed by short periods of release. Tensing and releasing various muscle groups serves to counteract the rapid decrease in blood pressure that occurs in many of these patients. Therefore, in contrast to other specific phobias in which it is recommended that relaxation skills be utilized only in preparation for exposure work and not during the course of the exposure itself, applied muscle tension is indicated for use as a coping technique during exposures for blood injury phobia (when patients experience feelings of dizziness, shaking, or fainting) (Ritz et al., 2014). As the patient gains confidence, it is possible that her need for the applied tension activities will reduce.

Visual/Auditory Exposures

Discuss and provide education on how the needle functions, what equipment is used, and how blood is taken (Willemsen, Chowhury, & Briscall, 2002).

Use and repeat words associated with injections (*needle, blood, shot, inject, syringe, immunization*). The therapist can use word games such as crossword puzzles, spelling bee challenges, hangman, word scrambles, or rapid naming to make this activity engaging for the child.

Create a tape with words repeated for child to listen to at varying intervals.

Draw a picture or have the child draw a picture of the equipment used, people in the room, and action of receiving an injection.

Read stories or children's books about going to the doctor or getting shots.

View videos clips of syringes going into a piece of fruit or another object. Move to pictures and then video clips of a person receiving a shot or getting blood drawn (Willemsen et al., 2002). Choose videos in which the child is coping effectively. Start video with audio off and move to audio on after the child's anxiety reduces.

Watch parts of TV shows that involve doctors and medical procedures (Antony & Watling, 2006) (examples: Elmo getting a vaccination, Sid the Science Kid receiving a shot, scenes from the TV series *Doogie Howser, MD*). Consider age and appropriateness of show content first.

Imaginal/Role-Play Exposures

Imagine an injection or a blood draw using a script that involves a standard routine. Walk through the following or similar steps: walking to the office, sitting in the waiting room, entering the examination room, sitting on the table, listening to the physician talk and examine you, watching the equipment being prepared by the nurse, and the procedure for receiving an injection: 1) lying down on the table, 2) pressing on arm to find a vein, 2) using tourniquet to wrap around arm, 3) swabbing the spot with an alcohol wipe and applying local anesthetic, 4) placing needle near the spot of injection, and 5) insertion of the needle (Ritz et al., 2014).

For those with a history of an event or trauma related to receiving an injection, develop a detailed script focused on that particular incident and read the script with a number of repetitions until anxiety reduces. Have the child then share the narrative with his parent.

Put equipment used for injections on the table (syringe or needle, tourniquet, alcohol swab or cotton balls, latex gloves, Band-Aids, blood collection tubes, and so on), plus fake blood. Allow child to look at, smell, and touch the objects (for example: hold needle or syringe with cap off, smell alcohol swab, place tourniquet on arm, press needle on arm) (Antony & Watling, 2006).

Role-play the procedure of getting blood drawn or receiving an injection (see procedure above in "Imaginal Exposure" section). Have the therapist serve as the patient first and the child as the doctor or nurse, and then switch to have the child as the patient. Start first without real props and use the point of a pencil as the pretend needle.

Role-play using real equipment and work through each step of the procedure at a pace that works for the child.

Coordinate with child's pediatrician to practice procedure within the pediatric office. Start in an empty room without the doctor or nurse present. If possible, have the nurse role-play with the child after the child habituates to role-play with the therapist.

In Vivo Exposures

Fill and look at a syringe with pretend blood (Antony & Watling, 2006).

Note: There are a number of recipes on the Internet for fake blood. Corn syrup, maple syrup, or hair gel can be mixed with water as a base. Red food coloring, as well as some drops of green or blue food coloring or chocolate syrup can create the right hue. Cornstarch or flour is often used as a thickener.

Look at blood drain off of a steak or other piece of raw meat.

When possible, have the child watch an adult receive an injection. She should watch someone who will cope well with the procedure.

Watch someone prick his finger using a lancet and look at the blood. Have the child prick her own finger using a lancet and squeeze out blood. Look at blood on finger (Antony & Watling, 2006).

Have child volunteer at a hospital with an adult or watch an adult donate blood.

Engage in actual blood draw or injection.

Reducing Safety Behaviors and Avoidance

Look at stimuli (for example, receiving the injection), rather than looking away (Antony & Watling, 2006).

Stand or sit up during the procedure, as opposed to lying down with legs elevated (Willemsen et al., 2002). (*Note:* Lying down may be helpful initially to reduce fainting sensations, but should be reduced over time as confidence increases.)

Reduce efforts at distraction that may be necessary initially (examples: playing a handheld video game, listening to music, using a muscle tension or relaxation exercise).

STORMS AND WEATHER EVENTS

Visual/Auditory Exposures

Use and repeat weather-related terms (examples: *hurricane, tornado, downpour, flood, rainstorm, hailstorm*).

Draw pictures of the feared weather event or past experiences with the weather event (example: standing in a thunderstorm at a park).

Look at photographs of a variety of storms and weather events. Start with ones that are mild and work up to ones that appear more intense.

Listen to audio recordings of storms (gusts of wind, downpour of rain or hail, tree branches swaying or snapping, thunder, rush of water). Slowly increase the volume of the sound. Make sure the bass of the speaker is on high so that you can detect the vibration created by the sounds of thunder.

Watch full video clips of storms and weather-related events. Start with mild weather-related events (examples: a storm brewing, a windy day, rain) and build up to more intense weather phenomena (full thunderstorm, hurricane, tornado). Watch lightning and turn off the sound of corresponding thunder to disconnect that conditioned response.

Listen to or watch video clips of news reports when bad weather is predicted or occurring. Include clips that have the emergency weather alert noise.

Imaginal Exposures

Create a detailed script and imagine the vivid sensory experiences of standing outside on a windy day, or in a rainstorm, thunderstorm, or other weather event, or have child imagine a specific weather event from the past that induced a fear response.

In Vivo Exposures

Practice opening a window on a rainy or windy day or a day when the sky is getting darker as a storm approaches. Have child move closer to the window or sit on a covered porch. Consider safety and do not conduct this activity if the storm is directly overhead or there are other safety recommendations to stay indoors.

Engage in outside activities near the home when weather is approaching (examples: shooting hoops, playing hopscotch, jumping rope).

Practice sitting outside without using distraction (instead, focus on noticing the sights and sounds) on a day when a weather event is approaching.

Take walks on days when it is windy, cloudy, or rainy, or there are other signs of a weather event approaching. (*Note:* Adults should consider safety related to likely weather conditions and any local recommendations to stay indoors.)

Engage in activities that require extended time periods in an open area—such as sporting events, long walks in the park, and hikes. Increase challenge by engaging in activities on a windy or rainy day.

Go to a mall or carnival that has a storm or tornado simulator. The child may benefit from an adult modeling or participating with him at first.

Reducing Safety Behaviors and Avoidance

Reduce use of the Internet, TV, newspaper, or other media to repeatedly check weather reports.

Avoid moving to an internal location or basement when a weather event is predicted or signs are present. Start moving closer to windows or other locations to view the weather event (as long as it's considered safe in the particular circumstance).

Have parent avoid providing repeated reassurance or answering repeated questions about whether she thinks a storm or other weather event may occur based on subtle cues such as wind or clouds. Teach parents to say to the child, "What do you think?" when he asks for reassurance, so he can learn to answer for himself.

Go places without carrying an umbrella, rain jacket, or other safety object.

Avoid changing plans as a result of predicted weather (unless safety recommendations suggest to do so).

WATER

Visual/Auditory Exposures

Draw pictures of water scenes. Have child describe what is happening in the scene. Have child draw a situation from the past involving water that scared her. Discuss the situation in detail and have child recall sensory experiences.

Look at and discuss pictures of various water scenes. Explore which scenes elicit greater tension and fear. Explore details in the scenes (examples: the color of a sailboat, the white tips of the ocean waves).

Play sound recordings of various ocean and water sounds. Generate a recording so that the child can listen repeatedly to the sounds.

Watch video clips of water scenes from animated films (example: *The Little Mermaid*). Start with scenes that are calm and happy, and work up to scenes where water is rough. Start with the audio off and build to having both video and audio on.

Watch video clips of calm scenes of a body of water such as a lake or ocean (examples: people riding in a sailboat, cruising on a yacht, or playing in a lake). Work up to watching video clips in which water is rough or storm is present. Watch people having fun and laughing while going on a raft through rapids.

Imaginal Exposure

Have child imagine a beach scene: *You are at the beach and your family starts to go into the water. You put your foot in and it's cold. As you stand there, your feet get used to the temperature and feel okay after a while. Go in up to your knees; stand there until your body is used to the temperature.* Continue imaginal exposure with child slowly putting more of his body into the water.

In Vivo Exposures

Bring in a plastic basin or tub and fill with 6 inches of water. Engage in water play and explore aspects of the water (example: making splashes, waves).

Put face in a tub of water. This behavior may need to be shaped by putting ear, hair, chin, or forehead in first, and building to larger parts of the face. Therapist should model each step first, including blowing bubbles with face in water. A transparent tub can be helpful if it is propped up so that the child can view your face while you are blowing bubbles from underneath the tub.

Have child wear goggles and practice opening her eyes while her face is under the water, using the plastic tub.

Increase time outside of session playing in bathtub, and the amount of water in the tub. (Consider age of child.)

Spray water on face with water bottle. Stand in shower without face submerged. Then slowly move closer until the spray of water is on the child's face.

Go to lake or pool and sit near the edge. Watch and describe the water.

Walk or have parents drive over a bridge with water under it.

Put feet in the water and play games in this location. Adjust to the sensation of water on the feet and discuss observations. Bring water toys that are easy to use in a small amount of water (examples: cups, pitchers, sponges) for younger children. For older kids, you might have them engage in a science experiment (examples: testing the water pH, collecting shells, identifying small creatures in the water).

Slowly immerse more of the body in the water. For younger children, be cognizant of swim capabilities and make sure work is done in the shallow parts of the pool, lake, or ocean.

Work on slowly putting various parts of the face in water and practice blowing bubbles. A swim instructor may be helpful at this step for guidance on the best methods for teaching a child to bob and blow bubbles. Use goggles to allow child to look under the water, or a snorkel mask to make it more fun!

Float in an inner tube or other flotation device, such as a boogie board, in shallow parts of the water.

Spend time sitting in a sailboat, paddleboat, motorboat, or other water vehicle without it moving, or even when it is not physically in the water. If possible, have child touch and play with water on the side of the boat.

Take a ride in a water vehicle that moves slowly and is on a calm body of water (example: paddleboat on a small lake). Have child use paddles or push pedals if possible.

Take a ride in a water vehicle that moves faster, or when waves are present.

Sit in shallow water at a lake, pool, or ocean.

Wade in a pool or clear lake where you can see to the bottom.

Wade in a lake that is muddy and you cannot see to the bottom.

Submerge face in water in lake, pool, or ocean.

Go to a water park and spend time in the wave pool, or attempt certain water slides if child has swim capabilities to do so.

Spend time standing in crashing waves at ocean, using boogie board or vest to ride the waves.

Swim in water for short distance (if child has swim skills).

Swim longer distances in a large lake or other body of water (for older children who are strong swimmers).

Reducing Safety Behaviors and Avoidance

Reduce avoidance of family or school trips that involve water (examples: water park, pool, ocean, aquarium, boat ride).

Reduce need to rely on alternate routes when anxious (example: refusing to allow parents to drive over bridge).

Reduce information seeking about dangers in the lake or ocean (example: whether sharks are present), and about harm or death related to water (example: news stories about drowning victims).

Reduce reliance on safety objects such as tubes or flotation devices (only when child has necessary swimming skills and location is appropriate).

Reduce reliance on safety person nearby.

Case Example

An 8-year-old boy presented for treatment due to a specific phobia of a famous male vocalist and his music. This child avoided all situations that would expose him to his image or music. He refused to allow music to play on the radio in his mother's car or attend family gatherings for fear that the singer's music would play. If he was in a situation in which he heard his music or observed his image, he panicked and attempted escape. Of note, in addition to the specific phobia, this client had a high verbal IQ and overall intelligence; however, he was generally rigid with his routines and preferences. He presented with an uncertainty about treatment, although he was interested in feeling less anxious.

After considerable work on helping him to understand the rationale for exposure and developing coping tools, exposure work started with a discussion about the singer, what he looked like, how he sounded, what the child did not like about his appearance and music, and so on. The therapist worked to slow down the pace of discussion, expressing curiosity about the client's thoughts and perspective. Once the child had successfully habituated to these discussions as indicated by low ratings on his fear thermometer, exposures proceeded to the therapist reading the singer's lyrics at a pace chosen by the child. The lyrics were first read in a monotone voice, without rhythm or inflection. The client then read the lyrics back to the therapist. The therapist then sang the lyrics, and then both therapist and child practiced singing the lyrics together. A tape was made of both therapist and child singing the lyrics for him to take home to listen to for homework. At the following session, an attempt was made to have this client listen to audio clips of the songs, sung by the artist. However, he refused to listen to the audio, even at low volume. The therapist then negotiated to start the exposure with the boy standing outside of the room, about one foot away from the doorway, with the door cracked and the audio on at low volume inside the room. While the audio was likely not audible to the child at first, the initial exposure gave him enough confidence to move closer to the doorway on the second exposure. Repetitions continued with this child moving into the room and eventually sitting next to the speakers, with audio of the song playing at low volume. This particular exposure with repetition took a full session. Subsequent sessions involved increasing the volume of the audio and listening to different songs. The client then practiced listening to the audio clips in the home setting, and a reward system was used to encourage his practice.

Exposures transitioned to working on his fear of the visual image of this singer. Initially, therapist and child spent time drawing pictures of the singer. Attempts were made to use humor to help him manage and participate in this work. Printed pictures of parts of the singer's body and wardrobe (hair, clothing, face, shoes, and so on) were shown to the client before attempting exposure to his entire image. When an attempt was made to view a music video of the singer, refusal was again encountered. Initial exposures involved watching his music video with no volume and at a physical distance from the computer. The therapist also set a time challenge that started with the goal of watching the video for 10 seconds, gradually increasing to the full 3-minute length of the video. Exposure work then progressed toward: 1) moving physically closer to the video, 2) watching the video while it played in its entirety, 3) incorporating sound and increasing volume, and 4) watching other music videos of this artist.

Each week the child and his parent were given homework to continue to practice exposures that he had been successful with during the session that week. Treatment lasted a total of eight sessions, at which time this child was capable of experiencing all visual and auditory aspects of this artist with minimal anxiety. Avoidance behavior dissipated and he achieved his goals of listening to the radio despite uncertainty regarding whether the singer's music would play, and listening to the singer's music in public settings. He was able to attend parties and other activities with minimal anxiety or attempts to control the music played. Parent and child were encouraged to continue to practice exposure exercises at varying intervals post-treatment to encourage maintenance of treatment effects.

Conclusion

Specific phobias in children and adolescents involve a persistent and pervasive fear of a specific object or situation that is endured with severe distress and active avoidance. Being in the presence of the feared object or situation often results in behavioral reactions such as crying, clinging to parents, refusing to participate in activities, attempting escape, and sometimes aggressive behavior in an effort to avoid the fear. For children and adolescents with specific phobia, exposure-based CBT is considered the most efficacious and promising treatment. This chapter reviewed diagnostic information, key treatment considerations, and implementation of exposure-based CBT for children and adolescents experiencing a variety of specific phobias. Samples of specific exposure tasks were provided for consideration in creating individualized exposure hierarchies with clients. Finally, case examples were used to illustrate the clinician's role in implementing general CBT skills and exposure tasks with real clients experiencing specific phobia.

CHAPTER 11

Exposure for Selective Mutism

In this chapter, you will find information related to exposure treatment for children and adolescents with selective mutism (SM). The chapter provides an overview of treatment considerations for this population related to CBT and exposure work, as well as a comprehensive list of exposure ideas and exercises. The information included is intended to support clinicians in creating and implementing an exposure hierarchy that is tailored to each individual client who experiences symptoms of SM.

Clinical Presentation and Causal Factors

SM is defined as a persistent failure to speak in specific social situations in which speaking is expected, despite speaking fluently in other situations (American Psychiatric Association, 2013). The lack of speech interferes with academic achievement or social communication and is not better accounted for by the presence of a pervasive developmental disorder, a communication disorder, or a psychotic disorder. Children with SM often experience problems such as peer rejection, difficulty making and maintaining friendships, difficulty completing verbal standardized tests, and poor social skills (Cunningham, McHolm, & Boyle, 2006). Estimates of prevalence suggest that between 0.47% and 0.76% of children in early elementary school have SM (Chavira, Stein, Bailey, & Stein, 2004; Elizur & Perednik, 2003; Bergman, Piacentini, & McCracken, 2002), with an average age of onset between 2 and 5 years (Garcia et al., 2004; Viana et al., 2009; Sung & Smith, 2009). In adolescence and adulthood, the disorder is considered exceedingly rare (Sharp, Sherman, & Gross, 2007). Most cases remit by this point, and rarely does SM present with a late onset.

Children with SM frequently present with co-occurring conditions. They have a higher prevalence of comorbid speech and language deficits, including deficits in phonemic awareness, auditory processing, and expressive and receptive language (Manassis et al., 2003; Steinhausen, Wachter, Laimbock, & Metzke, 2006), and higher rates of developmental delays (Kristensen, 2000), as compared to the population of children without SM. Early language difficulties and developmental delays may impact the subsequent development of SM (Reuther, Davis, Moree, & Matson, 2011). Evidence also suggests that the development of SM may be influenced by second language acquisition or the primary language spoken at home being different from that of the surrounding environment (Elizur & Perednik, 2003). In addition, children with SM are more likely to exhibit other internalizing conditions, including obsessive-compulsive disorder and social anxiety disorder, as well as somatic complaints, compared to children without the disorder (Cunningham, McHolm, Boyle, & Patel, 2004; Viana et al., 2009). SM and social anxiety/phobia significantly overlap in their symptomatology and temperamental precursors (Sharp et al., 2007; Silveria, Jainer, & Bates, 2004; Yeganeh et al., 2003); the comorbidity between these two conditions is estimated to be between 80% and 97% (Black & Uhde, 1995; Young, Bunnell, & Beidel, 2012). Recent research suggests that SM likely reflects a developmental variant of social phobia with an earlier age of onset.

In terms of risk factors, a behaviorally inhibited or "slow to warm" temperamental style is considered a precursor to the onset of SM (Ford, Sladesczek, Carlson, & Krochwell, 1998; Hadley, 1994). Children with this temperamental style tend to become withdrawn, shy, and avoidant. They also experience higher and more accelerated heart rates when in stressful or unfamiliar situations. While early studies of SM suggested that these children were also temperamentally difficult and oppositional, evidence now confirms that the noncompliant and stubborn behavior often observed in SM may be better understood as a behavioral response to feared situations rather than a reflection of general oppositional tendencies (Sharp et al., 2007).

Learning and reinforcement are believed to play a key role in the development of the disorder (Bergman, 2013). The expectation to speak in certain situations elicits anxiety, which causes the child to avoid speech. This avoidance leads to a reduction in anxiety. Thus, the child is negatively reinforced by the absence of the negative outcome (discomfort, anxiety, or embarrassment upon speaking). This pattern of avoidance then increases and expands over time due to its power to reduce anxiety. Well-intentioned adults in the child's life often inadvertently reinforce this behavioral pattern by speaking for the child with SM, providing excessive help or support, or offering alternative (nonverbal) means of communication. As the child's lack of speech increases in consistency, confidence decreases and response patterns become further ingrained.

Exposure Therapy for SM

This learning and behavioral conceptualization of SM speaks strongly to the need for an approach that directly targets behavioral avoidance and patterns of negative reinforcement. As such, exposure therapy is an ideal choice for creating a shift from avoidance to approach, unlearning negative behavioral patterns, and practicing new responses. In addition, the habituation in anxiety experienced during exposure work can help children with behaviorally inhibited temperaments build confidence in their ability to tolerate anxious situations. While published studies of the treatment of SM are limited, in large part due to the rarity of the disorder, research that is available supports the use and effectiveness of various cognitive behavioral techniques that emphasize exposure-based strategies similar to those applied in the treatment of children with SoP (see Cohan, Chavira, & Stein, 2006, for a review; Baskind, 2007; Bunnell & Beidel, 2013; Fisak, Oliveros, & Ehrenreich, 2006; Vecchio & Kearney, 2009).

Core treatment components include rapport building, shaping, stimulus fading and systematic desensitization, contingency management, and behavioral exposures. A number of preliminary studies also support the use of behavioral self-modeling techniques via audio and video editing to aid in the treatment of SM (Blum et al., 1998; Lang et al., 2011). Throughout all of these therapeutic techniques, there is a focus on generalizing speech and social gains to as many individuals, settings, and situations as possible and transferring the implementation of the intervention from therapist to parents, teachers, and other adults in the child's life.

Clinically Relevant Factors

Ongoing clinical assessment must focus on a clear and detailed understanding of the specific nature of SM-related symptoms and impairment in preparation for exposure therapy. As discussed in chapter 2, the environmental context within which the symptoms present, and the specific nature of the child's cognitions and behavioral responses, are critical considerations in the subsequent engineering of effective exposure exercises. Below we present typical fear triggers or cues, feared consequences, and avoidance and safety behaviors commonly occurring in children with SM.

Fear Cues

Fear cues or triggers are specific environmental factors or variables that typically elicit the child's or anxiety. These are the situations that activate the fear response due to the presence of specific stimuli that are perceived as dangerous or harmful in some way. The following fear cues commonly trigger anxiety in children with SM:

Locations or events where speaking may be expected that are outside of their comfort zone (examples: school, sports events, playgrounds, restaurants, stores)

Questions or social cues that create pressure to speak (typically from people other than close family members and friends)

Participating in activities or games that generally require speech

Physical sensations of anxiety during a social situation

Feared Consequences

Feared consequences are those environmental conditions and outcomes that the child expects will result from exposure to the feared stimuli. That is, the child's fear is initiated and maintained through his experience or his belief that these negative outcomes will occur. The following are common feared consequences for children with SM:

Others hearing their speech or sound of their voice

Not being able to get the words out (sometimes described as a knot in the throat or stuck feeling)

Uncomfortable physiological sensations when pressured to speak

Receiving attention from others (as in all eyes on them)

Receiving a negative reaction from others (example: *others will laugh at me or think I am dumb*)

Feeling embarrassed when speaking

Providing an incorrect response

Appearing nervous (blushing, stuttering, or shaking)

Inability to escape the uncomfortable situation

Being forced to speak

Avoidance

Children with anxiety commonly avoid the environmental stimuli and situations that trigger their anxiety because they perceive a high likelihood of their feared consequences occurring. The following are common avoidant behaviors observed in children with SM:

Refusal to participate in, or restricting participation in, activities that the child feels will require speech or even nonverbal communication

Refusal to speak, or limited speech, in any situation the child has designated as nonspeaking (examples: school, friends' homes, public settings)

Refusal to look at or approach individuals with whom the child has decided she will not speak, or has a history of not speaking with

Safety Behaviors

Children and adolescents with anxiety often rely on specific objects, individuals, or actions that they believe will protect them from the feared stimuli or feared outcome. Safety behaviors are any actions the child performs in an attempt to feel safe. The following are common safety behaviors displayed by children with SM:

Staying close to their "safe" person and using this person (often a parent or caregiver) as a physical barrier to interacting with others (for example, hiding behind or refusing to detach from the parent)

Making eye contact only with the safe person when asked a question, and expecting that person to respond for him, or speaking only to that person

Seeking excessive reassurance to confirm that she will not be required to speak in a given situation, or refusal to attend an activity when uncomfortable

Avoiding or limiting eye contact and facial expressions (examples: looking down, covering parts of face with hands, lack of smile, strained or serious facial expression)

Willingness to participate only in a part of an activity under certain conditions that make him feel safe (example: talking with the school aide when alone, but not around peers)

Tailoring Exposure Therapy for SM

This section is designed to serve as a primer for the implementation of exposure therapy specifically for children with SM. It builds on the guidance presented in earlier chapters by offering the therapist specific guidelines for what must be uniquely considered when carrying out this work with children with SM. That is, additional strategies and modifications to the treatment approach will be discussed that are of paramount importance to implementing exposure-based work with this group.

Exposure therapy for SM can be particularly tricky to implement because it requires the child to generate an active response that is very difficult for her (speaking). Many children with SM describe feeling that the words are stuck in their throat, or just won't come out. As such, the use of specific games and methods of interacting that reinforce speech and the inclusion of familiar people with whom the child typically speaks are important components of treatment. These considerations allow children with SM to reduce hypervigilance of their own speech and increase the likelihood of speech generation. They serve as starting points for treatment through which therapists gradually "fade in" or add new individuals to the play, as well as adjust environmental variables, one at a time, to increase the challenge as the child demonstrates success. These approaches are described in detail below, including recommendations for how parents, teachers, and the treatment team should respond to the child with SM at different stages of treatment and how to train and collaborate with the treatment team, generalize treatment gains, and transfer control of the intervention to the treatment team over time.

Development of the Fear Hierarchy

The development and implementation of a series of graduated exposures is a main focus in the treatment of SM (Bergman, 2013; Cohan et al., 2006; Kearney, Haight, & Day, 2011). Prior to exposure, a detailed list of the locations and settings in which (and individuals with whom) the child demonstrates varying degrees of speech should be elicited. Exposures are designed creatively and flexibly throughout the therapy process given parent and teacher input and observations of child responses. The major goals of behavioral exposures are to expand the variety of situations and conditions under which the child speaks, as well as to increase the quality of that engagement (for example, voice volume, elaboration, spontaneity, and self-advocacy). With this purpose in mind, the difficulty level of exposures is tailored to gradually increase in small, incremental steps based on the child's progress.

Building an appropriate exposure involves considering all of the building blocks or variables that may have an impact. Children with SM are typically unbending in their uniquely held rules for when they will and will not speak and highly sensitive to minor changes in the environment. Treatment must therefore target the expansion of these boundaries through challenges that are individually tailored. For example, a child may answer questions in a whisper at the desk of her math teacher, but may not speak at all with her reading teacher. In the former case, a daily goal may be to answer questions with increased volume at the teacher's desk or to answer questions in a whisper at different locations within the classroom. In the latter case, intervention may start with the reading teacher being incorporated into play sessions with the child and parent after school. For children with SM, the following is a list of environmental variables that will be considered for adjustment in expanding the variety of situations the child speaks in:

The specific individual(s) engaging with the child, and presence of other individuals in the room

The structure and type of activity (structured game, free play, playground play, table work, and so on)

The location (classroom, library, playground, clinic room, waiting room, other public setting)

The method of engagement for each adult and peer in the room (observation only, verbal commentary/reinforcing statements, or commentary and direct questions)

The physical proximity of various individuals in the room

The type of questions asked (forced-choice, yes/no, open-ended)

The explicit goals for child response (gesturing, mouthing words, whispering, low-volume talk, normal-volume talk, one-word versus sentences, and so on)

PROVIDING EDUCATION AND A COLLABORATIVE TEAM APPROACH

It is extremely common for individuals in the child's life (parents, teachers, coaches, family members, other adults) to inadvertently reinforce non-speech due to their attempts to reduce discomfort in the child and in themselves. For example, adults may speak for the child, allow the child alternatives to speaking—such as writing on a dry-erase board or pointing to his choices—or avoid asking the child questions at all. All individuals who come in contact with the child with SM should receive education and support designed to give them knowledge about how to interact effectively with the child with SM. If a teacher or parent struggles to encourage and coach verbal responses and willingly accepts all nonverbal means of communication, SM symptoms will be further reinforced.

Providing education on the nature of SM, behavioral treatment, and the role of parents, teachers, and other team members in the treatment process is critical for the success of subsequent treatment. A treatment team approach should be developed in which members collaborate to promote treatment goals and exposure work (Bergman, 2013). Education can be provided to the treatment team in the form of ongoing school meetings or videoconference sessions. Treatment will also be modeled by the therapist through implementation of fade-in sessions at the school and trainings provided to staff. Treatment team members should be composed of all individuals who interact with and come into contact with the child on a regular basis. This will encourage the generalization of speaking across environments (such as gym, art, music class, or soccer practice). The following are important principles for communication and collaboration within the treatment team:

Education on the nature of SM and the process through which avoidance and nonspeaking becomes learned and reinforced over time

Assessment of where, when, with whom, and in what context the child speaks and does not speak

Education on the treatment approach, including shaping and fade-in procedures, behavioral exposures, and the development of reward plans

Collaborative development of ongoing treatment goals/plans and careful design of exposure tasks

Education on when it is appropriate and necessary to expect and encourage a verbal response (for example, when the child has shown some demonstration of the desired behavior in that situation) versus when some accommodation is needed (for example, early on in treatment, and for higher-challenge scenarios in which the child is not yet ready to demonstrate a response in a specific situation)

STIMULUS FADING

In the treatment of SM, fade-in or stimulus fading procedures are an important component (Cohan et al., 2006; Richburg & Cobia, 1994). They are typically utilized during initial meetings with the child to encourage the initiation and transfer of speech from parent to therapist, as well as incorporated throughout therapy to transfer speech to teachers, peers, and other individuals. The overarching goal of stimulus fading is to integrate a new individual into the interaction and fade out a familiar individual. That is, the child is placed in a comfortable situation in which he typically verbalizes, with new individuals being "faded in" to the interaction slowly as the child's confidence increases.

In a typical format, you begin the session by leading the parent (or other individual the child speaks easily with) and child into a room (such as a clinic room or classroom) with a number of highly desirable play activities. We recommend that you leave the room for a while to allow the parent and child time to warm up together by playing with the toys. Stimulus fading continues with the therapist, teacher, or other target person slowly entering the room and gradually moving closer in visual and physical proximity to the child. For example, the target person might return to the room and sit at a desk in the far corner of the room (at a large distance from the play). To start, consider having this person engage in deskwork and avoid eye contact, as to reduce the challenge for the child at first. Gradually, the person to be faded in will start verbalizing during the play.

As the child shows increased acceptance of the target person's statements by continuing to verbalize to his parent in their presence, slowly increase the difficulty level of the exposure. There are various adjustments that can be made to add challenge to the interaction. The target person might move closer in physical proximity to the play (for example, watering plants, adjusting a desk clock, or erasing a board), while periodically continuing to make positive comments regarding the play. You can also adjust the difficulty level by beginning to add eye contact and facial expression, increasing the frequency of the comments made, or engaging in direct verbal interaction with the parent. Eventually, the target person will join the play by participating in a game or activity of the child's choice. During this time period, the target person is not yet asking any direct questions of the child, nor is she giving any instructions to the child.

PARENT CHILD INTERACTION THERAPY (PCIT) FOR SM

Preliminary research suggests that a specific protocol traditionally used for improving compliance and enhancing the parent-child relationship, parent-child interaction therapy (PCIT), can be adapted for use in the treatment of SM (Carpenter et al., 2014; Mele & Kurtz, 2013; Kurtz, 2012; Furr et al., 2012; Lynas, Kurtz, & Brandon, 2012). Traditional PCIT has been proven effective for encouraging positive child behavior and adult-child interaction in numerous large-scale studies (e.g., Eisenstadt et al., 1993). For the purpose of working with the child with SM, PCIT skills are utilized with the unique goals of sensitizing the child to the adult's presence, reinforcing the child's play and verbalizations, and minimizing factors that discourage verbal responding.

In the PCIT-SM approach, team members are specifically coached to utilize a high rate of reinforcing statements during interactions with the child. That is, they are encouraged to use skills that build positive interaction, including specific praise, behavioral descriptions of the child's actions, and reflections of the child's statements (Carpenter et al., 2014). This phase is referred to as child-directed interaction (CDI). Team members are coached to avoid leading the interaction through commands, criticism, or questions. Below are definitions and examples of each of these CDI skills:

Behavioral description: A specific description of a child's ongoing actions.

"You're coloring the dinosaur purple." "You're building a tall house."

Labeled praise: A specific positive interpretation of the child's actions or products.

"I love the colorful rainbow you drew." "Thank you for showing me your drawing."

Reflection: A summary or repetition of the child's verbal statements.

Child: "I want to play with the castle." *Parent:* "You want to play with the castle."

During a stimulus fading procedure as described above, the target person will begin to provide labeled praise, reflection, and behavioral description as she approaches the play (Carpenter et al., 2014; Mele & Kurtz, 2013). This potentially increases the child's awareness that the target person has heard him and builds tolerance to being heard. The parent is also coached to use CDI skills in combination with easy questions to maintain a high rate of child speech as the target person enters the room. The overall goal is to encourage the initiation of child speech by placing the child in a comfortable situation with a high likelihood of verbalization: that is, a focus on interacting with his parent or another individual he speaks easily with, who is providing reinforcing statements during the play and asking easy questions, with a gradual introduction to the presence of the target individual's statements.

INTRODUCTION AND TIMING OF QUESTIONS

In the treatment of SM, it is extremely important to carefully consider the timing and context of direct questions posed to the child and the behavioral responses of individuals who ask the questions. Inadvertent reinforcement of mute behavior is likely when questions are asked of the child in situations which, or by individuals to whom, the child is not yet ready to speak. Consistent with this, the utilization of direct questions must develop in a gradual fashion, starting with easier situations and building toward more difficult situations. The timing and context of questions will require ongoing consideration. As new goals are set with small adjustments in environmental variables, the lack of response to a question often indicates the need to return to the previous, easier goal for further reinforcement.

During stimulus fading, easy questions can be added once the child is successfully tolerating the target person engaging through physical proximity and verbal commentary. As the child successfully answers the target person's questions, this individual can increase the rate of her questions and slowly fade the parent or other familiar individual out of the play. For example, the parent might tell the child she needs to make a brief phone call and step out of the room, suggest that the child play the game with the target person while she observes, increase her physical distance from the child, or take a smaller role in the game (for example, serving as the score keeper.)

The PCIT-SM approach specifically utilizes an instructional phase known as verbal-directed interaction (VDI) to encourage speech (Carpenter et al., 2014; Mele & Kurtz, 2013). Through this approach, teachers and other team members are coached to ask specific types of questions once the child has become accustomed to the presence of the target person and their use of CDI skills, while continuing to verbalize to the parent. These questions are interspersed between the continued use of reflections, descriptions, and praise. Team members are taught to avoid rescuing the child by speaking for the child or jumping in too quickly. Specifically, target individuals are coached to wait 5 seconds for the child's response after asking a question; provide immediate, specific praise for verbal responding; and follow up with another question if the child has answered verbally (Carpenter et al., 2014). Alternatively, if the child does not answer, it is recommended to briefly return to the use of CDI skills or otherwise reduce the challenge of the task (for example, by modifying environmental variables) to increase the likelihood of success.

TYPES OF QUESTIONS

Questions that require easy, one-word responses may be the most beneficial and likely to elicit speech early on in treatment. The PCIT-SM approach suggests that forced-choice questions, in which the child is given two or more options, are one of the most effective options for prompting speech in the early stages of treatment. The following are examples of forced-choice questions:

Would you like the red or green marker?

Do you want to play with the blocks or LEGOs?

Do you prefer peanut butter and jelly or ham sandwiches?

Other types of questions may not be as effective for encouraging speech in children with SM in the early stages of treatment. For example, children with SM are likely to use physical gestures (head shakes and nods) in response to yes-or-no questions, reducing the likelihood of speech. The treatment team must be prepared with a response when physical gestures are used in response to questions, such as, "Please let me know yes or no." Clinicians might consider avoiding yes-or-no questions altogether until it is clear that the child will provide a verbal answer to this type of prompt. Open-ended questions (such as, "How was your weekend?") that require an elaborative response with multiple phrases or sentences are also likely poor choices for beginning treatment work. Similarly, learning-based questions that assess the child's knowledge of a given subject will also likely present a higher-level challenge for the child. That is, the child may be worried about getting the answer correct, which can add to the anxiety related to speaking. An exception to this may be the use of questions about facts or information the child has carefully rehearsed and mastered.

POSITIVE FEEDBACK AND REWARD SYSTEMS

At the outset of treatment, it is particularly important to reward the child with praise for every instance of verbal behavior observed. As treatment progresses and the child starts speaking naturally and fluidly with certain individuals, praise and points can be focused on current goals and areas that pose greater difficulty. We recommend that praise be delivered in a gentle, nonchalant manner for children who may withdraw from overly loud or enthusiastic displays. Some children may prefer the use of a hand gesture (such as a thumbs-up) or other discreet signal from the adult to encourage their success.

Positive feedback is also critical to provide for approximations of the end goal. If the child demonstrates effort toward a difficult goal (for example, whispering the words or stating part of a sentence), share what you heard the child say as a way to reinforce and validate that you heard her, and offer praise for her effort. If the child's speech was audible but unclear, rather than making corrective statements (such as, "I can't hear you. Can you please speak up?"), you might praise the child for answering or making an attempt to answer the question. (For example, "Thank you for answering my question. I appreciate you sharing with me.") These suggestions are consistent with the PCIT-SM approach, which encourages reflections and labeled praise to reinforce speech, as opposed to criticism or correction.

As with other anxiety disorders, establishing a reward system early on in the treatment process is critical for encouraging child motivation and interest in working on bravery-related goals. It is important that a reward system is developed that allows the child to earn desired commodities or privileges in the home and school settings. It can also be beneficial to add flexibility and increased opportunities for positive feedback by spontaneously awarding points when you "catch" the child being brave. These points are awarded for brave speech that is observed but is not the focus of a current goal. This encourages the child to take risks and consider brave speaking at times when she might not have otherwise. A star or box can be placed around the point to indicate that this is a special point. This means that the child did something above and beyond expectations, and the box can be designated as worth a greater number of points.

Structured Games and Play Tasks for Exposures

We also strongly recommend that you carefully consider the activity that will serve as a medium through which you facilitate speech-related, exposure goals. A simple prompt to practice a given goal (such as saying hello to a peer or answering a question) without the presence of an engaging activity is less likely to bring about success, especially early on in treatment. We highly recommended incorporating fun, engaging activities that motivate the child and encourage speech. Engaging activities can serve to relax the child, reduce pressure, and create enjoyment within therapeutic work. As a result, the child will have a greater desire to speak and the act of speaking may feel less daunting. The choice of activity should be made through considering child preferences, previous success with specific activities, and the type of response desired from the child. Specific games present different levels of challenges based on the type of verbal response that is required from the child. As children build to higher-level goals, practice can include questions during increasingly structured times, such as classroom didactics.

For example, games such as *Spot It!* and *Zingo!* require one-word responses: the child has to call out the name of an animal or object pictured. Other games, such as *HedBanz* or *20 Questions*, have the child ask questions to guess an animal or object. *Go Fish* requires that the child ask questions to obtain matching cards. Other games have the child report on his likes and dislikes (by doing a survey of the child's favorite food, sport, music, or superhero, for example). Card decks from various games (such as *Whoonu* or *American Girl 300 Wishes Game*) can be used to ask the child engaging, forced-choice questions about his interests (such as, "Would you rather be a ballet dancer or a magician?" or "Would you rather climb a mountain or scuba dive in the ocean?"). During scavenger hunts, the child tells the adult whether she is getting "warmer" or "colder" as she approaches the object that is hidden. Games that involve elaboration on the part of the child may be used for a more difficult challenge. For example, the game *Tell Tale* has the child tell a story using a series of picture cards. We recommend referring to the *Treatment for Children with Selective Mutism: Therapist Guide* (Bergman, 2013) for additional game ideas.

Frequency, Duration, and Length of Sessions

As described above, treatment focuses on a series of small approximations toward achievement of each goal, as well as efforts to generalize achieved goals to as many situations and settings as possible. Therefore, the clinician and treatment team will work collaboratively to develop goals that are at an appropriate level depending on the child's previous performance in that setting and to generalize speech within and across a variety of settings. Exposure work may therefore take place on the school playground; in the classroom, gymnasium, hallway, or lunchroom; on playdates; at family gatherings; in public places such as restaurants and stores; and during extra-curricular activities. As such, treatment duration will vary for each child and will depend on a number of factors, including the initial severity, duration, and expansiveness of the SM; comorbid conditions that impact treatment; and the extent of parent and teacher involvement and capability in implementing intervention components.

REPETITION, REINFORCEMENT, AND INCREASING DIFFICULTY

In terms of the frequency of exposure activities and length of sessions, repetition is extremely important in the treatment of SM. Repetition should occur within the context of an individual exposure session as well as across exposure sessions. Therefore, it is important to allow enough time for exposure work at the school or clinic to allow the child to repeat and reinforce specific goals. Consider increasing the difficulty level of a goal only once the child is demonstrating the desired response with sufficient consistency. For example, the goal might be to answer forced-choice questions as asked by the teacher at her desk with an 80% response rate. Reinforcement and repetition will continue until the child reaches this criterion. At this benchmark, additional challenges may be added. For example, the teacher may move other children physically closer to her interaction with the child with SM, or the teacher may ask the child with SM a more difficult type of question.

Warm-up activities are also important to consider from one exposure session to the next. Even though children may habituate to a task during the course of an individual exposure, it is extremely common for some anxiety to return during the same task at the outset of the next exposure session. During each new time period, the child will likely need warm-up time and repetition to build confidence in her use of previously mastered skills. Therefore, we generally recommend starting each new school day or exposure session with easy speaking goals that have been previously mastered and highly reinforced, in order to empower and encourage the child. For example, if the child increased her speech from single words to long sentences in the context of playing a game with the therapist and teacher, then at the start of the subsequent session, the child might warm up by playing a game that requires easy, one-word answers before open-ended questions are posed by the therapist and teacher. Continued shaping of behavior through repetition and reinforcement of easier goals will increase the likelihood that the child will build momentum and progress to higher-level goals during the course of the session. Repetition can be created by playing the same game, sitting in the same location, repeating the same type of question, or maintaining any other environmental variable with consistency from one exposure to the next.

FADING THERAPIST INVOLVEMENT, AND TRANSFER OF CONTROL

As treatment continues, the focus shifts to transferring responsibility for implementing the intervention from the therapist to parents, teachers, and other treatment team members (Bergman, 2013). Therapists should remain cognizant of the skills needed for these individuals to further progress. Psychoeducation for treatment team members should be integrated throughout therapy. It is important to model and discuss the techniques utilized with the child with each treatment team member. Over time, you will encourage parents and teachers to develop their own bravery-related goals, design successive exposures, and track and deliver rewards with your support and feedback.

Goal achievement can be reviewed with the therapist at subsequent clinic sessions with parent and child, during phone or video consultation with the school, and during observation and consultation directly within the school setting.

Cognitive Considerations

For many children, the cognitive piece of CBT will play a minor role in the treatment of SM, with a much greater emphasis on behavioral and exposure-based techniques. That is, young children are unlikely to understand and benefit from in-depth cognitive restructuring techniques, and in some cases it may be contraindicated. In contrast, young children may benefit from a tailored and simplified approach in which they are taught and practice basic coping thoughts (for example, *I am brave; It's okay to feel embarrassed sometimes*) and identify physical sensations and their connection to thoughts and feelings (*When I am anxious and think something bad will happen, my tummy hurts and my throat feels dry*).

Adaptations for Older Children and Adolescents

While a diagnosis of SM in older children and adolescents is considerably less common, it is important to consider developmental modifications that are essential when working with this subgroup. It continues to be critical to provide psychoeducation, develop a strong treatment team approach, and work collaboratively to set goals. One major difference between the treatment of children and the treatment of adolescents is that adolescents will have increased responsibility for collaborating on goal setting and the structure of the treatment program. Their feedback and ideas for achieving goals will be frequently solicited (once they have established speech with the therapist) and additional efforts made to help them feel empowered within the system. For example, they may work on self-tracking their goal achievement during the school day and reviewing with you in subsequent clinic sessions, or with a designated guidance counselor. Working within the school may also take on a different form. Allowing the therapist in the classroom may be developmentally inappropriate at times, and adolescents may be less inclined to allow it. Therefore, early treatment efforts may focus on transferring control of the intervention to school personnel who can provide support and reinforce effort discreetly.

Additionally, older children and adolescents can benefit from a greater cognitive emphasis in treatment. As treatment rapport and speech with the therapist is established, older youth can be taught to challenge maladaptive thought patterns and develop more constructive ways of thinking. Given a higher cognitive level, adolescents are also better suited to utilize mindfulness and relaxation skills to manage anxious sensations.

The specific choices for games and activities must also be developmentally appropriate. For example, an adolescent may prefer to engage with the therapist around a game such as *Mad Libs* or *Taboo*, as opposed to *Zingo!* or *Go Fish*. Finally, adults must take care to provide feedback in developmentally appropriate ways and reward meaningfully. For example, adolescents may be interested in earning desired privileges and additional freedom in the home setting for achieving goals in school and public settings. The provision of positive attention through the use of behavior descriptions, reflections and labeled praises may also require some tweaking. It will be important that statements be delivered in a natural and fluid way and at a rate that feels reinforcing to the adolescent.

Exposure Tasks and Activities Guide

Below, we present a list of exposure-related goals for building and generalizing speech and social interaction in children with SM across a number of settings. These tasks are loosely organized according to an increasing level of difficulty. However, many tasks (such as smiling while speaking, and reading aloud) do not fit easily into a defined place in this hierarchy and each child's needs are unique. We strongly recommend using clinical judgment and information from the treatment team in determining the most effective series of exposure steps for each individual child. Finally, while the therapist is used in these examples primarily as the person implementing the exposures, in real life cases, any member of the treatment team the child has established speech with (parent, teacher, guidance counselor or other school staff) can facilitate these interventions.

Transferring speech from parent to therapist in clinic (see stimulus fading procedure)

Speaking to therapist alone on school playground when no one else is present

Speaking and answering questions in the school hallways about various pictures, diagrams, and other objects displayed with therapist alone and peers at a distance

Speaking to therapist alone in school classroom while playing a game (starting with forced-choice questions and easier games such as *Uno* or *Spot It!* and transitioning to open-ended questions and games that require elaboration, such as *Tell Tale*)

Speaking to therapist in the classroom while playing games, with teacher observing from a distance and eventually approaching (see stimulus fading procedure)

Speaking to therapist in the classroom while playing games, with teacher using reinforcing statements to comment on the play (see PCIT-SM approach)

Answering forced-choice questions from the teacher in the context of the play, after the question has been repeated first by the therapist

Answering forced-choice questions from the teacher in the context of the play, when the question has not been repeated first by the therapist

Answering teacher questions, in a nongame context and with increasing question difficulty (for example, the teacher asks forced-choice questions about favorite activities or interests and transitions to open-ended questions such as, "What did you do for fun this weekend?")

Answering teacher questions related to academic topics (example: mock lesson with only teacher, therapist, and student present)

Speaking to teacher while playing games with one preferred peer (eventually include more peers)

Answering forced-choice questions directly from one or more peers in the context of the play

Responding with elaboration and providing information during the game (example: child is asked by teacher to explain the rules of the game to his peer)

Answering teacher questions during a mock lesson with one or more peers included

Answering teacher questions during transitions (example: teacher is standing near the doorway of the classroom or right outside of the classroom when peers are moving past the door)

Speaking to one or more peers and teacher in other locations within the school building (example: walking to gym class or the restroom)

Answering forced-choice and open-ended questions from the teacher at the teacher's desk or at a distance from peers in the classroom (with the full classroom of students present)

Answering forced-choice and open-ended questions from the teacher at the student's desk or table, or nearby the rest of his peers

Answering forced-choice and open-ended questions during circle time or other small group activities (example: "Is the weather cloudy or rainy today?")

Answering forced-choice and open-ended questions during whole class activities

Raising hand to answer these questions during small group and then whole class activities

Increasing voice volume from a whisper to low volume to fully audible voice during any and all of the above activities as needed (Use a voice meter application on a smart phone or an analogue sound level meter for a fun, visual way to enable the child to observe her current voice volume; alternatively, create a pretend volume meter: 1= soft whisper, 2= loud whisper, 3= soft voice, 4= normal or medium voice, and 5= loud voice.)

Asking questions of therapist, teacher, peers, and other school staff through surveys (Example: Create with the child a short list of questions he will then ask other peers or adults; questions should be geared toward the child's interests—such as, "Do you like Superman or Batman better?" Votes can be tallied to see which category is the most popular.)

Making verbal requests for help (examples: asking for needed work materials, requesting to use the bathroom, sharing when feeling ill)

Reading aloud to therapist, then teacher, then small group (examples: answering questions about what individual words are on the page; reading or sounding out individual words, then phrases, then full sentences)

Speaking spontaneously during any school activity

Giving a short presentation or reading aloud in front of the whole class

Making verbal requests in other public settings such as stores or restaurants (examples: ordering food, purchasing a snack or soda)

Using basic social skills (examples: saying "hi," "goodbye," "thank you," "please")

Smiling and making eye contact while speaking

Using various facial expressions while speaking (examples: playing games in which the child makes a face and the therapist must guess the emotion—and vice versa; modeling and having the child make silly faces into the mirror)

Speaking without covering mouth with hands

Singing, dancing, and using gestures and movement during music (examples: "The Itsy Bitsy Spider," "Head, Shoulders, Knees, and Toes"), playing songs that have the child repeat back different letter or phoneme sound combinations (examples: "Fee Fi Fo Fum," "Do Re Mi")

Speaking in the presence of friends' parents during playdates, leaders or coaches of extracurricular activities, extended family members, and so on

Making phone or video calls (examples: calling to ask the time a store is open or other general requests; practicing talking to a relative or friend on the phone or via FaceTime or Skype; practicing basic social skills; leaving a voicemail message)

Allowing adults to record voice while singing, reading, or answering questions (Child then allows teacher, peers, therapist, and others to listen to the recording in the child's presence. To slowly increase the challenge, adjust the volume of the recording, the physical distance of the person listening, and the duration the recording plays.)

Case Example

An 8-year-old child in second grade presented with a longstanding history of SM. This child spoke individually to select peers, but had never spoken with his teachers. Speech was initially transferred from parent to therapist during fade-in sessions within the clinic, which took approximately three treatment sessions. Treatment was then transferred to the school, where stimulus fading was conducted to transfer speech from the therapist to the school counselor. These sessions initially took place in the school counselor's office, where she transitioned closer to the play between therapist and child and eventually established speech with the child. The school counselor received training in SM treatment from the therapist, which allowed her to practice exposures daily during school.

As a next step, this student practiced speech in the hallways of the school with his counselor, such as answering questions about the bulletin boards or playing games at a table in the hallway or in the lunchroom at a distance from peers. Practice then transitioned to adding one preferred peer to the game playing in a variety of locations, including the lunchroom, counselor's office, and hallways of the school. Over a number of sessions, peers the child spoke less to were integrated into the play. Eventually, the practice was moved to playing games on the carpet in the classroom with the school counselor, with the teacher at a large physical distance. First, peers were incorporated into the game one by one. As this child mastered speaking to peers in the classroom with the teacher at a distance, the teacher was moved closer and coached to use CDI skills during the play. After the child became accustomed to the teacher's presence, she transitioned to incorporating forced-choice questions. After a number of successful sessions answering teacher questions on the carpet, subsequent work involved the school counselor talking to the child at the child's desk in the classroom with peers nearby, followed by having the teacher approach and listen to these conversations while reflecting, describing, and praising the speech she heard, and eventually asking forced-choice and then open-ended questions. Throughout treatment, the therapist provided guidance through a variety of methods, including phone calls, video consults, and in-person observation and training.

Summary

SM is defined as a persistent failure to speak in specific social situations in which speaking is expected, despite speaking fluently in other situations. Effective intervention is critical, given the host of problems that typically develop, including interference with academic achievement and social problems such as peer rejection and difficulty making and maintaining friendships. Specific CBT techniques including stimulus fading, shaping, and contingency management, within the context of a graduated series of behavioral exposures, are the most effective strategies available in the treatment of SM and are supported by research.

The major goals of behavioral exposures for children with SM are to expand the variety of situations and conditions in which the child will speak, as well as increase the quality of that engagement (voice volume, elaboration, spontaneity, self-advocacy). Exposures should be designed creatively and flexibly throughout the therapy process, while taking into account parent and teacher input and observations of child responses. As a therapist, you must give careful consideration to the environmental context of exposure tasks (location, people present, and methods of interaction provided and requested) in order to successfully facilitate speech. The use of engaging and fun activities can greatly facilitate the ability to achieve speaking goals. Development of a collaborative treatment team, provision of psychoeducation, and transfer of responsibility for delivery of daily interventions over time to the treatment team are also crucial steps in this process. Finally, careful consideration must be given to the need for developmental modifications based on age and cognitive ability.

CHAPTER 12

Exposure for Generalized Anxiety Disorder

In this chapter, you will find information related to exposure treatment with children and adolescents who have generalized anxiety disorder (GAD). The information included in this chapter is intended to support clinicians in creating and implementing an exposure hierarchy that is tailored to each individual client. Ideas for exposure tasks and activities are provided for consideration in creating individualized hierarchies. Finally, case examples are used to illustrate the therapist's role in implementation of CBT skills and exposure tasks with real clients who experience GAD.

Clinical Presentation and Causal Factors

Children and adolescents with GAD exhibit excessive anxiety and worry about a number of events that may shift during the course of the disorder. These children are typically described by their parents as "little worriers" (Albano, Chorpita, & Barlow, 2003). They often exhibit anxieties that are adult-like, such as concerns about punctuality, health and safety of self and family members, catastrophic events such as hurricanes or war, and finances. They may also worry excessively about more typical child concerns, such as their academic, social, or athletic competence. For most children, these types of fears manifest as a passing thought, but for children diagnosed with GAD, the worry is frequent, feels uncontrollable, and involves catastrophic thinking (anticipating the worst). Children with this disorder may be overly conforming and exhibit perfectionistic thoughts and intense behavioral reactions. They are often self-conscious and seek excessive reassurance. These tendencies result in impairment in their performance because they cannot move on from a task without constant feedback assuring them that they are doing well (Kendall et al., 2004). Primary physical manifestations of GAD are restlessness and mental exhaustion. Other common somatic complaints include muscle tension, stomachaches and headaches, difficulty concentrating, irritability, and sleep disturbance (American Psychiatric Association, 2013).

GAD is present in approximately 1% of children ages 9 to 12 (Costello et al., 2005) and 2% to 3% of adolescents ages 13 to 18 (Merikangas et al., 2010). Age of onset for GAD tends to be in later adolescence as compared to separation anxiety and specific phobias, in which most cases emerge prior to age 12 (Beesdo et al., 2009). Anxiety symptoms occur with higher frequency and at an earlier age in girls than in boys (Lewinsohn et al., 1998). However, both boys and girls diagnosed with GAD present with similar frequency, intensity, and quality of symptoms (Masi et al., 2004). Researchers have demonstrated that there are few developmental differences in the symptomatic profile of children and adolescents with GAD (Masi et al., 1999). However, younger children (ages 7 to 11) have been found to report a higher need for reassurance, while older children (over the age of 11) are more likely to endorse brooding and a higher number of physiological symptoms (Kendall & Pimentel, 2003). Additionally, children ages 10 to 13 are most likely to exhibit fears related to physical danger and death (Weems & Costa, 2005).

The research on the etiology of GAD is relatively sparse; however, evidence that does exist suggests an interplay between biological, familial, and environmental factors contributing to the development and maintenance of this disorder (see reviews by Hudson & Rapee, 2004; Newman et al., 2013). Specific risk factors for GAD include behavioral inhibition, adverse life events, cognitive biases, and parenting factors (for example, ambivalent attachment in infancy and negative parenting behaviors such as low maternal warmth or high maternal rejection).

The symptoms of GAD tend to be chronic, with waxing and waning throughout the lifespan (American Psychiatric Association, 2013). Individuals who develop symptoms earlier in life tend to have higher rates of comorbidity. Common comorbid conditions in childhood include other anxiety disorders, such as specific phobia, social phobia, or separation anxiety disorder (Keeton, Kolos, & Walkup, 2009), as well as ADHD, depression, and oppositional defiant disorder. There also exists age variation in comorbid diagnoses. Younger children tend to have a comorbid diagnosis of ADHD or separation anxiety disorder, whereas older children are more likely to have a concurrent diagnosis of specific phobia or major depression (Brady & Kendall, 1992).

The cognitive features of children with GAD include an overall attitude of apprehension and uncontrollable worry. Uncontrollable worries tend to encompass general life themes such as the future, past events, and competence in areas including school, sports, and peer relationships. Common cognitive distortions among GAD youth include catastrophic or "what if" thinking (as in, *What if I get a bad test grade and I fail the course, and then I won't get into a good college or have a successful career*), overestimating the possibility of harmful outcomes (for example, *My parents haven't answered my text, so they must have been in a car accident*), exaggerating anticipated consequences to a disastrous degree (*If I let a goal get past me during today's game, my entire team will hate me*), and undervaluing their own capacity to cope in adverse situations (*I can't handle it*) (Albano et al., 2003). One other common negative thinking process among both GAD and socially anxious youth is the fear of negative evaluation or embarrassment as a result of poor performance. This leads to high levels of self-consciousness and leads to avoidance behaviors in social or performance situations (such as a party, school, or a sporting event).

Exposure Therapy for GAD

Research findings demonstrate strong support for exposure-based CBT as an effective treatment for childhood anxiety disorders, including GAD. Furthermore, GAD is one of the most common anxiety disorders of children who participated in randomized controlled trials (RCTs) of evidence-based CBT protocols for anxious youth. These protocols are used in the context of individual (e.g. Coping Cat program; Kendall & Hedtke, 2006, and The C.A.T. Project; Kendall, Choudhury, Hudson, & Webb, 2002), group (e.g. the Cool Kids program; Hudson et al., 2009) and family treatment (e.g. the Building Confidence program; Wood et al., 2008). In these treatment protocols, approximately half of the treatment sessions involve exposure tasks, highlighting the importance of this treatment component with anxious youth, including those with GAD.

Treatment modifications can be applied to exposure-based CBT protocols to target the core features of GAD (such as physiological distress and uncontrollable worry about various events and activities). Exposure tasks for children and adolescents with GAD may involve more imaginal exposures, as many worries involve scenarios in which in vivo exposures are not possible (for example, cancer, natural disaster, or harm to a loved one) (Grover, Hughes, Bergman, & Kingery, 2006). Additionally, since youth with GAD tend to have a variety of worries at any given time, exposure tasks often involve exposure to their internal worry thoughts through the creation of a worry tape recording, as described later in this chapter. Relaxation and cognitive restructuring are also important components of CBT work with GAD youth and tend to be used prior to or following an exposure task to help them gain competence in healthy coping strategies for challenging their anxiety. For a more thorough overview of these CBT strategies, please refer to chapter 4.

Clinically Relevant Factors

Ongoing clinical assessment must focus on a detailed understanding of the specific nature of the child's anxious condition in preparation for exposure therapy. As discussed in detail in chapter 2, the environmental context within which the behavior presents, and the specific nature of the child's cognitions and behavioral responses, are critical considerations in the subsequent engineering of effective exposure exercises. As follows, we present typical fear triggers or cues, feared consequences, and avoidance and safety behaviors commonly occurring in youth with GAD.

Fear Cues

Fear cues or triggers are specific environmental factors or variables that typically elicit the child's anxiety. These are the situations that activate the fear response due to the presence of specific stimuli that are perceived as dangerous or harmful in some way. The following fear cues commonly trigger anxiety in children with GAD:

Physiological sensations (examples: stomachaches, headaches, muscle tension) in anticipation of entering an anxiety-provoking situation, or when thinking about that situation

Novel situations that would trigger fear of something bad happening, or uncertainty that is intolerable (Mahoney & McEvoy, 2012)

Thinking about, talking about, or hearing others talk about an unfavorable outcome (examples: hearing a news report about weather or recent burglary, nightmares about being kidnapped)

An activity in which there is the potential for negative peer evaluation or perceived personal failure (examples: academic test, dance performance, taking a turn to bat on a baseball team)

An activity or situation that involves uncertainty or unpredictability (examples: change in daily routine, decision that must be made)

Feared Consequences

Feared consequences are those environmental conditions and outcomes that the child expects will result from exposure to the feared stimuli. That is, the child's fear is initiated and maintained through her experience or her belief that these negative outcomes will occur. The following are common feared consequences in children with GAD:

Failure or inability to perform perfectly in school or extracurricular activities

Negative evaluation by others with regard to performance situations (examples: teacher being mad, disappointing teammates and parents)

Making a wrong or imperfect decision

A diagnosis of a chronic or fatal medical condition of self or loved one (example: *I have a headache; it must be a brain tumor.*)

Danger or death of self or loved ones (burglary, chronic or fatal illness, car accident). For example, a child might worry that *something bad must have happened because my parent is not answering the phone* or he picks up on subtle cues of potential danger. (*The car sounds funny; I heard a noise in the house; my throat hurts.*)

Damage or destruction (example: losing home in a fire)

Embarrassment or judgment

Inability to tolerate uncertainty or control the outcome of a situation

Avoidance

Children with anxiety commonly avoid the environmental stimuli and situations that trigger their anxiety because they perceive a high likelihood of their feared consequences occurring. The following are common avoidant behaviors observed in children with GAD:

Refusal to participate in situations predicted to be catastrophic. Examples might include avoiding school on days when there is a substitute teacher, not raising hand in class to answer a question unless 100% certain of the correct answer, refusal to try a new sport or after-school activity due to self-doubt about ability.

Use of somatic complaints to avoid tests or other evaluative activities (examples: baseball game, performance in school play).

Engaging in an all-or-nothing approach to completing an assignment. If they lack confidence in their ability to complete the assignment perfectly, they may avoid the assignment completely rather than tolerate the "bad" or good-enough grade.

Avoiding making decisions, or attempting to have someone else make the decision for them (examples: ordering food at a restaurant, picking an item from a store, deciding what activity to do with their friends).

Safety Behaviors

Children and adolescents with anxiety often rely on specific objects, individuals, or actions that they believe will protect them from the feared stimuli or feared outcome. Safety behaviors are any actions they perform in an attempt to feel safe. The following are common safety behaviors displayed by children with GAD:

Seeking constant reassurance from parents or other adults that nothing catastrophic will happen, prior to entering an uncertain situation or completing a task. For example, a child might ask a parent repeatedly if all the doors are locked before heading to bed, or if his homework assignment is completely accurate before being able to complete the task

Asking excessive questions about adult concerns—such as family finances, family relationships, and world or community events like war, terrorism, or political issues

Engaging in safety behaviors that involve frequent or excessive checking or information gathering. Examples include searching the Internet regarding car or plane safety, weather, or world events. For school worries, this presents as checking homework excessively for errors

Frequent visits to the school nurse, scheduling doctor visits more than is necessary, or engaging in excessive health care behaviors (examples: asking for medicine frequently when not needed, going to nurse to get temperature checked)

The need to make a schedule and follow that schedule exactly as it's written so as not to trigger anxiety around unknown future events

Using distraction in an attempt to cope during anticipation of, or experience with, the feared situation (examples: averting one's gaze from the feared stimuli, engaging in activities such as listening to music or playing an electronic game, or using relaxation skills to avoid facing the fear or situation in the moment)

Tailoring Exposure Therapy for Generalized Anxiety Disorder

This section is designed to serve as a primer for the implementation of exposure therapy specifically for children and adolescents with GAD. It builds on guidance presented in earlier chapters by offering the therapist specific guidelines for what must be uniquely considered when carrying out this work with GAD youth. That is, additional strategies and modifications to the treatment approach will be discussed that are of paramount importance to implementing exposure-based work with this group.

Exposure sessions for GAD must target specific fears and worries, but also the internal experience of excessive and uncontrollable worry. In order to design an effective exposure hierarchy, the therapist must conduct a functional analysis of the specific nature of the child's fear or worry. It is also important to evaluate the extent to which parental accommodation of the client's avoidance and use of safety behaviors maintains her anxiety. In an effort to be helpful and reduce their child's anxiety, parents allow children to avoid difficult tasks or situations (such as novel situations, school on the day a test is being returned, or hospitals). They also inadvertently rein-force the use of safety behaviors (for example, responding to excessive texting or phone calls, making decisions on their child's behalf, allowing excessive information seeking), which results in limiting the child's opportunity to develop age-appropriate independence. Parents will likely require guidance and skills training to decrease their accommodation of avoidance and safety behaviors. Other adaptations to expo-sure work for children and adolescents with GAD include imaginal exposures to worry-provoking situations and exposure to their internal worry loop of multiple, co-occurring worries.

Development of the Fear Hierarchy

Fear hierarchies for GAD youth must be tailored specifically to the child or ado-lescent. Many of the worries and fears that exist among GAD youth are difficult to treat with in vivo exposure tasks (for example, death or illness of a family member, being in a natural disaster, or local violence). When developing the fear hierarchy for these cases, imaginal or role-play exposures should be the primary focus. A 9-year-old boy who presented to our clinic with a fear of tornados put the following imaginary and role-play exposure tasks on his hierarchy: create a few different scripts of the tornado story from least to most fearful outcomes (for example, losing power, destruc-tion of home, harm to self or family members); imagine and role-play the tornado stories with therapist; imagine and role-play the tornado stories with family members; and listen to an audio recording of the tornado stories in between sessions. As another example, we worked with a 15-year-old girl who presented to our clinic with a fear of getting cancer, dying young, and missing out on many future life experiences. Her hierarchy had several imaginal and role-play exposures that included creating two different worst-case scenario scripts, each with one of her two feared outcomes: getting cancer and dying young. Rather than suppressing the feared emotional expe-rience, the exposures allowed her to sit with and practice tolerating emotion related to her fear. She then created a recording of each of these scripts and listened to them as part of her assigned homework.

Another important consideration when constructing a hierarchy with GAD youth is their often excessive and uncontrollable worry about a wide range of life events. In these instances, we have a few recommendations. First, it may be necessary to have the child construct more than one hierarchy, each with a separate worry theme (making decisions, health concerns, failure, novel people/situations). Another approach is to have clients rank the level of distress they experience around each of their worries and to start exposure work with the hierarchy of the worry that causes the most impairment. For some of our clients we recommend doing one hierarchy with exposure tasks that target multiple fears and worries. For example, an 8-year-old boy presented to our clinic with a fear of getting injured and a fear of failure. These fears impaired his academic functioning as well as his participation on his baseball team. We created one exposure hierarchy with tasks that addressed both his fear of failure and his fear of getting injured. Exposures started with doing an imaginal exposure to: *What if I get injured when I'm up at bat?* He read his imaginal exposure script each day until he habituated to and became bored by reading the script. In vivo exposures included playing baseball during therapy sessions, as well as going to the batting cage with his father on the weekends. There were also planned exposures for the number of times he would go up to bat at his practices. Completion of these exposure tasks helped this client to develop a higher tolerance for making mistakes during games and practices, as well as lower levels of anxiety around getting injured.

Frequency, Duration, and Length of Sessions

Factors such as frequency of exposures, duration of treatment, and length of sessions vary considerably depending upon the severity of symptom impairment. However, the typical treatment length for GAD is 10 to 16 weekly sessions (Keeton et al., 2009) followed by a gradual reduction in treatment frequency (for example, every other week followed by monthly) to monitor symptom reduction and implement relapse prevention strategies. For GAD youth, the first 5 to 8 sessions are typically focused on developing the fear hierarchy as well as introducing and practicing coping skills (such as relaxation, thought challenging, and replacement thinking) that will be useful prior to, during, or following exposure tasks. While weekly sessions are generally recommended for conducting the exposure work, it may be useful to have an individual exposure therapy session for the child as well as a parent-only session in the same week. This would be particularly helpful when exposure work is focused on flexibility or novel situations and the parent may require a more in-depth meeting to discuss her role in these exposures (for example, how to set limits on reassurance seeking in novel situations, or steps for implementing exposure involving changing up the child's routine). It is also an option to extend the weekly session in length in order to conduct the individual and parent session at the same time.

Cognitive Considerations

Therapeutic techniques that target the cognitive component of GAD will be of particular importance in the overall treatment of this disorder. As stated above, cognitive distortions that are most common among children and adolescents with GAD include: 1) catastrophic or "what if" thinking, 2) overestimating the possibility of harmful outcomes, 3) exaggerating anticipated consequences to a disastrous degree, and 4) undervaluing one's capacity to cope in adverse situations. Relatedly, children may hold mistaken beliefs regarding the value of their worry, including that worry helps motivate them, prevents bad things from happening, helps them solve problems, and protects them from their negative feelings. These misinterpretations should be addressed through cognitive restructuring work (detective thinking) as described in chapter 4, with the goal of helping the child build confidence in letting go of his worry, expecting more realistic or likely outcomes and an ability to manage those outcomes, and holding a more adaptive perspective when evaluating the actual threat in a situation.

Further, many exposures for GAD allow children to disconfirm the belief that worry benefits them by experimenting with a reduction in safety behaviors (such as excessive checking, redoing, list making, reassurance seeking, information seeking, and so on) and assessing the outcomes of those reductions. In most cases, children will realize that the worry did not vastly improve the situation or change the typical outcome, and that, in many cases, it caused additional problems (such as added stress and somatic complaints).

Additional therapeutic tools that are useful in reducing the level of distress caused by negative thinking patterns and uncontrollable worry include metacognitive therapy, daily worry time, and audio recordings of the worry loop. The application of these tools will lead to a reduction in avoidance and, in turn, facilitate increased compliance with exposure tasks.

METACOGNITIVE THERAPY (MCT)

Metacognitive therapy (MCT) focuses on teaching clients to identify more effective ways of responding to thoughts that trigger worry, in order to establish a sense of management over worry. Current research is focusing on adapting MCT to children and adolescents, including those with GAD (Esbjørn, Normann, & Reinholdt-Dunne, 2015; Ellis and Hudson, 2010). We strongly recommend that you refer to *Metacognitive Therapy for Anxiety and Depression* (Wells, 2009) prior to implementing any of the MCT strategies described below.

Detached mindfulness is an example of an MCT technique utilized with GAD youth. It involves becoming an objective observer of one's thoughts as opposed to analyzing or judging them. An example of this technique is the cloud image task, which involves the use of imagery to respond to a thought (Wells, 2009). During this task, the child is asked to identify a recent anxious thought. The thought would likely be one of her "what if" catastrophic thought statements. The child is then asked to imagine the thoughts typed out on clouds that are just passing through the sky and allow the clouds to be in that space, as it is impossible and unnecessary to push the clouds away or change their movements (Zucker, 2011). In detached mindfulness the thought is not changed, but rather it is observed as just a thought. Therapy homework involves spontaneous practice of this technique as anxious thoughts pop up throughout each day. This strategy will be particularly helpful to your client when she is working on delaying her worries until her scheduled worry time (described below). In summary, MCT techniques help youth with GAD become less reactive to their worries, regardless of their validity.

SCHEDULED WORRY TIME

Scheduled worry time is a therapeutic technique used to set limits on the constant, repetitive, and unproductive worries associated with GAD. It is also useful in the reduction of reassurance-seeking behavior. This task involves having the client set aside 10 to 15 minutes each day to write down or have a discussion with a parent about the worries that came to mind throughout that day. The goal is to teach the client to delay a worry that comes up earlier in the day until worry time. When a worry occurs outside of worry time, clients are instructed to either write down the worry and save it for worry time or practice a self-talk statement such as: *My anxiety is causing me to worry, but I will delay giving this worry any more attention until worry time later today.*

Younger children may benefit from a more tangible, physical reminder, such as a "worry box." This involves writing down worries throughout the day and placing them in the box, with the plan to open the box and review each worry with their parents during the scheduled worry time. Parents can support children in using this strategy by prompting them to write the worries down, reminding them of their coping self-talk statements, and making sure to incorporate daily worry time into their child's routine. Therapists should coach parents on how to handle their child expressing a worry outside of worry time. For example, parents might be encouraged to use statements such as, "That's something we can discuss during worry time, but we are not going to give that worry attention right now. Feel free to write down those worries so we can review them during worry time," or "That's just a worry, so let's save it for worry time."

Worry time sets limits on the amount of time and energy that is spent worrying each day, and eventually the habit of worrying starts to diminish in intensity and frequency. An added benefit is that children may discover that what they worried about earlier in the day (for example, running a few minutes late to school) is no longer an issue by the end of the day. Additionally, it allows for the process of worry to occur at more convenient times. For many children it is helpful to schedule worry time after school but at least a couple of hours before bedtime, so as not to interfere with their sleep routine. It's also encouraged to spend time focusing on worries while at home rather than at school, where children need to focus.

USE OF WORRY TAPES

Creating an audio recording that contains a sampling of worry thoughts is another strategy that can be helpful to children and adolescents with GAD. This form of exposure helps the child to habituate to hearing his worries or feared consequence and, in turn, feel less emotionally reactive when he notices this internal dialogue in the future. It also helps him to externalize the worries by hearing them outside of his own mind. The creation of the audio recording takes place in the therapist's office. It is helpful if the child has access to a smartphone or recording device. The child uses his voice to record the list or repeated loop of his worry thoughts (for example: *What if I don't know the answer? What if my friends laugh at me? What if my face gets red?*). He is then assigned homework, which is to listen to the recording for a prolonged period of time daily (about 10 to 15 minutes), until the recording no longer triggers an anxious reaction.

Family Education and Support

Family members, especially parents and caregivers, play an important role in exposure therapy for youth with GAD. Parents of GAD youth typically require education about avoidance, the importance of modeling healthy and nonavoidant coping strategies, and specific parenting behaviors, such as overprotection and accommodation, that exacerbate anxiety. It is also useful to educate parents about the challenges that may arise when doing exposures with their child outside of the clinic. It is often helpful for the therapist to model an exposure task in the session with the caregiver present so that she develops more competence in implementing the exposure task at home. Parents often want to protect their children and struggle to tolerate seeing them in an anxious state, especially when children exhibit more extreme externalizing behaviors (such as tantrums, anger outbursts, or refusal). They require support and guidance in order to understand that they are not harming their child by setting limits on reassurance seeking or supporting a reduction in avoidance behaviors. Further, it is important to communicate that reducing their accommodation sends an important message to their children regarding their confidence in the children's abilities to handle various life situations without the influence of anxiety. See chapter 4 for a detailed description of parental involvement in exposure.

ADDRESSING REASSURANCE SEEKING

Youth with GAD engage in an excessive amount of reassurance seeking from their parents as well as other family members. Therefore, exposure tasks that set limits on the frequency and quantity of reassurance provided are imperative. Parents should be educated and given skills to avoid giving responses such as, "It's all going to be okay," or "Everything is fine." Instead, parents should encourage children to seek their own answers through the use of cognitive techniques such as detective thinking. Another strategy we recommend to parents for setting limits on reassurance seeking involves having the child record his own thought challenge questions and statements for his worries in a journal. Each time the child has a worry, he would write it down along with his challenges for that worry. Then, when a worry arises, the parent can set limits on the anxiety by saying, "We have already answered this question, but you can check your journal if you're still feeling worried."

Exposure Tasks and Activities Guide

Below, we present a wide list of activities and ideas as a guide for clinicians' use in generating useful and creative tasks for a client's exposure hierarchy. The activities and tasks listed can be used in the context of targeting a variety of goals related to the multiple types of worries that encompass GAD. While some sections may be loosely organized according to an increasing level of difficulty, they are not meant to be utilized in sequence. Rather, the therapist should always use clinical judgment and parent and child input in determining the most effective next steps in any series of exposures and should strive to tailor tasks to the individual needs of each child. Some of the below exposures were adapted from the following sources: Abramowitz et al., 2011; Kendall et al., 2005; Peterman et al., 2015; Spencer, Dupont, & Dupont, 2003; Whitton, Luiselli, & Donaldson, 2006.

HEALTH (SELF AND OTHERS)

Audio/Visual Exposures

Read a developmentally appropriate book or article about the feared disease.

Conduct an Internet search regarding the facts of a given illness and correct misassumptions (regarding the prevalence rate, causal factors, symptoms, outcomes, and treatments for managing the condition, for example).

View pictures of individuals with the specific illness of concern. The child may need to start with less graphic pictures and work up to those that may be more distressing.

Listen to a worry loop with statements such as *I always could get cancer,* to address intolerance of uncertainty.

Imaginal/Role-Play Exposures

Conduct a *"What would happen if…"* role-play. For a child who fears that her mother will get cancer, the child and therapist would act out everything that would happen from beginning to end in this situation—including how she would feel, what she would be told when she receives the news, the changes that would occur in the family's daily routine, what her mother would look like as she went through chemotherapy, and so on.

Create and repeatedly read a written script about the child or a family member acquiring the feared disease. The child may require steps in this process that start with discussing aspects of having the illness and eventually lead to listening to a whole script from start to finish.

Imagine having symptoms of the illness (nausea, faintness, stomach pain, headache, and so on).

In Vivo Exposures

Sit in the waiting room of a doctor's office where people are sneezing and coughing.

Walk around a hospital, starting with sitting in the waiting areas and working up to walking up and down the halls of different floors of patients with varying levels of health conditions.

Conduct interoceptive exposures for feared physiological symptoms. (See chapter 7 for review of interoceptive exposure techniques.)

Reducing Safety Behaviors and Avoidance

Attend doctor visits only according to doctors' recommendations and exceptions that are determined by parents and doctor (examples: a fever that lasts for more than a couple of days, a broken bone, excessive vomiting, a scheduled yearly exam).

Attend after-school activities even when somatic complaints (such as stomachaches and headaches) are present.

Develop a plan parents can use for responding to somatic complaints (such as stomachaches and headaches). For example, they could use a simple prompt such as "Use your coping skills," followed by active ignoring.

Schedule periods of parent-child time that are not contingent on child's reports of distress, to avoid inadvertent reinforcement of stomachaches at bedtime.

Ask medical professional questions about an illness (for a child who is avoiding the topic).

For adolescents who take health class as part of their school curriculum, have them remain in class to learn about the feared topic rather than allowing them to miss that lesson.

Refrain from looking up symptoms online (when excessive information seeking is involved).

Reduce avoidance of people who may be sick, places where there may be sick people, touching surfaces in public places, and so on.

MAKING MISTAKES/FAILURE

Audio/Visual Exposures

Watch video clips of others making mistakes, starting with more mild mistakes and moving to more embarrassing ones.

Imaginal/Role-Play Exposures

Imagine making a mistake and tell the story of what would happen. Possible situations might include forgetting uniform on gym day, forgetting a book or assignment, or turning in homework without parents checking it.

Imagine failure in a given situation. Possible situations might include not getting a part in the school play, earning a D on a test, receiving critical feedback on a project, or being called to the principal's office.

Practice giving an oral presentation and pretend it is taking place in front of a class. Purposefully make several mistakes (for example, state a fact incorrectly or skip a word). Imagine peers chuckling, sleeping, or other related fear.

Therapist and child act out making mistakes in a performance situation (examples: striking out during a baseball game, messing up lines in school play, playing a couple of wrong notes during music recital). Use of props (such as baseball bat and glove, musical instrument, play script) would be helpful in creating a more reality-based scenario.

In Vivo Exposures

Do "silly" things (examples: wear a mismatched outfit to walk around the shopping mall, trip while walking up the steps at school).

Create drawings without erasing (use pen or marker).

Turn in an essay without first checking it for mistakes, or intentionally leave several spelling mistakes. (We suggest this task only for smaller-scale assignments that will not grossly impact the overall grade in the class.)

Do something minor to get in trouble (this type of exposure would be for children who are eager to please others).

Practice making a mistake in session (examples: Draw an object, perform math calculations, or state something incorrectly).

Make a purposeful mistake on a homework assignment (examples: don't cross "t" or dot "i," make a spelling or grammar mistake, skip a question on a worksheet) and turn it in to the teacher.

Pay for something with slightly less than the correct amount of money. Start with a friendly clerk and then move on to a less friendly clerk.

Give child a "fake" test in session and mark the test with negative comments (example: *Needs more details*) and Xs.

Raise hand in class to answer a question following these steps: 1) Raise hand to answer a question when there is a high probability (but not 100%) she will answer it correctly; 2) Raise hand when there is only a 50/50 likelihood of answering it correctly; 3) Raise hand to answer a question when there is a high probability of answering it incorrectly.

Write a letter or note with the child's nonpreferred hand and give it to another person without explaining the sloppy writing.

Give the child a difficult task, such as a test on something he has not yet learned, or a writing task with an impossible time limit.

Reducing Safety Behaviors and Avoidance

Identify situations in which a client unreasonably blames herself and have her refrain from apologizing (examples: standing too close to someone else, using a slightly angry tone of voice, bumping into someone else but so softly that it is barely noticeable).

Have parents refrain from answering their child when asked repeatedly, "Are you mad at me?"

Gradually reduce reassurance-seeking questions during homework completion. Begin by setting a limit on the number of questions that can be asked during assignment completion; work toward turning in homework without having parents check it the night before.

Assist adolescent in studying for a test or writing a paper without over-preparation. For example, gradually decrease the number of times he rewrites the same notecard, or reread and review an essay only once before turning it in to the teacher.

Have the child check her homework for completion only one time, or pack her backpack without checking again that all items are there in the morning.

Deny child's request to stay home from school due to not finishing all of the work that is due that day.

(Please refer to chapter 13 for additional ideas on exposures related to mistakes and fear of failure.)

SAFETY/DEATH (SELF AND OTHERS)

Audio/Visual Exposures

Talk about the word *death* and the thoughts and feelings that come up for the child when this word is mentioned—including how he envisions death (going to heaven, being put into the ground, and so on).

Write the word *death* on a dry-erase board and have the child stare at it for prolonged periods of time.

Read books and look at pictures of people from earlier time periods who have passed away.

Read an age-appropriate book about the topic of death.

Watch an age-appropriate TV show or movie about the topic of death. (It could also be a movie or TV show that has a scene in which the characters' safety is at risk and the child is avoiding the scene due to having an anxious reaction when she first watched it.)

Create and listen to a worry loop tape with statements such as "My parents could get into a car accident and die," to address distress around uncertainty.

Imaginal/Role-Play Exposures

Imagine various scenarios using a written script or audio recording of how one might die, including the impact on family and friends (examples: sudden accident, chronic illness, cancer, kidnapping).

Conduct a *"What would happen if…"* role-play around self or others dying. For a child who fears her parents dying in a car accident, the therapist and child would act out all aspects of this scenario including the child's affective experience, who would take care of her, where she would live, what would happen to her parents after they died, and what would happen to her brother and sister.

In Vivo Exposures

Walk around the outside of the house at night in the dark (only in safe areas).

Go into a part of the house (example: basement) in which there is a worry (such as fear that a burglar or kidnapper is hiding), stay in that location, and gradually increase amount of time the child remains there alone.

Walk around a public location where the child is exposed to a lot of strangers (example: shopping mall) and stand in close proximity to a stranger who the child labels as suspicious (with parents or therapist present).

Arrange with parents to not answer the phone when the child calls them to be picked up at the end of a therapy session. Parent would call the child back after 5 to 10 minutes.

Reducing Safety Behaviors and Avoidance

Gradually reduce parental overprotective behaviors and set limits on reassurance seeking. (Examples: limit responses to child's questions about whether a situation will be safe and have the child answer his own questions; give child reasons to enter feared locations in the home, such as bringing up laundry from the basement.)

Gradually reduce the number of texts or calls parents will respond to from the child. Different situations might warrant different limits.

Go into a room in the house and refrain from checking closets and corners to guarantee safety.

Spend time at a cemetery, or go to an antique store and touch old clothing.

Gradually reduce checking behaviors (such as checking the locks at night).

FLEXIBILITY

Imaginal/Role-Play Exposures

Create a written story and imagine some part of the child's day unexpectedly not going as planned.

Imagine staying calm instead of yelling or crying during a trigger situation (examples: sibling not playing by the rules of a game; friend doesn't want to play during recess; there is not enough time to finish a routine or complete steps in the preferred order).

In Vivo Exposures

Play a board game in which the therapist changes the rules in the middle of the game; also practice at home, first with family members and then with friends.

Break or bend minor rules at school (examples: calling out in class, coming into class a couple of minutes late, having one unexcused absence).

Ask the parent to be late when picking the child up from the therapy session: first anticipated, then unanticipated, and vary the duration.

Read only a portion of a book, or stop reading mid-way.

Switch up a part of the daily routine. For example, randomly assign family members to sit at different spots at the dinner table than is usual, have the child sit in a different spot in the car, take a different route to school, or have something different packed for lunch.

Assign a preplanned time the child is aware of in which there will be a "surprise" activity in the schedule. Start with pleasant activities, such as going out for ice cream or going to the movies, and move to more ordinary activities, such as running errands or picking sibling up at practice.

Watch a TV show and parent says ahead of time that she is going to pause the show at some point but the child will not know when.

Ask parent to make a plan for an activity that the child is aware of and then change it 15 minutes prior to the start of the activity. (Use a believable reason.)

Go to the mall, shop alone, or meet at a time and place that is not nailed down beforehand (example: text once at the mall to figure out the plans). This task is most appropriate for adolescents.

Have parent ask child to get in the car and start driving without a destination.

Conduct a "mystery exposure" during which a roll of the dice determines what the task for the session will be.

Reducing Safety Behaviors and Avoidance

Use reward programs to reinforce "go with the flow" or flexible behaviors (examples: calmly handling a schedule change, shifting from an enjoyable activity to a boring task without becoming argumentative, attending an activity the child is not excited about without resistance).

Have parent gradually reduce number of questions the child can ask prior to an event or activity, to encourage more of a "surprise" element (examples:

"Who is picking me up?" "What time will you be there?" "We are going to do that today, right?").

Reduce child's attempts to recheck instructions of a game, and play the game with the uncertainty of whether he is playing by the exact rules.

NOVEL SITUATION/ANTICIPATION

Imaginal/Role-Play Exposures

Imagine, or write a story about, what would happen in an anticipated situation (examples: applying to colleges across the country and possibly abroad, taking a driving test, going on a date or to a party, joining a new club or sports team, starting a new summer camp).

Imagine, or write a story about, the worst-case scenarios that could occur in an anticipated situation.

Role-play any situation around which there is anticipatory anxiety. The therapist plays the role of the child while the child plays the other person in the role-play (coach, peer, teacher) to model an appropriate way of managing anxiety in the situation, and then the roles are reversed.

In Vivo Exposures

Break attendance at an activity into small, manageable steps. For example, stand outside of the activity, observe the activity with parent from a distance, observe the activity with parent up close, participate in 5 minutes of the activity, participate in 10 minutes of the activity, and so on.

Have parent move farther away while child engages in the novel activity to increase exposure difficulty. For example, when dropping off the child at an activity, the parent would stay for an identified period of time and gradually reduce the length until the child immediately leaves the car to attend the activity independently.

Increase independence in completion of novel daily living activities. (For younger children: chores, making their own snack, inviting friend for playdate. For adolescents: walking home from school instead of parent picking them up, walking to a local restaurant with friends after school, or walking around the mall without parents.)

Start a conversation with a new person at school. Start with someone who is only mildly anxiety provoking and work toward speaking to an identified person labeled by the client as more difficult to talk to (example: adults versus same-age peers, nice versus mean teacher).

Participate in a class discussion and share an idea or opinion that differs from other ideas or opinions being offered. This exposure could also be done in novel settings, such as with an unfamiliar group of peers at a party or youth group event.

Go to a store the adolescent has never been to and have her go in by herself to make a purchase.

Join or start a club at school.

Do at least one, but ideally several, overnight visit at colleges (first local then out-of-state) the adolescent is interested in attending, during the spring and summer prior to their start date. For adolescents with GAD, the uncertainty and novelty involved in going away to college can be overwhelming, so these visits can help them feel more confident in being able to tolerate this new situation.

Reducing Safety Behaviors or Avoidance

Have parents set limits on the number of reassurance-seeking questions (such as "What is going to happen?") their child can ask about a new activity.

Limit text messages, phone calls, or other communication with the child or adolescent while he is in the novel situation, and graduate to the child attending the event in its entirety without contacting the parent.

Encourage independence with completion of tasks in the daily routine and not relying on or asking parents for help.

Reduce over-preparation for an event (examples: reviewing things to bring multiple times, checking and rechecking clothing and accessories).

Reduce excessive information seeking about the event or activity to increase certainty. (In contrast, if child is avoiding thinking about the event, you would encourage some reasonable information seeking.)

DECISION-MAKING

Imaginal/Role-Play Exposure

Do a "*What would happen…*" exposure around making the "wrong" decision. For example, a high school student imagines the worst-case scenario around picking the wrong college to attend.

In Vivo Exposures

Make a decision by flipping a coin and don't reverse it (example: which sports practice to attend if they fall on the same night and there is no preference expressed).

Make a minor decision within a specified time frame (example: a few minutes) and don't undo the decision.

Refrain from weighing pros and cons for a lengthy period of time before making a decision. Use self-talk statement such as, *I need to make a decision that is okay, not perfect.*

Make a more major decision (examples: which sleepaway camp to attend) within a specified but reasonable time frame to set limits on over-thinking and the number of parent-child discussions on this topic.

Have parent set up various small scenarios to practice quick decision-making outside of the session (examples: what color marker would you like, which dessert, what time to start an activity). Have parents set expectations and encourage child to make the decision within a specified time frame. (Use of a timer may be fun and helpful.)

Make decisions on a plan when hanging out with friends, rather than just allowing the friends to make all the decisions (examples: pick the movie or restaurant; suggest games to play or craft projects to work on).

Reduce Safety Behaviors/Avoidance

Instruct parents and other family members and peers to refrain from "rescuing" the child when she is struggling to make a decision.

Have adolescent refrain from making extensive lists of pros and cons for smaller or minor decisions.

Have youth refrain from reassessing his decision immediately after making it (example: deciding the other option would have been better).

WORLD EVENTS AND NATURAL DISASTERS

There will be wide variation among worries in this category. Examples include hurricanes, earthquakes, tornados, school shootings, and acts of terrorism. Refer to chapter 10 for additional exposure ideas.

Audio/Visual Exposure

Use the Internet to find news stories that relate to an anxiety-provoking topic; have client share her feelings about the stories and talk about the likely conclusions of each news story, as well as possible perceptions of the story.

Imaginal/Role-Play Exposure

Describe the feared situation in detail and create an imaginal exposure script. This type of exposure would be particularly helpful for natural disasters that are not likely to be experienced in the location in which the child resides (examples: earthquake, hurricane). A more difficult exposure might be imagining a natural disaster with a greater likelihood of occurring where the child resides.

Reduce Safety Behaviors/Avoidance

Parents use the resources they have available to them (parents of child's friends, police, local public health department) to determine reasonable versus unreasonable risk and together with the child, assess whether avoidance is warranted. For example, it would be a reasonable risk to go back to a shopping mall a couple of weeks after an isolated shooting incident.

Parents reduce responses to worry questions by encouraging the child or adolescent to answer his own questions once parents have already provided an answer.

Case Example

A very bright 10-year-old girl presented to treatment for anxiety related to academic performance and low self-esteem. She struggled to complete schoolwork, homework, and tests. Both her teachers and parents reported it was taking her excessive amounts of time to complete assignments. Oftentimes, she would avoid completing the work or leave certain parts of an assignment blank so that she did not risk answering something incorrectly or doing it imperfectly. This child experienced constant self-doubt and was hypersensitive to any form of corrective feedback from parents, teachers, or peers. She feared disappointing others, as well as any form of rejection.

Her safety behaviors involved seeking constant reassurance from parents and teachers. She asked frequent questions of her parents, such as "Are you mad at me?" or "Does this sound good?" The reassurance seeking delayed her bedtime as she would stay up late asking her parents questions and experiencing anxiety when they attempted to leave her room. Other safety behaviors included double- and triple-checking of her work, excessive erasing and rewriting, and rereading of words and sentences to ensure perfection. She avoided taking risks both in her academic performance and in other extracurricular activities. In school, she started to read books that were below her reading level and in gymnastics she avoided working on a back handspring because of fears of failure.

The first five sessions focused on identifying and challenging cognitive distortions around failure and embarrassment. We worked on developing self-talk notecards with helpful statements that challenged her cognitive distortions and addressed self-doubt as well as difficulty tolerating criticism. Additionally, a relaxation routine and worry journal was implemented to address nighttime anxiety.

Exposure work started with addressing the homework routine. Her school homework was used for in vivo exposures. The homework assignments that were the least anxiety provoking were identified as the starting point for exposures (math problems followed by writing assignments). The exposures followed this order: 1) working on an assignment for unlimited time with an unlimited amount of reassurance-seeking questions, 2) working on an assignment for unlimited time with a limited number of reassurance-seeking questions (gradual reduction of questions), 3) working on an assignment for limited time (according to teacher's guidelines) with limited questions, 4) working on an assignment for limited time with questions only once the assignment was completed. Additional exposures with homework involved purposefully turning in imperfect homework assignments to the teacher (leaving a question or problem blank, writing less, or making a grammar or spelling mistake), turning in an assignment after the deadline, and reading without rereading.

This client was initially resistant to the exposure work. Not only did she express reluctance around in vivo exposures, she also exhibited significant distress with discussing her anxiety symptoms (anxious thoughts and somatic symptoms). To increase motivation and treatment compliance, a reward program was introduced in which she could earn points for participation in the therapy session, practicing coping strategies in between therapy sessions, and completing imaginary and in vivo exposures. Additionally, this child's parents met with her teachers and developed some temporary accommodations around work completion both inside and outside of school. Knowing that her teachers were on board with her treatment plan and having the reward system in place resulted in an increased willingness to engage in the treatment process and start to complete exposures.

The exposure work transitioned from homework to addressing this child's avoidance of hobbies she previously enjoyed, such as knitting, soccer, and reading. Books that were at her reading level were gradually reintroduced, and she eventually started to read more quickly and spend more time engaging in this hobby. Additionally, she started to write stories and joined a children's knitting club. Throughout the treatment process, the child and her parents were assigned homework in between sessions to continue to practice exposures that had been successfully completed in the session that week. The client attended weekly sessions for 5 months, followed by twice a month for 2 months and then once a month for 3 months, to encourage maintenance of treatment effects and relapse prevention.

Conclusion

This chapter reviewed the diagnostic information, key treatment considerations, and implementation of exposure tasks for children and adolescents with generalized anxiety disorder. Research findings demonstrate strong support for exposure-based CBT as an effective treatment for childhood GAD. Exposure sessions for GAD must target specific fears and worries, but also the internal experience of excessive and uncontrollable worry. In addition to situational exposures, exposures to internal worry thoughts are conducted through the creation of worry tape recordings. Samples of specific exposure tasks were provided for consideration in creating individualized exposure hierarchies with clients. Finally, a case example was used to illustrate the clinician's role in implementing general CBT skills and exposure tasks with real clients experiencing GAD.

CHAPTER 13

Exposure for Social Phobia

In this chapter, you will find information related to exposure treatment with children and adolescents who have social anxiety disorder, also referred to as social phobia (SoP). The information included in this chapter is intended to support clinicians in creating and implementing an exposure hierarchy that is tailored to each individual client. Ideas for exposure tasks and activities are provided for consideration in creating individualized hierarchies. Finally, a case example is used to illustrate the clinician's role in the implementation of CBT skills and exposure tasks with real clients who experience SoP.

Clinical Presentation and Causal Factors

Social anxiety disorder is characterized in the *DSM-5* (American Psychiatric Association, 2013) as excessive fear or anxiety about one or more social situations in which the child or adolescent is exposed to possible observation or scrutiny by others and fears acting in a way that leads to negative evaluation by others (either stemming from his own behavior or from showing physiological anxiety symptoms). Feared negative evaluation typically includes embarrassment, humiliation, rejection, or offending others. For youth to meet *DSM-5* criteria for social anxiety disorder, the anxiety must be present in situations involving peer interactions, in addition to adult interactions. These feared social situations are typically avoided or endured with intense anxiety. Crying, clinging, tantrums, freezing, shrinking, or failing to speak in social situations are behavioral expressions of anxiety in socially anxious youth. Physical symptoms such as stomachaches, headaches, trembling, blushing, and even panic attacks are often present for youth with social anxiety. It should also be noted that the fear and anxiety experienced in these situations is considered to be disproportionate to the actual threat that exists.

Social anxiety disorder is associated with impairment in academic and interpersonal functioning, with higher numbers of social fears being indicative of higher levels of detrimental impact if left untreated (Beidel, Ferrell, Alfano, & Yeganeh, 2001). In some cases, social anxiety results in such severe amounts of distress for the child or adolescent that it leads to school refusal. Unlike children with externalizing disorders, socially anxious children have a strong desire to attend school but their anxiety causes them to feel paralyzed and unable to attend.

The age of onset for SoP is late childhood into early adolescence (Beesdo et al., 2007; Beesdo et al., 2009) with a lifetime prevalence rate of approximately 7% to 9% (American Psychiatric Association, 2013; Burstein et al., 2011; Merikangas et al., 2010). The best predictor of recovery is a later age of onset, as the development of social fears prior to age 11 predicts non-recovery in adulthood (Davidson, Hughes, George, & Blazer, 1993). High levels of comorbidity exist between SoP and other specific anxiety disorders (such as specific phobia, agoraphobia, panic disorder, separation anxiety disorder, GAD, and PTSD), as well as oppositional defiant disorder (ODD), depression, and, in adolescence and adulthood, substance abuse disorders (Ruscio et al., 2008). As is the case with other anxiety disorders in the general population, SoP occurs more frequently in females, and this difference is more pronounced in adolescents versus children.

A great deal of heterogeneity exists among children and adolescents with SoP. Variation exists in the types of people, places, and situations that evoke fear. Most social fears fall into one of the following three categories: interactional (initiating and maintaining conversations with peers, unfamiliar adults such as store clerks, or authority figures such as teachers or coaches), observational (situations involving embarrassment or being the center of attention, such as eating in front of others or attending a school party), and performance (speaking up in class, giving an oral presentation, performing in front of a group of people such as at a dance recital) (Beidel & Turner, 2007; Burstein et al., 2011).

In terms of causal factors, there are a host of intrinsic and environmental variables that contribute to certain children and adolescents being more vulnerable than others to the development and maintenance of social anxiety disorder. Behavioral inhibition, cognitive biases, poor social skills, over-controlling and intrusive parenting styles, aversive social experiences (such as teasing, bullying, or rejection), as well as an early history of abuse and neglect all play a role in predisposing a child or adolescent to the development of SoP (see review by Spence & Rapee, 2016).

Exposure Therapy for Social Phobia

Children and adolescents with SoP experience significant impairment in many areas of functioning. They tend to have few friends, lower academic achievement and attendance, and limited extracurricular activities (Khalid-Khan, Santibanez, McMicken, & Rynn, 2007). Exposure-based treatment is an effective method for helping children and adolescents confront their social fears, thereby decreasing the level of distress they experience in social situations and improving their quality of life. The current research literature demonstrates strong support for CBT with an exposure component as an efficacious intervention for treating children and adolescents with social anxiety. These evidence-based treatment programs include Cognitive Behavioral Group Treatment for Adolescents (CBGT-A; Albano et al., 1995; Hayward et al., 2000), Social Effectiveness Therapy for Children and Adolescents (SET-C and SET-A; Beidel, Turner, & Morris, 2000), Therapy for Adolescents with Generalized Social Phobia (Intervencion en Adolescentes con Fobia Social Generalizada-IAFSG; Olivares & García-López, 1998), and CBT plus Parent Involvement (CBT-PI; Spence, Donovan, & Brechman-Toussaint, 2000). One of the most studied empirically-supported CBT protocols for youth is the Coping Cat program (Kendall & Hedtke, 2006), an individual therapy treatment protocol that was intended to target socially anxious youth, as well as those with GAD and separation anxiety. Researchers have demonstrated that each of these treatment interventions resulted in significant short- and long-term outcomes, including improvements in self-esteem, higher levels of social engagement, reduction of social anxiety symptoms, and improvements in academic, family, and social functioning (García-López et al., 2002; García-López, Olivares, & Hidalgo, 2005; Kendall et al., 2004; Spence et al., 2000).

Exposure-based treatment for SoP differs from other areas of anxiety treatment in that it is often conducted in a group format. The group therapy context provides participants with a double exposure opportunity in that they complete exposures on their individual hierarchies while also participating in role-play exposures for other group members' hierarchies (Antony & Swinson, 2008). See the *Tailoring Exposure Therapy for Phobia* section for a more detailed description on the benefits and drawbacks of group therapy with SoP youth.

Social skills (such as initiating and maintaining conversations, giving and receiving compliments, and establishing and maintaining friendships) and assertiveness training are additional treatment components that are specifically targeted in exposure-based treatment protocols for SoP and will be described in more detail later in this chapter. Additionally, relaxation training, parent and school involvement, cognitive restructuring, and in-between session homework are emphasized in the CBT model for social anxiety. For a more thorough overview of these CBT strategies, please refer to chapter 4.

Clinically Relevant Factors

In preparation for exposure therapy, ongoing clinical assessment must focus on a detailed understanding of the specific nature of the child's anxious condition. As discussed in detail in chapter 2, the environmental context within which the behavior presents, and the specific nature of the child's cognitions and behavioral responses, are critical considerations in the subsequent engineering of effective exposure exercises. As follows, we present typical fear triggers or cues, feared consequences, and avoidance and safety behaviors commonly occurring in youth with SoP.

Fear Cues

Fear cues or triggers are specific environmental factors or variables that typically elicit the child's anxiety. These are the situations that activate the fear response due to the presence of specific stimuli that are perceived as dangerous or harmful in some way. The following fear cues commonly trigger fear in children and adolescents with social anxiety disorder:

Certain types of people (examples: authority figures, a potential romantic interest, unfamiliar peers or adults)

Internal experience of somatic symptoms that can be easily observed by others (examples: flushed face or blushing, body trembling, sweating)

A situation in which an audience is present or observing (examples: working out at the gym, attending dance class, eating lunch in the school cafeteria, doing homework in front of others, using public restrooms while others are present)

Performance-based social situations (examples: going up to bat during a baseball game, raising hand to speak in class, doing a presentation in front of the class, singing with the class during a school performance)

Initiating and maintaining interpersonal interactions (examples: asking a romantic interest on a date, starting a conversation with a less familiar peer, joining a conversation with a group at a party)

Situations in which an action might inconvenience others (examples: returning food at a restaurant or an item to a store, requesting help from a teacher or asking a teacher to recheck a test because she marked something incorrect that was really correct)

Feared Consequences

Feared consequences are those environmental conditions and outcomes that the child expects will result from exposure to the feared stimuli. That is, the child's fear is initiated and maintained through his experience or his belief that these negative outcomes will occur. The following are common feared consequences in children and adolescents with social anxiety disorder:

Being negatively evaluated, ridiculed, criticized, or rejected

Offending others

Being stared at by others

Appearing anxious, "crazy," "weird," foolish, weak, or unintelligent to others

Losing control, or inability to complete an activity or goal

Inability to escape the social situation when distressed

Avoidance

Children with anxiety commonly avoid the environmental stimuli and situations that trigger their anxiety because they perceive a high likelihood of their feared consequences occurring. The following are common avoidant behaviors observed in children and adolescents with social anxiety disorder:

Pervasive avoidance of specific feared social situations

Refusal to speak to anyone other than individuals identified as "safe," or to make eye contact with anyone other than these individuals

Engaging in acting-out behaviors, such as whining, demanding, crying, or full temper tantrums, in attempts to escape or avoid attending social activities or events

Complaints of feeling sick to avoid events such as attending school on the day of a presentation in front of the class

Arranging to be picked up early from event or activity

Refusal to share grades or schoolwork with family and friends or to share personal information or vulnerabilities, due to fear it may lead to criticism, rejection, or overt attention

Safety Behaviors

Children with anxiety often rely on specific objects, individuals, or actions that they believe will protect them from the feared stimuli or feared outcome. Safety behaviors are any actions that are performed in an attempt to feel safe. The following are common safety behaviors displayed by children and adolescents with social anxiety disorder:

Speaking very softly or quickly and avoiding eye contact

Excessively rehearsing or over-preparing for conversations or presentations

Seeking excessive reassurance regarding what to say to others in specific social situations or at times when assertiveness is appropriate

Escaping to a quiet place when feeling anxious in a particular situation (examples: bathroom, nurse's office)

Staying busy with distracting activities while in an anxiety-provoking situation (examples: talking to the aide at recess instead of attempting to play with other kids)

Sitting in the back of the class or as close to the outside of a group gathering as possible, so as not to draw additional attention

Talking to or attending an event only with "safe" people (examples: a parent, a close friend)

Covering face with collar, hair, or hat

Covering up different parts of the body to hide anxious reactions, such as trembling or blushing (examples: wearing heavy makeup or turtlenecks to hide blushing, or hiding hands in pockets)

Drinking water due to fears of dry throat or other physiological sensations

Wearing extra antiperspirant to decrease risk of sweating through clothing

Acting unusually polite and accommodating to avoid criticism

Listening to music with headphones or reading a book instead of engaging in conversation with others (example: on bus ride to school)

Using alcohol or other drugs (such as marijuana) to reduce anxiety symptoms and facilitate more relaxed conversations in social settings

Tailoring Exposure Therapy for Social Phobia

This section is designed to serve as a primer for the implementation of exposure therapy specifically with the population of children and adolescents with SoP. It builds on guidance presented in early chapters by offering the therapist specific guidelines for what must be uniquely considered when carrying out this work with children and adolescents with social anxiety. That is, additional strategies and modifications to the treatment approach will be discussed that are of paramount importance to implementing exposure-based work with this group.

Exposure sessions for SoP typically involve the child or adolescent gradually approaching and engaging in feared social situations, eliminating the use of safety behaviors in those situations, and through these experiences collecting information that corrects maladaptive beliefs about feared outcomes. Parent and school involvement are additional treatment components that lead to successful exposure therapy with this population. There is a great deal of heterogeneity among social fears. Therefore, to design an effective exposure hierarchy, it is critical that clinicians conduct a functional assessment to understand the specific nature of the child's fear. The social skills deficits that often exist in socially anxious youth are another area that is critical to target in exposure therapy. It is important to integrate social skills training and practice into the treatment protocol for children and adolescents with SoP to enhance social competence and increase engagement in social interactions.

Development of the Fear Hierarchy

As with any solid fear hierarchy, a hierarchy for SoP youth must be tailored specifically to the child or adolescent. As stated above, there is a great deal of heterogeneity in the fears of socially anxious youth. As such, the fear hierarchy for a child who struggles to make friends due to worry about rejection will be fundamentally different from the hierarchy for an adolescent who experiences anxiety in larger group situations out of fear of embarrassment.

Treatment for SoP youth is often conducted in a group format. The group format provides opportunities to utilize other group members for completion of role-play, social skills practice, and in vivo exposure tasks. In these groups, we recommend developing both individual and group hierarchies. The group hierarchy is a list of feared situations that is challenging for most of the group members, while individual hierarchies focus on each child's unique social fears. Throughout the group, members take turns completing exposure tasks on the group hierarchy list (for example, starting and maintaining conversations, texting each other, making mistakes), as well as work on their own individual hierarchies. In addition, exposure field trips provide opportunities to get exposure practice in a real-life setting (such as at a restaurant, bowling alley, or shopping mall).

While the benefits of group therapy with SoP youth is clear, there are also considerable advantages to implementing exposure tasks in the context of individual therapy for this population. At the beginning of treatment, it is important to evaluate which of these treatment approaches would best fit your client. This decision should be based on factors that include symptom severity, treatment goals, logistics (such as affordability, proximity, and scheduling), and client preference. Children and adolescents with SoP may be fearful of participating in group therapy, especially at the outset of treatment, and they may have a negative and avoidant response at the mention of a group intervention. Therefore, initially in treatment, it can be more effective to work through a fear hierarchy within individual therapy until they feel more comfortable and confident doing exposures that are more difficult (such as participating in group therapy). Many of our SoP clients are very successful working through their fear hierarchies in the context of individual therapy alone. It is also important to note that there is not always a group treatment option that is available or convenient for the client and their family, so group treatment may not always be a feasible treatment option.

It is imperative that hierarchy development for SoP youth targets the specific safety behaviors that maintain anxiety and diminish the effectiveness of the exposure. Socially anxious youth are often forced to engage in their feared social situations on a daily basis (for example, in social interactions throughout the school day). Despite this repeated exposure, they continue to experience the same or worsened levels of distress when in these situations. This is because they often cope with anxiety-provoking situations through the use of safety behaviors (distraction, over-preparation, checking and reassurance-seeking, substance use, and so on). For example, a child who always has to sit in the back of her classes to avoid judgment by peers would have some items placed on her fear hierarchy to gradually eliminate this safety behavior (for example, to gradually sit closer to the front of the classroom with the ultimate goal of sitting in the middle seat of the front row). For an adolescent who spends excessive amounts of time grooming his hair due to his fear of being perceived by his peers as ugly, a step on his fear hierarchy would involve reducing the amount of time he spends engaging in this safety behavior.

Socially anxious youth often experience somatic symptoms of anxiety and fear that others will notice and judge their physiological response (such as blushing, trembling, or sweating). Hierarchy exercises that systematically and purposefully generate the feared somatic symptoms while in the presence of the feared social situation will be an important component of the exposure work. (See chapter 7 for a review of interoceptive exposure techniques.) For an adolescent who fears that others will notice her shakiness and anxiety during an oral presentation, tasks on the exposure hierarchy would begin with interceptive exposures that generate the physiological experience of shaking. Once habituation to the shaking alone is achieved, a more challenging exposure task might involve generating shakiness while engaged in a mock presentation in the clinic, prior to an actual presentation.

Finally, tailoring exposure work for children and adolescents with SoP should also address fear of situations in which social mistakes or blunders actually do occur. In contrast to exposures in which the feared consequence or social catastrophe does not occur, social mishap exposures prepare youth for managing and tolerating situations in which evaluation or negative consequences from social mishaps do exist. These exposures are considered an important component of the fear hierarchy for socially anxious youth (Hofmann, 2007; Fang, Sawyer, Asnaani, & Hofmann, 2013).

Social mishap exposure tasks involve asking the child to intentionally create the feared negative consequence of a feared social situation. Purposefully engaging in these social blunders helps clients to realize that the long-lasting negative outcomes they anticipated do not actually occur. This process of correcting maladaptive beliefs and gaining increased competence in coping with these types of situations leads to an interruption in the avoidance cycle. In the case of an adolescent who fears appearing stupid to her classmates, she might complete an exposure task that involves raising her hand in class and giving the incorrect answer. By doing so she learns that even if there are some short-term negative consequences of making the mistake (such as the teacher saying she is incorrect, or classmates whispering something like, "That was such an easy question"), these are all temporary consequences that have no significant permanent impact. Imaginary exposures to making mistakes are also extremely useful to practice prior to the in vivo exposures, as they allow youth to work on tolerating the thoughts and feelings that arise prior to entering the feared situation.

Considering the Safety of Exposure Tasks

It is always important to consider safety while engaging in exposure tasks. Exposure functions best when tasks are manageable and appropriate given the youth's current level of progress and momentum. Occasionally, clients may threaten self-harm when overwhelmed by anxiety or in an effort to avoid an anxiety-provoking situation. They may believe that parents will back down once these statements are made and they will be allowed to avoid the feared situation. These threats should always be taken seriously, but without abandoning the exposure hierarchy. For example, discussing a gradual exposure option that the youth finds more tolerable may be warranted. If a teen threatens extreme behavior, the clinician or parent should state that safety is a priority, and if the teen cannot guarantee safety, he will be taken to a crisis center or hospital. Clearly state, however, that after safety is reestablished, the exposures will continue. The adolescent needs to understand that threatening harm to himself is not a successful avoidance tactic, and parents should respond with clear limits rather than abandoning the request and enabling such behavior.

Frequency, Duration, and Length of Sessions

The average length of treatment for this population is 10 to 12 weeks (Beidel et al., 2001). However, it should be noted that factors such as symptom severity, existing comorbidities, and treatment compliance may extend treatment duration. A child who only fears public speaking will require fewer sessions than a child who is struggling to attend school due to a pervasive fear of embarrassing herself throughout the school day. With SoP, the specific treatment plan is dependent upon the level of impairment the anxiety is creating. Generally, the more frequent the exposure sessions, the faster progress will be. We recommend (when feasible for the family) holding a parent-only session in addition to the child's exposure session on certain weeks, to give parents a separate time to learn the appropriate tools for exposure work with the child. It is also a possibility to extend the weekly session in length in order to have the parent and child sessions at the same time. Finally, when undertaking exposure tasks that are longer in duration (such as visits to a crowded mall or eating out at a restaurant), therapists might consider allotting 60 minutes or more for the therapy session so that they have enough time for habituation and repetition of any tasks involved.

Cognitive Considerations

There are several types of thinking errors that are common in children and adolescents with SoP, including: personalization (example: *My classmates are whispering and looking my way, so that must mean they think I'm weird*), catastrophizing (*What if I ask my teacher a question that she has already answered and then she will think I don't care about her class and she will hate me*), all-or-nothing thinking (*I messed up a couple of my lines for my part in the school play; I'm such a failure!*), "should" statements (*I should be able to make friends more easily*), and disqualifying the positive (*George asked me to the dance just to be nice, and because there was no one else to ask.*). Through cognitive restructuring, children and adolescents are trained to be more aware of these maladaptive patterns of thinking and to challenge and correct these thoughts with rational and reality-based statements that encourage coping and social approach.

Other Treatment Considerations

Social skills training and school collaboration are two additional treatment components that lead to successful exposure work with children and adolescents with social anxiety. Below is a description of how each can be integrated into exposure therapy with this population.

SOCIAL SKILLS AND ASSERTIVENESS TRAINING

Social skills training is a process of learning to improve communication and social behaviors to increase and enhance interpersonal relationships. With children and adolescents, this process involves identifying social behaviors that impede the child's successful social interactions and creating a specific list of the skills that need remediation. Social skills deficits common among SoP youth include perspective-taking, assertiveness, talking on the phone, utilizing appropriate greetings and introductions, initiating and maintaining conversations, listening, and joining groups. Skills training involves practicing the targeted skill in a variety of settings, including alone in front of the mirror, with those deemed "safe" (such as parents or siblings), and in the locations or situations in which anxiety is present. Role-playing the skills during therapy sessions can also be effective. Please refer to Beidel and Turner (2007) and Albano and DiBartolo (2007) for specific guidelines on implementing social skills and assertiveness training for SoP youth. It should be noted that while children and adolescents with SoP tend to overestimate their social skills deficits, engaging in social skills training is a beneficial component to treatment for many, with positive outcomes of increasing competence and confidence in use of the skills to elicit more positive social interactions.

SCHOOL COLLABORATION

The school environment is a useful setting for exposure work, as it provides an array of social opportunities. For socially anxious youth, we strongly recommend the clinician contact teachers and school counselors to gather additional information on how the child's anxiety is impacting his academic and social functioning. Further, it is often beneficial for the clinician to have ongoing communication with school personnel as exposure work begins. For example, clinicians might consider communicating to teachers their weekly plan for exposure tasks. This helps the teachers be aware of what the child is working on and provides the child with support in facing his fears while in the school environment. As exposure work progresses, however, it may be helpful to refrain from giving teachers a heads-up about exposure tasks so that the child has the opportunity to learn to tolerate the natural consequences of his actions (for example, that raising his hand and answering a question incorrectly may result in a mildly negative response from teacher).

School counselors can also be a helpful resource in encouraging and helping a socially anxious youth commit to social interactions, such as joining a new lunch table, introducing herself to a new student, or joining an extracurricular activity that matches with her interests. Children or adolescents may be more open to suggestions from their school counselor, as opposed to their parents. With the help of the therapist, the counselor can work through small fear hierarchies related to a given goal. For example, joining an extracurricular activity might include items such as gathering information about the club or activity (such as day, time, location, and frequency), attending the activity with limited participation, and eventually taking on increased participation or a leadership role.

Family Education and Support

Parents and caregivers play an important role in supporting their socially anxious child in exposure treatment by reinforcing social skills practice and exposure task completion. Parents can support their child in setting up real-life, exposure-based social activities outside of therapy sessions (such as setting up playdates or encouraging their adolescent to attend an upcoming school event or sign up for extracurricular activities with a social interaction element). As with other anxiety disorders, parents often accommodate anxiety by allowing their anxious child to avoid participation in social activities outside of the regular school day. With socially anxious youth, it is imperative that parents be educated about their accommodating behaviors, especially those that involve allowing their child to avoid potentially anxiety-provoking social interactions. Additionally, parents should be educated about the value of modeling proactive coping strategies in handling their own social fears. For example, they might model for their child how to handle nervousness about an upcoming event. (For example: "I am nervous to go to your father's work holiday party because there are a lot of people I'm not familiar with, but I'm still going to attend because it will be nice to get to know his coworkers better, and I am not going to let my anxiety win.") It should be noted that parental involvement is likely to be a more primary treatment component for younger children. For adolescents, discussion and expectations should be set early on in treatment regarding the amount of parent involvement that is appropriate and desired.

Exposure Tasks and Activities Guide

Below, we present a wide list of activities and ideas as a guide for clinicians' use in generating useful and creative tasks for a client's exposure hierarchy. While some sections may be loosely organized according to an increasing level of difficulty, proposed tasks and activities are not designed to be utilized in sequence. Rather, the therapist should always use clinical judgment, as well as parent and child input, in determining the most effective next steps in any series of exposures, and should strive to tailor tasks to the individual needs of each child. The exposure tasks below are categorized into the three main types of feared situations that are most common among children and adolescents with social anxiety: interactional, observational, and performance-based situations. Some of the exposure tasks below were adapted from Abramowitz et al., 2011; Albano and DiBartolo, 2007; Antony and Swinson, 2008; Dixon et al., 2015; Peterman et al., 2015; Sisemore, 2012.

SITUATIONS INVOLVING INTERACTING WITH OTHERS

Audio/Visual Exposures

Watch TV show clips of kids having conversations, to reinforce conversation skills.

Create an audio recording of a role-played conversation between the client and therapist that child will listen to in between sessions, starting with an easy conversation that flows well and working up to recording a more complicated conversation that involves a disagreement or sharing a differing opinion.

Imaginal/Role-Play Exposures

Imagine getting a negative reaction during a conversation (example: waiter rolls eyes when a change is made to an order, being teased when trying to join a conversation with a group at lunch, getting yelled at by a teacher when asking for help).

Role-play different conversation scenarios during a therapy session (see in vivo exposures for examples of types of conversations).

Role-play conversation scenarios with parents and siblings in session or as homework.

Conduct a *"What would happen if…"* role-play: For a child who fears a negative reaction by a waiter when she returns food at a restaurant, the role-play might first involve what is likely to occur in that situation (example: the wait staff is kind and says "Okay"), followed by the feared negative response (example: eye rolling, yelling, or a statement such as, "I can't believe you are doing this!"). The therapist and child can take turns playing the roles of the wait staff and the person ordering the food.

Conduct a mock job interview with an adolescent who is looking for a part-time job during the school year or a summer job. The role-play would involve having the therapist act as the interviewer and asking questions with increasing levels of difficulty.

In Vivo Exposures

Start a conversation with a peer (example: someone the child sees often in class) and gradually work up to starting a conversation with a less familiar person, but someone the child wants to get to know (example: an unfamiliar peer or romantic interest). Set a weekly goal, such as saying, "Hi, how's your day going?" to the same peer in math class at least three times during the week and asking at least two follow-up questions in each conversation.

Start a conversation with an authority figure (examples: coach, teacher, dance instructor); ask an easy question (examples: "What grade did I earn on _____?" or "What time is practice on Tuesday?") and gradually work toward asking a question that involves receiving some form of feedback (examples: "What can I do to improve my current grade?" "Can you tell me how to study for the upcoming test?" "Are there other things I can do to improve my batting swing?"). Assert self by sharing an opinion, asking for help, or making a request (examples: ask to use the bathroom during the middle of class; ask a teacher to recheck a test because she marked something incorrect that was actually correct; share idea for group project that differs from the majority).

For younger children: Practice conversations by conducting surveys. The child walks around the clinician's office and interacts with staff and others in the waiting room. Or the child might conduct the survey with peers on the playground (sample questions: "What's your favorite food?" "What's your favorite sport?").

Give or receive compliments. Offer someone else a compliment (examples: peer, teacher, coach, stranger); receive compliment by saying "thank you" rather than being dismissive or making self-deprecating comments.

Join an ongoing conversation with peers who are engaged in a discussion on a topic of interest (example: during lunch at school, during extracurricular activity, at a party); set goal to wait for a pause in the conversation and then ask one question or share one opinion.

Join in and offer ideas or opinions while working on a group project; set a goal to make a certain number of statements during each meeting.

Participate in a "lunch bunch" with the school counselor to practice social skills and enhance self-efficacy.

Identify a target number of peers and ask for their phone numbers.

Respond and initiate text conversations. Conversation topics might include asking a question about a homework assignment, mentioning something funny that happened in a class, or asking about making plans for the weekend. Some adolescents may first need to work on increasing the frequency with which they respond to text messages, as they often feel anxious about saying the "right" thing. Once they have mastered this, the focus can switch to initiating texts with peers they are more comfortable with and working toward expanding their texting network, maybe even joining and responding in group chats.

Use a social media platform (examples: Facebook, Instagram, Snapchat) to initiate and maintain conversations with less familiar or unfamiliar peers (when developmentally appropriate).

Initiate small-talk conversations while engaging in online video game play.

Make telephone calls. Start with phone calls that require little time or thinking on the spot (examples: asking a store for directions or their hours) and work up to phone calls that have the potential for negative reactions (examples: answering a phone call for a parent, scheduling an appointment, or ordering food and then calling back to cancel the order).

Invite a friend over for a get-together. This task typically involves the social skills training component and teaching the child or adolescent the steps involved in making plans outside of school (identifying location, activity, day, time, and so on) and addressing barriers so that plans don't fall through (examples: making plans ahead of time, making sure to confirm the specific day and time, responding in a timely manner to text conversations about the plans).

Ask a romantic interest out on a date. Start by saying hi and making small talk, followed by calling or texting, and eventually asking the person out on a date.

Talk to strangers. Walk around the mall for an hour and ask a certain number of strangers for the time, or for directions to a particular store in the mall.

Talk to a cashier or sales clerk. Make eye contact and say "hi" while checking out, make small talk while checking out (example: commenting on the weather). More challenging tasks might include asking for advice, such as, "How does this shirt look with these pants?" or exchanging an item.

Order food at a restaurant. Gradually increase level of difficulty through varying the context and requirements (examples: order at the counter versus at a table), or start with ordering something the way it is stated on the menu, then make one or two small changes to the order, and work toward sending food back once it's received, telling the waiter the order was prepared incorrectly).

Express an opinion that is different from the majority, starting with situations where there are likely to be few negative consequences (example: opinion about a movie or TV show) and working up to intentionally sharing an opinion when it is known that there will be strong disagreement from others (example: political views).

Say no when a classmate asks to copy the homework or assert self in other situations in which a boundary or limit is desired (example: not wanting to share grades when peers ask, speaking up when asked to do more work than others on group project, saying no when a peer asks to switch seats on a school bus ride).

Join school-based clubs that align with the client's interests. Start with gathering information about the club, then attend meetings, and eventually work up to increasing participation and involvement at the meetings.

Attend a job or college interview. Try to arrange it so that the adolescent can do multiple interviews that occur close together, in order to create frequent and repetitive exposure.

Reducing Safety Behaviors and Avoidance

Make a phone call or start a conversation without use of a "what to say" script.

Attend a high school party without engaging in the use of alcohol or drugs.

Go into a store without parent present. (This may be more appropriate for preteens or adolescents.)

Make good eye contact and look up during conversations instead of speaking with head down and diverted eye contact.

Text or make phone calls without seeking reassurance from parent first (examples: "What should I say?" "Is it okay if I say _____?").

Invite a friend to participate in an activity that facilitates conversation (examples: painting pottery, bowling, mini golf, walking around a shopping mall, eating at a restaurant) rather than going to a movie, during which there is little opportunity to converse.

Attend a high school club meeting and participate, instead of attending but sitting quietly in the back.

Say hello and make eye contact when spontaneously running into acquaintance-level or closer peers or adults in public (examples: at the grocery store, shopping mall, sibling's soccer game).

SITUATIONS INVOLVING EMBARRASSMENT OR BEING THE CENTER OF ATTENTION

(Refer to exposure tasks under "Making Mistakes/Failure" in chapter 12 for additional ideas.)

Audio/Visual Exposures

Watch video clips of others being the center of attention (examples: receiving an award, assisting in a magic show or other live performance, being called out for praise or reprimand in front of the class).

View images of people speaking, singing, and dancing in crowded public places (examples: concerts, sporting events, festivals).

Watch video clips of others making social mistakes (either in real life or in TV shows or movies).

Create a video recording of the therapist making a social mistake and watch with the client, then make the same recording with the client making the mistake and watch for a prolonged period of time.

Imaginal/Role-Play Exposures

Imagine being called to the front of the class for various reasons (examples: to answer a question, to accept a reward, to receive a reprimand).

Imagine or role-play a friend or parent bragging about the client to other individuals.

Imagine or role-play being ignored or teased in various social situations, or someone telling the client that he looks funny.

Imagine or role-play the teacher giving corrective feedback or receiving criticism from teacher or parent.

Imagine or role-play walking into a school dance, party, or other social event and not knowing anyone.

Imagine "worst-case scenario" consequences of making a social mistake (examples: losing friends, not being able to make any friends, never having a boyfriend or girlfriend, letting the whole team down).

Role-play a scenario that involves making a social mistake in front of others (see examples under the following in vivo exposures section); have the therapist and client take turns playing the part of the individual making the mistake, so that the client has the opportunity to experience both roles.

Role-play anxious reaction (example: sweating) in front of someone the client fears will see the reaction (example: when on a date or when trying to have a conversation with a romantic interest).

In Vivo Exposures

Use a public restroom; take an excessively long time in the stall.

Have picture taken in a public place; show the picture to family, close friends, or those in a group or class.

Post pictures on some type of social media platform (examples: Instagram, Facebook), varying the length of time pictures remain posted. Start with group pictures or what the client identifies as a "good" picture of herself and then move to more challenging tasks (example: post pictures in which the adolescent is not perfectly groomed or is doing something silly or mildly embarrassing).

The therapist should help the adolescent consider what is an appropriate picture for public posting.

While playing online video game, intentionally make a mistake during the game at the expense of your own team.

Go up to the front of the class and solve a math problem on the board, or read aloud to the class; as a higher-level challenge, mispronounce words or skip words while reading aloud.

Practice exercising in front of others. Attend an exercise class at the gym; start by participating in the back row and gradually move up to the front.

Stand up in the cafeteria, gym, or other crowded location to shout or cheer about something.

Share an art project with someone else; work up to sharing with multiple people and then in front of a class.

Do homework or draw while someone watches.

Raise hand in class to ask or answer a question with the goal of gradually increasing the number of times raising hand throughout the school day. Start with answering questions when the response is highly likely to be correct, and work toward raising hand when there is more uncertainty and potential to produce an incorrect response.

Intentionally answer a question incorrectly in class.

Go to school or another public location with some kind of fashion mishap; wear a gaudy shirt or a piece of clothing inside out and keep the outfit on all day long.

Eat a messy meal in front of friends; make funny noises while eating.

Intentionally drop something from backpack when walking in the school hallway, and then stop and pick it up.

Intentionally elicit an anxious response immediately prior to entering any of the above fear-provoking situations.

Reducing Safety Behaviors and Avoidance

Arrive a few minutes late to class or an extracurricular activity to increase the likelihood of being noticed when entering the room.

Purposefully yell out something silly in the middle of class or ask the teacher a "stupid" question.

Make eye contact in a public place.

Attend a concert or sporting event and stay for the whole time.

Speak loudly when in a public place, rather than the usual whisper or low volume.

Eat lunch in the school cafeteria and sit with a large group, instead of alone in a teacher's classroom or at a quiet table.

Speak up and share opinions when working on a group project.

SITUATIONS INVOLVING SPEAKING OR PERFORMING IN PUBLIC

Audio/Visual Exposures

Watch video clips of different types of public performances with large crowds (examples: presidential speeches, athletes performing in front of large stadium crowds, concerts, theater performances).

Find clips of others making mistakes while performing in public (examples: professional sports bloopers, microphone malfunctioning during musician's performance, speeches in which mistakes in word choice or delivery were made).

Read articles about performers and how they deal with making mistakes during performances and overcome performance anxiety.

Interoceptive Exposures

Place heat pack on cheeks for 2 minutes or drink a hot beverage within 2 minutes to elicit blushing and sweating.

Do as many push-ups as possible in a minute, or tense arms and hands to create sensation of trembling or shakiness. Start with interoceptive exposures during the therapy session, followed by assigning daily practice for homework. Initially, the client should do these tasks in the absence of feared social situation. More challenging exercises would involve creating the physiological sensation in the presence of the fear cue.

Imaginal/Role-Play Exposures

Conduct a *"What would happen if…"* role-play for making a mistake during opening night of the school play, or another performance-based situation. Create a detailed script of what goes on immediately before, during, and after the mistake occurs, and include specifics about the thoughts and emotions experienced in this situation, as well as the predicted negative reactions received by others.

Conduct an imaginal exposure to a worst-case scenario performance situation (examples: making a large mistake during the performance, being laughed at by peers, getting kicked out of the drama club).

Conduct an imaginal exposure of a performance that has not yet occurred. Have the child or adolescent create an audio recording of the script so that he can read or listen to the script in between sessions.

Conduct imaginal exposure of having an observable anxious reaction (examples: trembling, sweating, blushing) in any feared performance situation.

In Vivo Exposures

Practice a presentation several times in front of different people and gradually increase the size of the group (examples: in therapist's office in front of therapist, in therapist's office with parents present, at home in front of parents and siblings, at home with family and close friends). Ask for feedback after each practice.

Practice the presentation with an audience appearing bored or frustrated (example: rolling their eyes, averting glance, putting head in hands).

Practice the presentation while purposefully making mistakes (examples: mess up wording, skip words, pause for a long period of time, drop papers).

Sign up for a drama or music class outside of school, for which there is a time-limited, high frequency commitment (example: summer camp) instead of the entire school year.

Participate in a school-sponsored or extracurricular activity that involves some form of public performance (examples: band, chorus, school play, cheerleading). Most of these activities are either daily or a few times a week, which provides the repetition needed for a good exposure.

Volunteer to go first to give an oral presentation in front of the class.

Play a musical instrument in front of the therapist, followed by family members, and work up to playing in front of gradually increasing numbers of peers (examples: small social gathering, school-sponsored event such as a talent show).

Perform in a dance or music recital with the possibility of doing this on multiple occasions.

Join drama club, debate team, or another extracurricular activity that specifically targets performance fears, and engage in the activity for an extended period of time (at least one season or school year).

Run for a position in the student government association and give a speech in front of the whole school (for younger children, in front of the grade).

Purposefully exhibit an anxious reaction in any of the above performance situations (example: immediately prior to doing an oral presentation, place heat pack on face for 2 minutes).

Reducing Safety Behaviors and Avoidance

Tell a joke or a funny story to a group of friends in a public setting (examples: cafeteria, party, school dance).

Intentionally mess up a part of a speech in front of the class.

Wet forehead prior to presentation or performance to simulate sweating.

Do a short speech in front of the class without practicing ahead of time.

Say the announcements over the loud speaker at the beginning of a school day.

Instead of getting permission from the teacher to do an oral speech during lunch, do the speech at the same time as the rest of the class.

Case Example

A 16-year-old girl presented to the clinic with difficulty initiating and maintaining conversations with less familiar peers as well as interacting with strangers or adults in an authority role. The majority of her peer-related anxiety stemmed from her participation in a youth group outside of school, as well as a summer program in which she was participating for the first time. This client experienced anticipatory anxiety on days when she had her youth group meeting, and there were several occasions when she convinced her parents to allow her to avoid attending. She struggled to join in on group conversations, felt that she never knew what to say, and worried that she would experience rejection due to appearing weird or awkward if she said the "wrong" thing.

In school, this adolescent had a small group of friends, and while she had a desire to make more friends, she felt her anxiety held her back from accomplishing this. In addition, her anxiety around interacting with authority figures and unfamiliar adults occurred within situations such as setting up and completing driving lessons with an instructor, interviewing for a summer job, and going on college tours and interacting with unfamiliar people. Safety behaviors included only participating in extracurricular activities with at least one close friend, talking fast, and rehearsing in her mind what to say next in a conversation instead of following the conversation. She presented to treatment at this time due to feeling that her anxiety was interfering with her social functioning, and she expressed concern that if she did not figure out ways to manage her anxiety now, it would impact her college experience.

Treatment began by establishing rapport and helping this client feel comfortable in treatment. Two separate fear hierarchies were created—one for peer interactions and the other for interactions with adults. In addition to developing the fear hierarchies early on in treatment, relaxation and cognitive restructuring strategies were introduced. Homework assignments included daily relaxation practice and daily practice of self-talk notecards to challenge the cognitive distortions.

The exposure tasks were primarily comprised of role-plays and in vivo tasks. Many of the role-play exposures took place in the office to help prepare her for the real-life experiences. For example, each week prior to attending her faith-based youth group meeting, at least part of the therapy session would focus on setting an exposure goal for the upcoming meeting and then doing a role-play of that task in the session (for example, saying "hi" as she entered the room, sitting next to a different person than usual, or joining in on a group discussion). Another role-play exposure completed in session involved doing mock college and job interviews. This involved first allowing the client to prepare responses to the interview questions, followed by having to answer questions on the spot, without any preparation. In vivo exposures that took place in session included sending emails to teachers, texting less familiar peers, and making phone calls (for example, to set up driving lessons, get information from a store, or set up a college tour).

Each week she was assigned in vivo exposure tasks to complete in between therapy sessions. For example, she was given the exposure task to have a back-and-forth conversation with a couple of the girls in her summer program three to four times during the week with the eventual goal of getting their phone numbers and initiating a get-together. While some of the exposures focused solely on experiencing real-life situations, other exposure tasks centered around eliminating safety behaviors (for example, speaking more slowly in conversations and interviews, attending extracurricular activity without a close friend, and getting together with someone new outside of school), as well as intentionally making and tolerating social mistakes in these situations (for example, asking a "stupid" question when calling to set up driving lessons, dropping something as she entered the youth group meeting, and making a small mistake in an email to a teacher).

Another aspect to this adolescent's treatment involved social skills training. Her main challenges included maintaining one-on-one conversations, joining a group conversation, active listening, and assertiveness. The social skills training and practice was incorporated into her fear hierarchy. For example, one of the role-play exposures involved sharing a differing opinion in a group conversation in an assertive rather than aggressive way. On a different occasion, she was asked to practice having more spontaneous and less rehearsed conversations. One exposure task involved being introduced to a few different clinicians in our clinic and being instructed to practice small-talk conversations while actively listening to what they were saying, instead of planning what to say next.

There was minimal parent involvement with this treatment case, as this adolescent was very motivated and compliant with doing the assigned exposure work in between sessions, and since she was going away to college in the next year, it made sense for her to take ownership of her own treatment. Her parents were, however, given guidance regarding strategies for reducing accommodation of her avoidance behaviors (for example, allowing her to miss her youth group meetings, stepping in to schedule appointments that were her responsibility to take care of, or interacting with store clerks on behalf of her needs).

At treatment's end, the client expressed feeling much more comfortable with participating in extracurricular activities without a close friend. Additionally, she was taking steps to broaden her social circle and had identified a couple of clubs she planned to join even if her close friends didn't join. She had also started to attend college tours with lower levels of anxiety, and was in the process of scheduling college interviews. Additionally, she successfully completed a couple of summer job interviews. She shared that while there continued to be some social situations that evoked anxiety, she felt confident about being able to handle these situations and worried less about negative evaluations from others.

Conclusion

Children and adolescents with social anxiety experience significant impairment in many areas of functioning. They tend to have few friends, lower academic achievement and attendance, and limited extracurricular activities. Exposure-based treatment is an effective method for helping children and adolescents confront their social fears, thereby decreasing the level of distress they experience in social situations and improving their quality of life. It may be conducted in group or individual format, and often includes additional treatment components involving school collaboration and social skills training. This chapter reviewed diagnostic information, key treatment considerations, and implementation of exposure tasks for children and adolescents with social anxiety disorder. Samples of specific exposure tasks were provided for consideration in creating individualized exposure hierarchies with clients. Finally, case examples were used to illustrate the clinician's role in implementation of general CBT skills and exposure tasks with real clients experiencing social anxiety.

CHAPTER 14

Exposure for Obsessive-Compulsive Disorder

This chapter focuses on exposure therapy—specifically, exposure and response prevention (ERP)—with children and adolescents who have obsessive-compulsive disorder (OCD). We set the stage by describing the clinical presentation of pediatric OCD before going on to explain why exposure therapy is used as a first-line treatment. Next, we present assessment considerations and clinically relevant factors. We go on to discuss how to develop fear hierarchies and tailor exposure tasks to target the particular needs of each child. Then we provide a detailed guide on specific exposure tasks for various types of OCD, including ways to reduce safety behaviors and avoidance. Overall, this chapter is intended to present you with guidelines to help you understand, design, and implement successful exposure therapy for pediatric OCD.

Clinical Presentation and Causal Factors

The clinical presentation of OCD in children and adolescents involves the presence of obsessions and/or compulsions, defined in the following ways within the *DSM-5* (American Psychiatric Association, 2013): Obsessions are persistent and recurrent thoughts, images, or urges that are unwanted and intrusive (for example, fears of death or illness to self or loved ones), usually causing significant distress or anxiety; attempts are made to suppress or neutralize the obsessions with other thoughts or actions (such as compulsions). Compulsions (or rituals) are repetitive behaviors (such as checking, cleaning, or ordering) or mental acts (counting, repeating words in head, praying) that a person feels compelled to perform in response to an obsession or following rigidly applied rules. These are performed to reduce obsession-related distress levels or prevent feared outcomes—although the compulsions are either clearly excessive (such as checking the door 25 times to be sure it's locked) or are not realistically connected to the feared outcome (such as counting things in multiples of eight to prevent harm to a parent). In order to meet diagnostic criteria, the obsessions and compulsions must either be very time-consuming (for example, more than an hour per day) or cause significant levels of distress or functional impairment in daily life. There is a wide range in the content of obsessions and compulsions, as discussed later. Youth with OCD often have multiple obsessions and compulsions, and types of symptoms may change over time.

The development of OCD has been linked to biological, behavioral, and cognitive factors. Heritability estimates for OCD range from 27% to 65%, with the most robust study to date reporting 48% (Browne, Gair, Scharf, & Grice, 2014). Neuroimaging studies indicate atypical structure and function in various brain regions of youth with OCD, including fronto-striatal-thalamic networks (Bernstein et al., 2016; O'Neill et al., 2012). Behaviorally, both classical conditioning and operant conditioning (such as negative reinforcement) are likely at play in the development and maintenance of OCD (Mowrer, 1960). From a cognitive perspective, there are common patterns of misappraisal associated with OCD, including an inflated sense of responsibility for harm, an overestimation of the threat level connected with thoughts, a heightened intolerance of uncertainty, an overestimation of the anxiety level that will be experienced without rituals or avoidance, and an underestimation of coping ability (Rahman et al., 2011).

The prevalence rate of OCD in children and adolescents is estimated between 1% and 3% (Rapoport et al., 2000; Zohar, 1999). Age of OCD onset in youth varies, with a mean onset of 8 to 11 years old (Piacentini, Bergman, Keller, & McCracken, 2003), although OCD has been noted in children as young as 2 years of age (Coskun, Zoroglu, & Ozturk, 2012). Moreover, up to half of adults with OCD report age of onset prior to 18 years old (Attiullah, Eisen, & Rasmussen, 2000). In children, males may be affected at a higher rate than females (Geller et al., 2000; Masi et al., 2005), although the gender distribution appears to equalize by adulthood (Mancebo et al., 2008). There is a high rate of comorbidity—up to 75% to 80%—in children and adolescents with OCD, with the most common comorbid conditions including anxiety disorders, mood disorders, externalizing disorders, and tic disorders (Geller et al., 2000; Langley et al., 2010). It is important to highlight that OCD in youth can impede psychosocial development and have a significant detrimental impact in functioning across multiple domains, including home/family, school/academic, and social (Piacentini et al., 2003; Valderhaug & Ivarsson, 2005). Accordingly, time and effort dedicated to mitigating OCD symptoms through ERP is clearly warranted.

Exposure Therapy for OCD

Exposure therapy used to address OCD symptoms is called exposure and response prevention (ERP) and is the principal component of cognitive behavioral therapy (CBT) for OCD (Bolton & Perrin, 2008). ERP involves gradually and repeatedly exposing individuals to feared stimuli that underlie their obsessions ("exposure"), while having them refrain from engaging in associated rituals or compulsions ("response prevention") used to reduce related anxiety. The behavioral mechanisms underlying ERP may include habituation, among others (Benito, Conelea, Garcia, &

Freeman, 2012). More specifically, the process of experiencing anxious arousal in a sustained and repeated way during exposures to obsessional stimuli typically leads to a decreased anxiety response to these stimuli—or habituation—over time. At the same time, preventing clients from engaging in compulsions to reduce their anxiety level disrupts or weakens this negative reinforcement cycle, contributing to a reduced frequency of both compulsions and avoidance over time. Cognitive mechanisms of change may also be at play during ERP (Foa & Kozak, 1986): exposure to feared stimuli without feared consequences occurring, or exposure to feared situations with adequate coping ability experienced (despite not engaging in compulsions), may shift a client's beliefs about his obsessions and his need to engage in rituals.

There is a strong research base that supports the success of ERP-based CBT for treating pediatric OCD. This includes both randomized, controlled efficacy studies (e.g., Bolton & Perrin, 2008; Watson & Rees, 2008) and community-based effectiveness studies to establish generalizability (e.g., Torp et al., 2015). Recent meta-analyses of CBT, CBT + SRI (selective reuptake inhibitor) medication, and SRI medication alone, found the largest effect sizes for CBT and concluded that the combination of CBT + SRI did not yield better outcomes than CBT alone (e.g., Ivarsson et al., 2015; McGuire et al., 2015; Öst et al., 2016). These studies found that CBT not only had the best treatment efficacy, but also led to the highest rates of treatment response and symptom/diagnostic remission. Moreover, a recent meta-analysis reported that most acute gains made in CBT remained during follow-up periods from 3 to 9 months (Franklin et al., 2015). Thus, data from research studies to date indicate that CBT is an empirically supported treatment for pediatric OCD and a superior treatment option over medications. However, medications may be indicated in a number of cases—for example, severe cases of pediatric OCD that are initially unresponsive to CBT (Geller et al., 2012).

It is important to underscore that ERP is believed to be the cornerstone of CBT for OCD. Along with exposure therapy, a cognitive behavioral model of treating pediatric OCD may include psychoeducation, parent training, positive reinforcement, cognitive restructuring, and other anxiety management techniques (such as relaxation skills). However, many of these are predominantly used to complement and support ERP, with exposure considered key to CBT treatment of OCD (Freeman et al., 2014): larger effect sizes are seen in studies that focus on ERP, and even those that emphasize cognitive strategies still include exposure components within behavioral experiments. Furthermore, studies that have examined the efficacy of ERP alone (e.g., Bolton & Perrin, 2008) have found it to be significantly effective in symptom reduction, reinforcing the notion that ERP is a (or potentially *the*) critical active ingredient in CBT for pediatric OCD.

Dishearteningly, despite the strong statistics mentioned above, there is a huge gap between the number of youth with OCD who could benefit from CBT-based exposure therapy and the number who receive it (Franklin et al., 2015). Along these lines, Geller and colleagues (2012) reported survey results that indicate only one-third of clinicians treating pediatric OCD "regularly" use exposure techniques, another third "sometimes" use them, and the final third "rarely or never" use them. It is our hope that this chapter will help to mitigate some of these factors and provide a framework for the successful application of ERP with children and adolescents who have OCD.

Clinically Relevant Factors

Clinical assessment must focus on a clear and detailed understanding of the specific nature of the child's obsessions and compulsions in preparation for exposure therapy. The context within which obsessions and compulsions present, and the specific nature of the child's cognitive and behavioral triggers and responses, are critical considerations in the subsequent design of effective exposure exercises. Below, we discuss specific fear cues (triggers that activate obsessions), feared consequences, avoidance behaviors, and safety behaviors (rituals/compulsions) often seen in youth with OCD. The examples are subdivided into some of the common OCD categories seen in children and adolescents: contamination, harm/catastrophe, and symmetry/"just right." We also highlight related safety assessment considerations.

Fear Cues

Fear cues, or triggers, are specific variables that typically elicit the child's anxiety and activate obsessions. These may be situations, objects, or thoughts that activate the fear response (or cause feelings of disgust or discomfort) because they are perceived as dangerous, harmful, or distressing. The following fear cues commonly activate obsessions in children with OCD.

Contamination

Any object or surface that several people may have touched (examples: doorknobs, hand-railings) and may be internalized as "dirty" or "contaminated" regardless of visible signs of dirt or contamination

Any object or surface that objectively or visibly appears to have dirt or unknown substances on it (examples: park bench, countertop)

Thinking about, talking about, hearing, or seeing someone sneeze, cough, get sick (vomit), or have other potential signs of illness (example: stomachache)

Exposure to urine, feces, saliva, or blood

Experiencing physical sensations (stomachache, nausea, dizziness) that could be associated with illness

Any enclosed public space where germs could be spread through the air or on surfaces (examples: movie theater, mall, public restroom, hospital or doctor's office, airplane, metro or subway)

Any food that appears "not fresh" due to brown spots, specks, wilting, potential mold, and so on. This can include foods that have little specks in them naturally (example: multigrain crackers) but child is unsure if the specks indicate dirt or mold.

Any food with an unknown expiration date (examples: yogurt not in original container with date stamp)

Any food for which the preparation method is unknown (example: at a restaurant) and child is uncertain if the food might be poisoned or rancid

Any plates, utensils, or cups that the child is unsure are clean (example: cup with water spots)

Clothing, objects, pets, or people that may be "contaminated" because they may have touched something the child views as a source of contamination (example: child's friend at school went home sick and now backpack and outfit child wore to school that day are viewed as "contaminated")

Environmental contaminants, such as asbestos, chemicals, or poison—even if not direct exposure (examples: asbestos under floor tiles; fruit that may have touched fertilizers or pesticides)

Furniture or rooms that the child believes are "contaminated" because either someone the child believes is "contaminated" used it, or it had a potential source of contamination in or on it at one time (examples: couch because brother sat on it when he had a cold; pantry because it had moldy potatoes in it one time; science room at school because of chemicals used in lab experiment)

Harm/Catastrophe

Thinking about, talking about, hearing, or seeing any object that could lead to a catastrophic event (examples: candles, stoves, or fireplaces could be connected to house burning down; door locks could be connected to burglary)

Doubt about having completed a routine task (examples: locking the door, blowing out a candle) or about having done something wrong (example:

adolescent in car drives over bump in road and is plagued with doubt about whether she might have hit an animal or person)

Thinking about, talking about, hearing, or seeing something related to a terminal illness or death (examples: cancer awareness events, a movie in which someone dies of cancer, a news article about cancer)

Being in an enclosed area or alone with loved ones (people or pets) where something could potentially harm them

Being near potentially "dangerous" objects (examples: knives, razors, other sharp objects; metal or wood bats; sports racquets) that could be used to harm self or others

Household cleaners, or other products that have warning signs (examples: nail polish remover), that could lead to harm if misused

Any little objects—such as toys with small parts (example: LEGOs), board games with little pieces (examples: *Life, Battleship*), or tiny household items (examples: paper clips, staples)—that could accidentally be swallowed

Being in potentially "dangerous" situations (examples: near busy traffic, near open window, on a balcony) that could lead to harm of self or others

Symmetry/"Just Right"

Anything that *looks* asymmetrical or not "just right" (examples: a disorganized desk, bookshelf, or backpack; a "messy" room, hairstyle, or clothing appearance)

Anything that *feels* uneven or not "just right" (examples: tightness or placement of clothing, shoes, or hairstyle; doing an action with only one side of the body)

"Sensory phenomena"—physical or mental sensations (example: perceptions of "incompleteness")

Feared Consequences

Feared consequences are the outcomes that the child worries will result from exposure to the feared stimuli. Obsessions and compulsions are maintained through the belief that these negative outcomes could occur. It is important to determine the child's ultimate feared consequences in order to adequately expose him to his core fears during ERP. The following are common feared consequences in children with OCD. (Some that span across all types of obsessions are presented at the end.)

Contamination

Child will get sick or die (examples: will contract a cold or flu virus; will eat something "bad" and vomit; will get poisoned and die).

Family member, friend, or pet will get sick or die.

Harm/Catastrophe

Child will be harmed in some way, get a terminal illness, or die. Often the fear is that this harm will be self-inflicted. For example, the child fears she may hurt herself if she holds a knife, or fears she will run into the street if near busy traffic, or fears she will jump if she is on a balcony.

Family member, friend, or pet will be harmed in some way, get a terminal illness, or die. Often the child's fear is that he will cause the harm to others. For example, he fears he will hurt his baby sibling if left alone together, or fears he will push a friend into busy traffic, or fears he will be responsible for a parent getting cancer.

Child will miss or overlook something important that could have a catastrophic outcome: damage or destruction will occur to home (burglar will get into house because door is not locked; house will burn down because she left candle burning) or other place child cares about (school, grandparents' house); or injury to another person or animal (she will fail to notice animal in street and run it over in car).

Symmetry/"Just Right"

Child will feel uncomfortable, incomplete, or not "just right" forever (examples: if shoes not tied with correct level of tightness, if desk isn't organized the "right" way).

Child will miss or overlook something important (example: will miss something critical in book chapter if he doesn't reread everything ten times).

There will be a terrible negative outcome if things are not done "just right" (example: will fail class if assignment is not written in perfect sentences).

Across OCD Categories

Something "extremely bad" will happen. (Child may not be able to specify exactly what will happen, but experiences an overarching sense of doom.)

Child will lose control or be emotionally overwhelmed by (and unable to handle) the physiological symptoms of anxiety, disgust, or distress experienced.

Child will be unable to tolerate uncertainty.

Avoidance Behaviors

Children and adolescents with OCD commonly avoid the environmental stimuli and situations that trigger their anxiety because they perceive a high likelihood of their feared consequences occurring, or are intolerant of the uncertainty, even with a very low likelihood of occurrence. The following are examples of avoidant behaviors commonly observed in children with OCD:

Contamination

Avoids touching surfaces or objects that she thinks may be "contaminated" or dirty (examples: doorknobs, hand railings, counter or tabletop at home, tables in cafeteria, notebook or binder), or uses a barrier to avoid direct contact (examples: shirt sleeve, paper towel).

Avoids eating anything that could potentially be "contaminated" (rancid, expired, poisoned, nonorganic). May include any food that appears "not fresh," any food with unknown expiration date, any food with unknown preparation method or food handler.

Avoids using plates, utensils, or cups that appear "dirty" or that he is unsure are clean.

Avoids talking about anything that relates to illness.

Avoids people who show or mention any signs of potential illness (example: person who sneezes, coughs, or mentions having a stomachache), or people who the child labels as "contaminated" for any reason (example: avoids classmate who got sick at school three months ago).

Avoids social interactions in general—may be due to perceived likelihood of germ exposure or fear of embarrassment if peers or others notice OCD-related behaviors.

Avoids going to certain places due to fear of exposure to germs or other contaminants (examples: doctors' offices and hospitals, movie theaters, malls, public restrooms, airplanes, metro or subway).

Refuses to participate in certain activities that might lead to exposure to germs (example: won't play basketball because she doesn't want to touch the basketball that might be dirty).

Avoids wearing certain articles of clothing that child believes may be "contaminated" (example: avoids ever wearing the outfit he had on the day his friend got sick at school).

Avoids using furniture or spending time in certain rooms that child believes may be "contaminated" (example: avoids sitting on the couch that her brother sat on when he was home sick, or avoids the family room altogether).

Harm/Catastrophe

Avoids talking about, reading books about, or viewing movies related to catastrophic events, terminal illness, or death (examples: conversations, books, or movies that involve fires, burglary, or cancer).

Avoids certain social situations or group activities that could involve topics related to catastrophic events, terminal illness, or death (example: doesn't want to go on camping trip because there might be bonfire at night that could burn down tents, or he could push someone into the fire).

Avoids using objects that could lead to catastrophic events (example: does not want candles in the house, does not want parents to have a fire going in the fireplace, avoids use of stove or toaster oven).

Avoids being alone with a person who she fears harming (example: refuses to be alone with baby sibling because she is afraid that she might hurt the baby).

Avoids being near potentially "dangerous" objects (examples: knives, razors, other sharp objects; metal or wood bats, sports racquets).

Avoids being in potentially "high-risk" situations (examples: near busy traffic, near open window, on a balcony, driving).

Avoids household cleaners, or other products that have warning signs (example: nail polish remover).

Avoids using toys or household objects that have tiny parts.

Symmetry/"Just Right"

Avoids doing activities (examples: homework, shower) because of the time it would take to complete these in a way that would feel "just right."

Avoids environments that look asymmetrical, imbalanced, or "messy" (example: avoids going over to friend's house because it is too messy; avoids play area because it is too disorganized).

Avoids wearing certain articles of clothing, jewelry, or hair accessories, because they feel uneven or not "just right."

Avoids people who are disorganized or wear clothing in an imbalanced way.

Safety Behaviors

Along with avoidant behavior, children with anxiety often rely on specific objects, individuals, or actions that they believe will protect them from the feared stimuli or feared outcome. Safety behaviors are any actions that are performed in order to feel safer. In OCD, these are the compulsions or rituals exhibited in response to obsessions, usually done in a repetitive way, to reduce anxiety levels. Below are examples of compulsions and rituals commonly displayed by youth with OCD:

Contamination

Spends an excessive amount of time washing hands at the sink or washing body or hair in the shower. This can include washing repeatedly, slowly, in a specific order, or using a lot of soap, as well as counting or performing other mental rituals while washing. In some cases, these behaviors get so extreme that they cause dermatological problems (skin lesions, rash, redness); however, youth are usually more distressed by the obsessions, so dermatological issues typically do not mitigate washing behaviors.

Uses cleaning products in off-label ways to clean himself or objects (example: rubbing hand sanitizer all over body, using household disinfectant spray on body, using either of these on stuffed animals).

Desires clothing, towels, or other objects to be laundered excessively; either does the wash herself (because she doesn't want anyone else touching stuff for fear of "contamination") or asks parent or caregiver to do it. In some cases, child may attempt to wash things that would not usually be laundered (example: puts backpack and school binders in washing machine and dryer).

Uses barrier methods to touch things he views as "contaminated" (example: uses shirt sleeve, tissue, or paper towel to open doorknob or pick up "dirty" book).

Engages in reassurance-seeking behaviors, such as conducting extensive Internet searches for answers regarding symptoms.

Repeatedly checks or inspects objects, surfaces, or foods (item of food itself, expiration date, or package), for any indication of "contamination."

Harm/Catastrophe

Counts or does things a certain number of times in an attempt to prevent something "bad" from happening (examples: touching or tapping things, breathing or blinking repeatedly). For example, a child blinks 10 times whenever the thought of cancer comes into his mind, so that someone he cares about doesn't get cancer.

Prays, or repeats words or phrases (silently or quietly), in an effort to prevent "bad" things from happening. For example, a child may repeat the phrase "I love my baby brother" several times in her head whenever the thought of hurting her sibling comes into her mind, in order to neutralize the thought.

Checks self or others for any evidence of harm. For example, if a child fears self-harm, she may check arms and legs for any cuts or scratches that could indicate she hurt herself.

Checks things repeatedly that could be connected to "catastrophic" situations. For example, a child worried about burglary may check the door several times to be sure that it is locked. A child worried about burning the house down may check the toaster oven and stove repeatedly to be sure they are off. A child concerned with ingesting household cleaner may check to be sure that the level of cleaner in the bottle has not changed since it was last used. A child worried about swallowing little things may repeatedly check to be sure that none of the pieces of a board game are missing.

Symmetry/"Just Right"

Organizes or arranges things in a very specific, usually symmetrical, manner. For example, a child may systematically organize all toys or books on shelves, all things on desk or in backpack, or all toiletries in bathroom by size, color, or distance between objects.

Performs actions a certain ("good" or "balanced") number of times or engages in unnecessary counting of items. For example, a child might touch or tap things, take steps, breathe, or blink, in even numbers to attain a sense of balance, or reread each page in a book 10 times before going to the next page, or say "Good night, I love you" to parents 4 times before bed or before leaving for school.

Engages in unnecessary counting of things or does things a certain "good" number of times, in an attempt to prevent something "bad" from happening (examples: touching or tapping things, breathing or blinking repeatedly).

Demands that parents or others do things in a certain way, or a certain number of times.

Repeats actions ("redoing") over and over again until they look or feel "just right" or "complete." (Here the exact number of times the action is repeated may not be the focus, but rather continuing to do it until the child achieves a "just right" feeling.) A child might re-tie shoes over a dozen times until they "feel right."

Engages in tasks in a very specific sequence in an attempt to achieve the feeling of "just right" or "completeness." For example, a child may wash body parts in the shower in a very particular order.

Repeatedly checks things to be sure they were completed fully and done well. For example, a child may check over homework several times to be sure all letters and numbers look neat, punctuation is correct, and so on.

Across OCD Categories

Repeatedly asks reassurance-seeking questions to parents, caregivers, teachers, or others (examples: asking whether things are clean or if food is safe to eat; asking if he did anything "bad" or hurt anyone; asking if things were done the "right" way or to completion). These can include indirect questions (example: child who fears she has swallowed tiny piece of board game may ask her dad if all pieces of the game are still there), or apologizing to elicit a reassuring response ("No need to apologize, you didn't do anything wrong…").

Safety Assessment

Along with the above clinically relevant factors, it is of critical importance to evaluate whether there are any safety concerns in the clinical presentation of each client. Especially in cases in which a child's obsessions include self-harm or harm to others, it is crucial to determine whether the child has any real intent or desire to harm himself or anyone else. This includes evaluating whether the child experiences pleasure or relief, versus significant distress, in response to thoughts of harm. The former is not usually present if harm thoughts are OCD-related; the latter, however, might be present in both cases. Within the context of OCD, the child usually does not desire to hurt himself or others, but rather fears this, or is plagued by enormous doubt about whether he wants to act on such thoughts, or experiences feelings of guilt for having such thoughts. If a child or adolescent states a clear desire or intent to engage in self-harm or harm to others, with or without a significant level of distress, this likely goes beyond OCD and is cause for concern regarding safety. It might be helpful to consult resources such as *The Imp of the Mind* (Baer, 2001), which explicitly addresses obsessive "bad thoughts," to aid in differentiating OCD-related versus actually dangerous thoughts of harm. In unclear cases, the child should be taken to a crisis center or hospital.

Tailoring Exposure Therapy for Youth with OCD

This section is designed as a primer for the implementation of ERP with youth with OCD. It builds on guidance presented in earlier chapters by offering the therapist specific suggestions for what must be uniquely considered when carrying out this work with pediatric OCD. Please review chapter 5 for a detailed discussion of the step-by-step process for structuring and implementing exposure sessions.

Development of the Fear Hierarchy

As is true for exposure therapy with all anxiety disorders, fear hierarchies used in exposure and response prevention for OCD must be tailored specifically to the child or adolescent at hand. The ERP hierarchy should be created using information collected during the assessment and functional analysis. It is important to take into account each child's connections between obsession triggers, feared consequences, avoidance behaviors, and compulsions. For example, the hierarchy for a child who takes 2-hour showers because she fears her arms got contaminated and is scrubbing her arms repeatedly to clean them will be fundamentally different from a child who takes 2-hour showers because she fears her mom will get cancer unless she performs each step in the shower 25 times. Of note, children across subtypes of OCD may fear being emotionally overwhelmed by (and unable to handle) the physiological symptoms of anxiety or distress experienced when faced with exposure tasks. In cases in which the experience of somatic sensations becomes one of the primary fears, the hierarchy should include interoceptive exercises to help the youth learn to cope with and habituate to such physiological sensations (see chapter 7).

Development of the ERP hierarchy should be a collaborative process with the child. You will probably need to help him come up with specific exposure tasks with the goal of having each one be realistic and attainable at that step in the hierarchy.

Importantly, in the context of OCD, each exposure task should also include the response prevention piece (for example, "Touch the doorknob for X minutes and don't wash your hands afterward"). Although the aim of ERP is to have clients participate in the exposure task and not perform their compulsive responses at all, sometimes children may be unable or unwilling to engage in ERP if you try to cut the compulsions out completely from the outset. Thus, you may need to work up to that goal in one or more of the following ways.

Reduce the frequency, intensity, or duration of repetitive behaviors in steps. The amount to reduce it by depends on baseline frequency or duration levels. For example, reduce hand-washing time in a single episode from 10 minutes to 4 minutes, or reduce the amount of soap pumps used from 5 to 1.

Change the way the ritual is being performed before fading it out. This could include changing the number the child focuses on when engaging in counting rituals (for example, having the child count in multiples of 5 instead of multiples of 4), or changing the sequence of events in rituals typically performed in an exact order (for example, doing a shower sequence in a different order or skipping one step).

Delay the urge. Have the child increase the amount of time between the exposure task and the compulsive response. For example, if a child would usually immediately wash his hands or use hand sanitizer after touching a doorknob, have him touch the doorknob and then wait X minutes afterward before washing or sanitizing his hands. You can explain to kids that they can talk back to the OCD ("Mr. Worry") to practice validating and delaying the urge: "I hear what you are saying, Mr. Worry, and I know you are upset, but I have to wait 15 minutes." You can tell the child: "Sometimes Mr. Worry might initially get louder because he wants you to listen, but if you stay strong, then eventually he will quiet down and might even go away on his own, and you might forget about the worry thoughts. If he is still there in 15 minutes, try telling him you need to delay things another 15 minutes." Continue to lengthen the time of the delay until the child is able to refrain from engaging in the compulsion at all.

Model the Task. Another way to encourage children and adolescents to engage in exposure tasks at the beginning of treatment may be for the therapist to model the desired ERP task. For example, during contamination ERP, model touching a doorknob for 5 minutes and then picking up a cracker with your hands and eating it, without washing or sanitizing your hands. It is best to use modeling only at the beginning of the therapy process and to fade it out as quickly as possible. This is because you do not want the child to become willing to engage in an ERP task only if the therapist first demonstrates it to be safe. In other words, you don't want the modeling to become a relied upon reassurance behavior. Rather, you want to help the child learn to engage in brave behaviors without therapist involvement.

Throughout ERP, it is essential to track progress and change, and to implement a positive reinforcement system. While detailed guidelines for these are in chapter 5, the following points are highlighted with regard to applying these principles with youth who have OCD. In cases in which OCD symptoms involve rigid focus on order or completing things a certain way, the ERP hierarchy should be approached in a flexible manner with ERP tasks sometimes completed out of sequence. When using a "feelings thermometer" to track ratings during exposures, the way this is specifically labeled may vary from the typical "fear/anxiety" and should match the primary feeling experienced by the child (for example, "discomfort thermometer" for "just right" exposures; "disgust thermometer" for contamination exposures). Moreover, which scale to use—numerical (such as 0 to 5), categorical (such as low to high), or visual (such as facial expressions)—may also depend on the OCD symptoms at hand. For example, if counting rituals or fears of "bad" numbers are part of the clinical presentation, then a numerical rating scale should be avoided, as these symptoms may interfere with accurate ratings. Finally, positive reinforcement has been shown to increase youth participation in exposures during OCD treatment, whereas punishment yields no clinical benefit (Geller et al., 2012).

Considering the Safety of Exposure Tasks

Care must be taken in the design of exposures to be sure that the child is not put in a dangerous situation, while also making sure not to avoid exposures that have minimal levels of risk. Although any exposure task that involves even minimal levels of risk may elicit your own feelings of discomfort, it is important not to avoid inclusion of these in the ERP plan, because doing so will only reinforce the child's OCD. This issue often comes up when considering appropriate exposures for children who have obsessions with contamination or obsessions with self-harm or harm to others. In general, exposures should be planned in a way that they would not cause the child to experience any greater level of risk than would be ordinarily experienced in daily life. However, there is often some level of minimal risk inherent to many daily tasks of living, and these should not be avoided in exposures. For example, exposing a child with contamination obsessions to the germs present on a doorknob and having him refrain from washing his hands might possibly result in the child coming down with a cold, but this is an appropriate exposure task. On the other hand, asking a child to handle feces and then put her fingers in her mouth would present an unusually high level of risk and would not be an appropriate exposure task. In another situation, having a child with self-harm obsessions hold a butter knife next to her wrist during an exposure involves a utensil used regularly by kids that would be unlikely to cause significant harm even if accidentally dropped, and is an appropriate exposure task. However, having a child hold a very sharp chef's knife that a child would not usually be allowed to handle would not be an appropriate exposure task.

Frequency, Duration, and Length of Sessions

The timing of sessions—regarding frequency, duration, and length—will vary based on multiple factors, including the severity and complexity of clinical presentation, the motivation and commitment of children and parents, and logistical considerations with scheduling sessions. As a range of reference, successful CBT-based treatment outcome studies of pediatric OCD have typically included approximately 14 sessions, 60 to 90 minutes each, delivered weekly over 12 to 14 weeks (Storch et al., 2007, March et al., 2004). In addition, CBT for OCD has been delivered successfully in more intensive formats: 10 sessions, 60 to 90 minutes each, 1 to 3 times per week over 4 to 7 weeks (Bolton & Perrin, 2008); 14 sessions, 90 minutes each, 4 to 5 times per week over 3 weeks (Storch et al., 2007). It is of note that although ERP was central to the above CBT treatments, it was not included in every session—some sessions were dedicated to psychoeducation, cognitive restructuring, other relaxation techniques, and so on, and these were often presented prior to the onset of ERP sessions. Interestingly, a study on the timing of exposure in CBT for pediatric anxiety disorders concluded that exposures can be successfully introduced earlier in treatment than manuals may suggest, and it might not be necessary to introduce other anxiety coping strategies prior to the onset of exposures (Gryczkowski et al., 2013).

Cognitive Considerations

Cognitive restructuring (see description in chapter 4) to help children build confidence and motivation to engage in ERP is a skill that must be used carefully in the OCD treatment process. During the actual exposure, use of this skill should be minimized or avoided, as it may become a ritual itself and might prevent the youth from fully experiencing the feared stimuli (see chapter 5 for detailed explanation). Importantly, a moderate level of anxiety or discomfort *should* be experienced by the youth as part of the ERP process in order for it to be successful (Benito et al., 2012). Thus, during the exposures, children should be directed to attend to negative thoughts related to their feared OCD outcomes, rather than trying to escape these thoughts. For example, while a child with contamination obsessions is touching a doorknob, she should be directed to think about the fact that the doorknob probably does have germs on it. This is necessary for children to habituate to their core fears and learn that they can survive their most feared situations. Similarly, you need to be careful not to inadvertently provide cognitive reassurance during exposures. In other words, refrain from saying things like, "It's okay, this isn't very dirty," or "You'll be fine" during an exposure. Rather, you can validate the difficulty of the task while continuing to focus attention on the feared stimuli—for example, "I know this might be a challenging exposure because there could be lots of germs on that doorknob and I can see you are working really hard."

Along these lines, a key cognitive piece to address in OCD treatment is intolerance of uncertainty (IU). Rather than focusing on the improbability of a child's feared consequences, a more helpful treatment goal is to help the child learn to live with the uncertainty that feared consequences may occur. To this end, it is important to help the child realize that his attempts to be 100% certain are futile, that such efforts result in significant losses of time, energy, and relationships, and that it is more constructive to plan how to cope with feared consequences that could result from ERP (e.g., Grayson, 2010; see also chapter 4).

Another useful cognitive consideration is the potential benefit of externalizing the OCD for children (in other words, saying, *It's the OCD talking,* when they have OCD thoughts or urges). For younger children, this may mean calling the OCD a name like "Mr. Worry" or "the Fear Monster," and drawing a picture to animate it. Externalizing the OCD provides a way to conceptualize the ERP process as "the youth" versus "the OCD," with you rooting for the youth to "win" by not giving in to OCD's deceptive tricks and requests. In this way, you can help empower the child to be stronger than the OCD.

Family Education and Parental Involvement

Although well intentioned, parents frequently inadvertently reinforce their child's OCD symptoms through accommodating behaviors they carry out to reduce their child's level of distress. Indeed, a CBT study designed to examine family accommodation in pediatric OCD reported that it was present in 88% of cases (Merlo, Lehmkuhl, Geffken, & Storch, 2009). The following are some common examples of accommodation in OCD.

Supporting or enabling avoidance by performing the child's avoided tasks. For example, for kids who fear contamination with germs, parental accommodation may include touching door handles (or other potentially "dirty" things) for kids, or wiping for them after they use the toilet (for older children who refuse to wipe themselves).

Behaving in line with the child's OCD rituals. For example, parents may agree to everyday washing of "contaminated" clothing or towels, or actively avoiding public restrooms for a child with contamination obsessions; or redoing things for kids several times, such as re-tying shoes until the child feels it has been done in a way that feels "just right."

Providing verbal reassurance by repeatedly answering their child's reassurance-seeking questions. For example, a child who fears harming a pet may ask the parent repeatedly how the pet is doing and whether it is hurt in any way, and the parent might routinely reassure the child that the pet is fine. Or a child with contamination fears might ask a parent if food is safe to eat before every meal or snack, and the parent might routinely reassure her that it's safe to eat.

Parental accommodation can impact the degree to which—and how quickly—ERP for OCD is effective. Merlo and colleagues (2009) found that higher family accommodation levels were associated with more severe child OCD symptoms at baseline, and decreases in family accommodation during CBT were predictive of positive treatment outcome. Thus, it is very important to work with parents to identify accommodating behaviors at the outset of therapy and to address these throughout the treatment process. Please refer to chapter 3 for a detailed discussion of how to help parents tolerate child discomfort during exposures, refrain from engaging in accommodations, appropriately encourage their child's efforts, and provide positive reinforcement.

Exposure Tasks and Activities Guide

Below, we present a wide list of activities and ideas as a guide for clinicians' use in generating creative and beneficial tasks for a child's exposure hierarchy in ERP for OCD. These examples are not designed to be utilized in sequence, as each may or may not apply to the client, and they are not organized by difficulty level (which also varies by client). Rather, you should use clinical judgment, as well as parent and child input, to tailor tasks to the individual needs of each child and to determine the most effective order of steps.

CONTAMINATION

Visual/Auditory Exposures

Draw pictures of people touching "dirty" things and then pictures of the same people touching their faces or eating with their dirty hands. (You can also make a "flip-book" with a series of these pictures to "animate" the person).

Draw cartoon-type pictures of little bacteria or viruses; give them facial expressions and silly names.

Look at pictures (online, in magazines, in books) of people touching "dirty" things or engaging in unsanitary behaviors (example: jumping in mud puddle).*

Look at up-close pictures of bacteria or viruses.*

Create a collage of images related to contamination and disgust (examples: feces, blood, vomit, dirt) and look at it repeatedly.*

*You can use exposure pictures to make a matching-pairs "memory game" to play with the child: Print or photocopy duplicates of each image, then scramble all the pictures and turn them upside-down on the floor. Take turns flipping over two images at a time, trying to find a matching pair). Habituation can also be bolstered by hanging up exposure pictures in the home, where they will be seen frequently (although it may not be appropriate, depending on the images, who else is present in house, and so on).

Watch a video clip (from the Internet or a movie), or listen to an audio clip (from a book on tape), of someone engaging in feared contamination-related behaviors (for example, a person eating something dirty, falling into a portable toilet, or vomiting).

Imaginal Exposures

Write out detailed feared contamination scenarios on paper or the computer. Include uncertainty scripts or statements that the feared consequences *might* happen (versus *will* happen). Read silently and aloud. Make an audio recording of these and listen to it as frequently as possible.

Imagine any of the below in vivo scenarios. (You can ask the child to vocalize the details as he is envisioning them.) Alternatively, read a feared scenario to the child while he closes his eyes and imagines it.

While using the scenarios below, have the child imagine that there are little germs all over the surfaces she is touching, germs on the foods and drinks she is consuming, or germs on the plates and utensils she is using. Have her envision the little germs crawling onto her hands or going into her tummy. Ask her to tell you what types of germs could be on the surfaces (example: "I might be touching a flu virus that could make me sick.").

In Vivo Exposures

Touch potentially "contaminated" surfaces around the office building, such as doorknobs (to office, bathrooms, stairwells, exits), tabletops, elevator buttons, banisters in stairwells, and so on. Similar exposures can also be done in other public places, such as the mall (touching handrails on escalators or balconies around the mall).**

Shake hands of staff around the office.**

Go outside and touch objects such as picnic benches, mailboxes, and parking lot signs.**

Go outside and touch things in nature that might be naturally "unclean"— such as trees, plants, grass, and dirt.**

**Following any of these activities, as a more difficult step in the hierarchy, have the child touch his face or eat a snack without washing his hands beforehand.

Touch a stuffed animal to "contaminated" surfaces and then touch, hug, or play with the stuffed animal. Have the "dirty" stuffed animal "cross-contaminate" other things, like the car, or the bedroom.

After child touches "contaminated" things herself, go to other settings (examples: bedroom in house, desk at school, seats in car), or to other people, and "cross-contaminate" them.

Wear "contaminated" clothing around the house, or to school.

Use furniture items or spend time in rooms that are believed to be "contaminated" (example: sit on the couch that brother sat on when he was home sick).

Drink from a public water fountain (at a mall, gym, school, park).

Spend time in places with a high likelihood of germ exposure (examples: sit in waiting room at doctors' offices or hospitals, ride the metro or subway, use public restrooms); in these locations, touch door handles, handrails, magazines, and so on, as further exposures.

Participate in peer-based group activities that could lead to exposure to germs (example: play basketball with shared ball).

Eat fruit that does not look fresh (examples: a banana with brown spots, a pear with bruises) without washing or wiping it off.

Drink from cup that therapist provides (so client is unsure where it came from, when it was last washed, and so on); to increase challenge, use cup with visible water spots. Eat food from plate (and with utensils) that therapist provides; to increase challenge, add crumbs to plate ahead of time to make it look dirty.

Eat food without knowing the expiration date.

Eat food that therapist provides and has been previously unwrapped (example: a cheese stick) so child does not know where it came from, who has touched it, and so on.

Go to movie theater and get popcorn from hand-serviced machine, then eat it.

Create or purchase and hold fake vomit, feces, blood, or urine (recipes online).

Touch toilet seats and bathroom floors at home and in public. To increase challenge, follow this with eating a snack.

Recontamination. This is an additional step often used as part of the exposure process in contamination-related OCD. After any decontamination procedure (a daily routine such as showering, or any "cleaning" action performed in response to touching an item not yet mastered in exposures), have the child immediately touch the "contaminated" object, surface, or person that he is currently working on mastering (or touch something that it has touched—such as a towel that was rubbed on a public hand railing and likely has germs on it). This method ensures the child is never completely free from contamination from that object, surface, or person.

Reducing Compulsions, Safety Behaviors, and Avoidance. Refrain from having child wash hands or body, or change clothing directly following exposures. This includes using hand sanitizer or any other cleaning product. Specify the amount of time you want to elapse after the exposure and before such behaviors are allowed to occur.

Practice reducing frequency, time, and quantity related to activities the child engages in to "get clean" during a regular day. For example, reduce number of times allowed to wash hands or shower, reduce duration of washing hands or showering, reduce amount of soap or shampoo used, leave one item of "contaminated" clothing on after returning home from school, and so on.

Intentionally leave out steps in the showering process. For example, get hair wet but leave out step of shampoo or conditioner; or omit washing certain body parts. Alternatively, change order of operations in showering process (example: instead of washing from head to feet, wash starting at feet up to head).

Reduce the frequency with which clothing, towels, or other objects are washed, and, if applicable, shift person who does the washing. (Example: if child usually wants to do it herself, have parent do it instead.) Refrain altogether from washing things that would not usually be laundered (examples: backpack, binders).

Reduce or eliminate barrier methods (examples: shirt sleeve, tissue, paper towel) the child uses to touch things he views as "contaminated," or that the child uses to keep already "contaminated" body areas from touching "noncontaminated" things (example: paper towel to hold food so he can eat it without the food touching dirty hands).

Reduce ability of child to check or inspect objects, surfaces, or foods (item of food itself, expiration date, package), to look for any indication of "contamination." For example, black out expiration dates on food packages.

Have parents and others refrain from answering reassurance-seeking questions (or providing unprompted reassurance) regarding: cleanliness level (examples: door handles, banisters), objects related to eating (plates, utensils, cups), clothing and furniture, food quality or safety. Parents can acknowledge the difficulty of the situation and provide appropriate responses as noted in chapter 3.

Have parents and others refrain from engaging in accommodating behaviors, such as opening doors for kids, checking food expiration dates for them, doing extra laundry for them, wiping for them after bathroom use, and so on.

HARM/CATASTROPHE

Visual/Auditory Exposures

Look at pictures (online, in magazines, in books) or draw pictures related to "terrible" thoughts—but that do not involve actual death or harm (examples: person standing on a balcony, person with cancer running a race, fire burning in a living room fireplace). You can use exposure pictures to make a matching-pairs "memory game" (see * earlier in chapter). It may also be helpful to hang up pictures in the home, where they can be viewed frequently.

Watch a video clip (from Internet or movie), or listen to an audio clip (from a book on tape), related to "terrible" thoughts—but that do not involve actual death or harm (examples: a person lighting a candle then walking out of the room, a person using knives in the kitchen).

Write out feared "terrible" words or phrases several times on paper or the computer (example: write *My mom could have cancer* repeatedly for 1 to 3 minutes). Read this out loud repeatedly (example: for 1 to 3 minutes).

Record (on the phone or voice recorder) child saying "terrible" words or phrases repeatedly for 1 to 3 minutes; practice listening to the recording both during and between sessions.

Imaginal Exposures

Make detailed uncertainty scripts or statements that the feared consequences *might* happen (versus *will* happen). Record and listen to these as frequently as possible.

Imagine any of the following in vivo scenarios. (You can ask child to vocalize the details as she is envisioning them.) Alternatively, read a feared scenario to the child while she closes her eyes and imagines it.

In Vivo Exposures

Light a candle, blow it out, then immediately leave the room or house. Turn on a toaster oven or stove then leave the room or house for X number of minutes.

Practice calling or texting parent to check in (attempted reassurance-seeking to see if parent is "okay") and have parent not pick up call and not respond to text. (Build up amount of nonresponsive time.)

Hold a butter knife up to child's wrist (if fear of hurting self) or to your wrist (if fear of hurting others).

Sit next to an open window; then stand next to the window (modify difficulty level by first using a window with a screen for both, then a window without a screen for both, and so on). Practice sitting and standing on a balcony or bridge.

Write the "terrible" thoughts on a slip of paper and keep it in the child's pocket all day, or give the slip of paper to other family members and have them carry it in their pocket or bag all day.

Make a wristband with "terrible" words or phrases written on the underside of it (example: write in a narrow line on paper, laminate or cover with clear tape, cut out strip, attach Velcro to either end) and wear it around during the day or in bed at night.

Practice thinking "terrible" things while looking at people (or pictures of people) the child cares about.

Practice saying the "terrible" thing out loud to a person the child cares about (example: saying to therapist, "You might get cancer," or "You might get in a car accident").

Wear "terrible" or "unlucky" (such as "cancer causing") clothing around the house or to school.

Go to places associated with feared thoughts. (Example: if the child has a fear of himself or family member getting cancer, go to a cancer treatment center and sit in the waiting area, or attend a cancer awareness event.)

Engage in social situations or group activities previously avoided due to stimuli related to "terrible" thoughts. (Example: go on a camping trip knowing a bonfire is planned.)

Practice tolerating being near or holding containers of household cleaners, or other products that have warning signs (example: nail polish remover), that could lead to harm if misused.

Practice using objects that have tiny parts: play with toys that have small parts (example: LEGOs) or board games with little pieces (examples: *Life, Battleship*), or use tiny household items (examples: paper clips, staples).

Practice tolerating parents having a fire going in the fireplace.

Practice being alone with the person who the client fears harming.

Reducing Compulsions, Safety Behaviors, and Avoidance

Reduce or eliminate counting behaviors or doing things a certain "good" number of times or certain multiples of numbers. This may include touching or tapping things, or breathing or blinking repeatedly. Practice doing things a "bad" or "unlucky" number of times instead, as a first step. Sometimes a child views it as "more okay" to do this if the therapist is telling him the number of times to engage in behavior; thus, it can be helpful to write down "bad" or "unlucky" numbers on slips of paper, put these into a hat, and have the child pick a number out of the hat to determine which number to use for each exposure.

Refrain from (or at first reduce frequency of) repeating words or phrases (silently, quietly, or out loud). To help with practice, have child engage in a mental task (such as a complex math problem) that would be nearly impossible to do at the same time as the mental ritual due to competing executive functioning resources. However, be careful not to replace current mental rituals with new ones, and not to distract the child too much from the feared stimuli.

Reduce or eliminate child's behaviors related to checking self or others for any evidence of harm. For example, have child wear pants and long sleeves so she cannot regularly check arms and legs for any cuts or scratches.

Reduce or limit child's behaviors related to checking things repeatedly that could be connected to "catastrophic" situations. For example, refrain from letting the child: check the door several times to be sure that it is locked; check the toaster oven and stove repeatedly to be sure they are off; check the level of cleaners in bottles to be sure they have not changed since last used; check that no small toy parts are missing.

Have parents and others refrain from answering reassurance-seeking questions (or providing unprompted reassurance) about the safety or health of them or others. Parents can acknowledge difficulty of the situation and provide appropriate responses as noted in chapter 3.

Have parents and others refrain from engaging in accommodating behaviors, such as promoting avoidance related to fears (examples: never using candles or fireplace in house, never leaving child alone with sibling).

SYMMETRY/"JUST RIGHT"

Visual/Auditory Exposures

Look at pictures (online, in magazines, in books) of asymmetrical things or "messy" scenarios (examples: a very disorganized desk or room, a crooked picture hanging on a wall). You can use exposure pictures to make a matching-pairs "memory game" (see * earlier in this chapter). It may also be helpful to hang up exposure pictures in the home, where they can be viewed frequently.

Draw pictures of asymmetrical things or people doing things in a "not just right" way. (You can also make "flip-book" with a series of these pictures to "animate" the person).

Watch a video clip (from the Internet or a movie), or listen to an audio clip (from a book on tape), of someone doing something in a disorganized or "not just right" way (example: someone putting on shoes and not tying the laces correctly, or putting up hair in a messy, lopsided way).

Imaginal Exposures

Write out scenarios about disorganized, asymmetrical, or "not just right" scenarios on paper or the computer. Include uncertainty scripts or statements that the feared consequences *might* happen (versus *will* happen). Make an audio recording of these and listen to it as frequently as possible.

Imagine any of the following in vivo scenarios (you can ask child to vocalize the details as he is envisioning them). Alternatively, read a feared scenario to child while he closes his eyes and imagines it happening.

In Vivo Exposures

Tilt pictures around the room in an uneven way, or rearrange furniture or objects in the room in an imbalanced way, and leave them like that the entire session until after the client leaves.

Tie shoes, wear clothes, or style hair in a "messy" or lopsided way or a way that doesn't feel "just right"; wear this way for increasing amounts of time throughout the day.

Intentionally make mistakes while writing sentences (examples: spell words incorrectly, use grammar incorrectly), by hand or on the computer.

Practice handwriting in a messy way. To aid in "response prevention" if the child has difficulty not going back to fix letters along the way, you can hold an index card down on the page to cover the words just written by the child.

Make binder or backpack messy or disorganized and go to school with it that way.

Mess up books on shelf (or papers on desk) in therapist's office or at home and leave them that way throughout session (in the office) or for hours or days (at home).

Practice reading pages in a book (and sentences within each page) only once, by using a blank piece of paper to cover each sentence after reading it (slowly covering up whole page so child cannot look back to reread sentences). After reading each full page, use a large binder clip to hold pages together that have already been read (to inhibit flipping back to reread pages).

Coordinate with teachers at child's school to have child turn in an "imperfect" homework assignment.

Say "I love you" (or other typically repeated phrase) only once at night before bed, before leaving for school, and so on.

Shift sequence of completing activities that the child usually does in a very specific "just right" order, or intentionally leave out steps in these processes. For example, have the child get dressed in an unusual order, or get hair wet but leave out step of shampoo, or omit washing certain body parts during shower.

Reducing Compulsions, Safety Behaviors, and Avoidance

Put a time limit on activities that child gets stuck on doing until they "feel right." For example, limit duration of getting dressed, doing hair, taking shower, and so on. It may be helpful to use a timer so the child can see how much time is left and try to "beat the buzzer."

Put a frequency limit on activities the child gets stuck on doing. For example, limit number of times allowed to change outfits, retie shoes, or redo hair.

Refrain from organizing or arranging things in specific or symmetrical ways, especially following related exposure tasks.

Reduce or eliminate repeatedly checking things to be sure they were completed fully or done well.

Reduce or eliminate counting behaviors or doing things a certain "good" number of times. This may include touching or tapping things, or breathing or blinking repeatedly. Practice doing things a "bad" or "unlucky" number of times instead, as a first step (example: odd numbers instead of even). As noted above, it can be helpful to write down "bad" or "unlucky" numbers on slips of paper and have the child draw these from a hat to determine which number to use for each exposure.

Have parents and others refrain from answering reassurance-seeking questions about whether something looks "good" or "perfect," or whether the child did a "good" or "perfect" job at something. Parents can acknowledge the difficulty of the situation and provide appropriate responses as noted in chapter 3.

Have parents and others refrain from engaging in accommodating behaviors, such as retying the child's shoes until they feel "just right."

Case Example

A 10-year-old male presented with fears of exposure to chemicals and getting cancer. These originated from a warning label he saw on a new couch in their family room that stated it may contain chemicals linked to cancer and birth defects. The child viewed most of the house as "contaminated," since he had sat on the couch and touched many things for several days before reading the label. Other family members were viewed as contaminated as well, with his mother considered the most highly contaminated because she had recently sprained her ankle and spent significant time on the couch.

The child avoided not only the couch and family room, but any physical contact with other family members (as they continued to use the couch) or with objects recently touched by them. (For example, he avoided sitting in kitchen chairs regularly used by family members.) He got into many heated fights with his siblings and parents at home if they touched him or his stuff. He engaged in extensive cleaning rituals each day—such as aggressively washing his hands if he came into contact with "contaminated" surfaces, objects, or people, and taking 75-minute showers in the morning before school. He did laundry himself every day, as he did not want his mother to touch his clothing or towels (and he refused to use anything she washed). Several family accommodation behaviors were ongoing. For example, his parents would "reserve" his specific seat at the dinner table, and would direct his siblings to sit in other seats and not touch his chair. They also let him watch TV in the guest room so he didn't have to go in the family room. His parents regularly answered his reassurance-seeking questions directly—telling him no chemicals were present and he was not going to get cancer, and so on.

The child also took measures to prevent "safe" places (such as his school) from getting contaminated. He showered extensively immediately before going to school, and would not sit on or touch anything around the house before leaving. He refused to bring his backpack or any schoolwork inside the house for fear of contaminating them, and he avoided the computer (contaminated from sibling use). Thus he often did not complete homework assignments, and his teachers noted he was falling behind in classes.

After building therapeutic rapport, providing psychoeducation on OCD, and discussing cognitive reframing (including addressing his intolerance of uncertainty, and externalizing the OCD as "the Worrymeister"), an exposure hierarchy was developed collaboratively. During all exposures, he was instructed to think about the fact that there might be cancer-causing chemicals on whatever was the focus of the exposure, and he gave "worry thermometer" ratings before, during, and after exposures. Parental accommodation behaviors were targeted early in treatment: parents were coached on how to handle reassurance-seeking questions (for example, reflecting back uncertainty about the presence of cancer-causing chemicals: "I don't know, maybe.") and how to refrain from feeding into the child's avoidance behaviors and rituals (allowing him to watch TV only in family room, for example, and allowing his siblings to sit anywhere).

From the first office visit (during which the child spent some time in the waiting room while his mother was inside the office), the child was clearly anxious about which seat his mother had been sitting in, so he sat on the floor. Thus, initial exposure sessions occurred in the office with the child practicing sitting for increasing periods of time in various seats that his mother might have sit in. "Contaminated" items from home (laptop, blanket, couch pillow) were brought in to practice using these items and to further "contaminate" the office environment. Next, exposure work included having him bring his backpack and schoolwork to the "contaminated" office. He initially brought his binders in a plastic bag, and gradually worked toward placing the binders in various contaminated places around the office (on the chair where his mother had been sitting, for example), then opening them, touching the pages, and so on.

Ritual reduction was also incorporated into treatment from the outset of exposure work. A key target was the extensive cleaning ritual of a 75-min shower before school. The amount of soap used in the shower was gradually reduced, the duration was progressively shortened, and the amount of time between showering and leaving the house was increased, with recontamination exposures added after the shower (for example, sitting in a kitchen chair used by his mother). The washing of objects and hand-washing after touching "contaminated" surfaces, objects, or people, was gradually eliminated. Furthermore, his mother was incorporated into the laundry process. For example, one step was having her take items from the washer and put them in the dryer—thus "recontaminating"—then he would remove items from dryer. The child also practiced wearing articles of clothing or using towels washed by his mother (first practiced after school, then prior to school). Excel charts were used to track between-session ERP goals; he earned points toward small prizes and larger fun activities (trampoline park, mini golf). The child also received regular positive reinforcement from the therapist and his parents in the form of verbal praise for his efforts.

Imaginal exposure work included recording an uncertainty script related to potentially being exposed to chemicals and developing cancer. He earned points for listening to this frequently between sessions. Another exposure task involved printing out copies of various warning labels related to chemicals known to cause cancer. He was instructed to put these in places where he would regularly see them at home (such as on the bathroom mirror, the door, or the bedside table); to put one inside each school binder; and to put one in his pocket and carry it around with him throughout the day. The therapist also conducted exposure sessions in both the home and school environments—these were extended sessions, 2 to 3 hours each. In the home, exposures focused on having the child touch contaminated areas (working up to sitting or lying on the primary source of contamination—the couch) then cross-contaminating throughout the house (for example, to all chairs, bathroom, and bedroom). Next, his school backpack and binders were brought into the home and used in various locations around the house.

Following an extended home visit, videoconferencing with the therapist was briefly used to support the child in initiating continued exposure practice at home. The school exposure session was coordinated with the school counselor and took place during after-school hours. His mother came to school with him and brought a pillow from the couch. Exposures included having his mother and the pillow touch his locker, his books and binders, his desk in each classroom, his table in the lunch room, and various areas of the gymnasium, auditorium, and library. The school exposures were the most distressing for the child (his mother was coached to remain calm and slowly proceed with the exposures), but also led to the greatest jump in improvement and highest child-reported feeling of accomplishment.

After 5 months of continued ERP practice, the child reported that worry thoughts still occasionally entered his mind and elicited mild anxiety, but the "Worrymeister" now had a very soft voice that he could easily not listen to. He was using the family room and couch regularly, playing with his siblings, and interacting normally with his mother. He no longer engaged in excessive cleaning rituals—he took brief showers at night and let his mom do his laundry. His proudest accomplishment was improved performance at school because he brought home schoolwork every day, got back on track with classes, and subsequently raised all his grades.

Conclusion

OCD is a highly prevalent disorder in childhood and adolescence that can have a significantly detrimental impact on functioning across social, academic, and home life. Current treatment outcome research on pediatric OCD indicates that exposure-based CBT is most effective in reducing symptoms and leading to long-term improvement. This chapter reviewed the role of exposure therapy in treating OCD, diagnostic information, clinically relevant factors and assessment considerations, key components in ERP treatment, and methods of designing and implementing ERP tasks for youth with OCD. Across various types of OCD, samples of specific exposure tasks and ways to reduce safety behaviors were provided for consideration in creating individualized exposure hierarchies. It is our hope that the information conveyed in this chapter will help increase the number of mental health providers who feel comfortable and competent in delivering the highly effective method of ERP to children and adolescents with OCD who could benefit greatly from such treatment.

CHAPTER 15

Exposure for Emotion Tolerance

In this chapter, we review key assessment and treatment considerations and the implementation of exposure-based therapy for children and adolescents who struggle to manage and tolerate distress or intense emotions. The information included in this chapter is intended to support clinicians in creating and implementing an exposure hierarchy that is tailored to each individual client. Ideas for exposure tasks and activities are provided for consideration in creating individualized hierarchies. Additional treatment strategies that address the cognitive and physiological components of this problem are also highlighted. Finally, case examples are used to illustrate the clinician's role in implementing exposure tasks with real clients with these concerns.

Clinical Presentation and Causal Factors

Emotions are central to the human experience. Research suggests that highly emotional situations underlie our most salient memories and are the easiest to recall. Emotions also influence the way we perceive our world, and provide important information about our environment. For example, fear might tell us that we are in a dangerous situation and need to escape. Sadness often conveys that we are overwhelmed or overburdened and encourages us to slow down and withdraw. Anger is associated with threat and prepares us to fight. Happiness suggests that what we are doing may be good for us and we should keep doing it.

Some emotions are also directly linked to our "fight-or-flight" response (as discussed in chapter 4). When we feel scared, threatened, or otherwise distressed, our body's sympathetic nervous system is activated, preparing us for action. This system leads to increases in our heart rate, blood pressure, and respiration; a slowing of our digestive system; and pupillary dilation. These are often the sensations we most closely associate with strong emotions, such as anger and anxiety. Conversely, our parasympathetic nervous system serves to slow down our bodies. When this system is activated, our muscles loosen, our pupils contract, our heart rate and breathing slow, and our digestion speeds up. Thus, it is the parasympathetic nervous system that is associated with relaxation and a subjective state of calm.

While we often label an emotional response with a feeling (as in, "I came across a bear and felt frightened"), in reality, an emotional response usually also includes physical sensations, thoughts, and behavioral urges. A person's feeling about a situation (also known as "affect") consists of her own perception of emotions, such as "I feel sad now," or "I am afraid." Physiological sensations associated with the sympathetic nervous system are also intrinsically linked to these feelings—like the experience of clammy hands or a racing heart when anxious. Accompanying these feelings and sensations are often emotion-driven thoughts. These thoughts may shift, maintain, or exacerbate the feeling, as in, "I'm sad and I'm never going to feel better," or "I shouldn't be angry about this." Finally, specific behaviors, or urges to act, often also accompany feelings. These may include urges to escape from frightening situations or urges to lash out at people who we feel make us angry. Taken together, our affect, physical sensations, thoughts, and behavioral urges compose a complete emotional experience and direct our subsequent behaviors (what we choose to say, do, or think next).

Emotions and emotional responses play a critical role in mental health disorders and are often targets of change in therapy. Over the past decade there has been a marked increase in research on emotional vulnerabilities that underlie psychopathology, and a growing understanding that emotional distress is present in the majority of mental health disorders. Emotion-intolerant children may have difficulty recognizing the thoughts and behavioral urges associated with their emotional distress, and instead make general complaints of feeling intolerably upset, or broadly present as irritable. Often, children attempt to suppress these emotions or channel the distressing feelings into violence or aggression. Alternatively, they may engage in cognitive avoidance techniques, such as rumination (Nolen-Hoeksema & Morrow, 1993). Research suggests that people who ruminate avoid the actual experience of the emotion by engaging in a repetitive thinking process without having to experience the distressing feeling directly (Giorgio et al., 2010). Counterintuitively, attempts to control or avoid these emotions often serve to make them more salient and long-lived (e.g. Spinhoven et al., 2016). Thus, increasing emotional distress tolerance is now recognized as an important target for mental health treatments across diagnoses (e.g., Boisseau et al., 2010; Linehan, 1993).

Exposure Therapy for Emotion Tolerance

The goal behind exposure-based approaches for youth with heightened intolerance for emotions is similar to treating other forms of anxiety disorders. Specifically, by being exposed to a feared emotion, the child will gain a sense of acceptance of these feelings and learn that affect is temporary. Like most physical pain a child might be familiar with (such as getting a splinter or stubbing a toe), mental pain can come on quickly and strongly. However, it recedes and disappears over time. It may be helpful to review with a child that strong emotional feelings are like jumping into a cold pool. At first, he will feel extreme discomfort and want to escape by getting out of the water. But, over time, his body temperature will adjust and the unpleasant feeling will go away. Attempts to avoid experiencing emotional pain inhibit the child's ability to acclimate to the affect and, in turn, prevent it from fully dissipating.

Currently, exposure-based methods for increasing distress tolerance are utilized as part of several CBT-based treatment packages for adults, such as the Unified Protocol for the Treatment of Emotional Disorders (UP; Barlow et al., 2011), Dialectical Behavior Therapy (DBT; Linehan, 1993) and Acceptance and Commitment Therapy (ACT; Hayes, Strosahl, & Wilson, 1999). While these approaches have been shown to increase emotional tolerance and reduce negative mood states (e.g. Ellard et al., 2010), they are primarily used alongside other distress-reducing techniques. Research examining the effect of emotional exposures alone is limited, and only recently have these approaches been extended for treating distress intolerance in younger populations (e.g. Seager, Rowley, & Ehrenreich-May, 2014). Though still emerging, early evidence indicates that emotion-intolerant youth can benefit from exposure-based methods.

Clinically Relevant Factors

The environmental context (both internal and external) within which the child feels distressed, and the specific nature of the child's cognitions and behavioral responses, are critical considerations in the subsequent engineering of effective exposure exercises. Special attention should be paid to any history of engaging in experiential avoidance or other maladaptive behaviors associated with distressing feelings. Please refer to chapter 2 for more detailed discussion of broad functional assessment strategies. Below we present typical fear triggers or cues, feared consequences, and avoidance and safety behaviors commonly occurring in children with emotion and distress intolerance:

Fear Cues

Fear cues or triggers are specific internal or external environmental factors that typically elicit the child's distress. These are the situations that activate the fear response due to the presence of specific stimuli that are perceived to be dangerous or harmful in some way. The following fear cues commonly trigger distress in children with intolerance for emotions:

Internal feelings and strong negative mood states—such as anger, sadness, fear, shame, or embarrassment

Being confronted with people or situations that the child does not think she can handle or that she associates with negative mood states

Specific physical reactions associated with perceived internal discomfort (physiological changes associated with activation of the sympathetic nervous system), such as a racing heart or muscle tension; or more diffuse, unpleasant sensations, such as stomachaches or headaches

Memories of distressing emotional reactions (for example, thinking about previous periods of sadness, or being in situations that remind the child of times he had difficulty tolerating his emotions)

Requests from others to talk about situations that elicit the undesirable emotional experience

Feared Consequences

Feared consequences are those environmental conditions and outcomes that the child expects will result from exposure to emotional distress. That is, the child's distress is initiated and maintained through her experience or her belief that these negative outcomes will occur. The following are common feared consequences in children with intolerance of emotions:

Losing control or being overwhelmed by emotion

"Going crazy"

Experiencing physical harm from intense emotional experiences

Being judged negatively by others

Being incapable of completing or participating in an activity or situation

Avoidance

Children with intolerance of extreme emotional states commonly avoid the environmental stimuli and situations that trigger their distress because they perceive a high likelihood of their feared consequences occurring. The following are common avoidant behaviors observed in children with intolerance of emotions:

Rumination, or dwelling on the causes and consequences of distressing feelings and the accompanying negative affect

Emotion suppression, or portraying a false emotional reaction to a situation

Refusal to acknowledge or discuss difficult emotions or situations that elicit difficult emotions

Use of distraction, or refusal to be present with an emotional experience

Engaging in aggressive or risky behaviors, such as hitting, kicking, or breaking things

Substance use

Self-harm behaviors (such as cutting, scratching, or hitting one's head against the wall)

Withdrawal from other people or activities for fear they will trigger the emotions

Safety Behaviors

Children who have trouble tolerating distressing emotions often rely on specific objects, individuals, or actions that they believe will protect them from the feared stimuli or feared outcome. Safety behaviors are any actions that are performed in an attempt to feel safe. The following are common safety behaviors displayed by children and adolescents with intolerance of emotions:

Seeking out reassurance from a parent or trusted adult that the child will be okay and that he won't be upset by an upcoming event

Keeping adults in close physical proximity in case the child needs to be soothed

Engaging in distracting activities to avoid thinking about the feeling

Keeping an object with her as a safety mechanism (such as a phone or stuffed animal)

Tailoring Exposure Therapy for Distress-Intolerant Youth

This section will explore specific concerns related to implementing exposure therapy for distress-intolerant and emotion-avoidant youth. It builds on guidance presented in earlier chapters by offering the therapist specific suggestions for what must be uniquely considered when carrying out this work with youth experiencing challenges tolerating, managing, regulating or expressing emotions such as sadness, anger, frustration, and embarrassment. Additional strategies and modifications to the treatment approach that are of paramount importance to implementing exposure-based work with this group are discussed as follows.

Exposures, as well as cognitive challenges, should be tailored to the needs of the child and based on information gathered from assessment. Similar to exposures in the treatment of anxiety, the goals of exposure-related exercises for addressing other emotions—such as frustration, sadness, and embarrassment—are the development of increased tolerance of the overall emotional experience, habituation to physical cues, and improved cognitive efficacy in the ability to discuss and manage these emotions. A hierarchy will be developed that focuses on the emotional experience that is currently avoided or difficult to manage. For example, a series of increasingly frustrating tasks may be engineered in session to build frustration tolerance. For sadness, a script may be created of a particularly sad event in the child's life and read repeatedly in stages until the sadness becomes more manageable.

Development of the Fear Hierarchy

Following an initial review of the rationale for exposure therapy, the child should understand that experiencing a variety of emotions, with varying intensities, are part of the typical human experience. It may be helpful to remind the child that emotions are often experienced like a wave crashing against the shore: "The wave may come on strong, and may briefly envelop us; but, with time, the wave will recede and go back into the ocean." Sitting with the emotion will allow the child to experience the analogous onset, cresting, and eventual receding of strong feelings.

As with other exposure techniques, close monitoring of the child's distress will be important in order to help him pay attention to the varying degrees of intensity of an emotional experience. In this case, you may help the child develop an intensity rating scale with different levels of the scale anchored to concrete descriptors. For instance, in developing an anger rating scale, the child should identify examples of varying degrees of the emotion, ranging from when he feels "just a little angry," which may be a number 2 on the scale, up to feeling like he is "exploding," which may be a 5 or a 6. Using examples of times from the child's life when he had these feelings will allow the therapist to more reliably assess the intensity of the emotion. It will also be important to help the child understand the accompanying facial and bodily expressions of each emotion that correspond to the different degrees or intensity of a feeling. With this goal in mind, therapists might consider taking photos of the child expressing different intensities of an emotion to display alongside the verbal descriptors. The resulting scale that is developed collaboratively with the child should be used to take emotion ratings every 1 to 2 minutes during an exposure, helping the child to chart the increase, plateau, and eventual decrease in distressing feelings.

In contrast to many of the exposure plans discussed elsewhere in this book, exposure hierarchies for increasing emotional tolerance will largely emphasize imaginal and role-play experiences in order to bring about the distressing feelings we want the child to habituate to. Thus, helping the child identify and accept these upsetting internal states, and understand the gradations in their emotion, is critical for measuring treatment progress. In addition, because many children struggle with overwhelming physiological sensations as they imagine, discuss, or role-play an experience associated with the targeted emotion, interoceptive exposures (as discussed in chapter 7) are often a helpful component of treatment, promoting increased tolerance of the physiological states they are avoiding. Finally, a reward system developed for use in the office or at home may focus on reinforcing the child's acceptance of an emotion or the expression of a feeling in a healthy and adaptive way. For example, a child could earn a sticker on a sticker chart for saying "I feel really angry," instead of kicking the wall or stomping away from a distressing situation.

Considering the Safety of Exposure Tasks

Very rarely, children may experience extreme emotional distress taking part in exposures designed to increase emotion tolerance. Although it's uncommon, therapists should be ready to address any potentially unsafe reactions to taking part in these activities. There are a number of potential obstacles to conducting exposure exercises both inside and outside of the office with distress-intolerant youth. These obstacles, presented in the following paragraphs, require careful planning and coordination with both the parent and the child.

BECOMING OVERLY EMOTIONALLY ENGAGED IN THE EXPOSURE

On occasion, a child may become overly engaged in an emotional experience to the point of seeming "stuck" in her own emotional reaction. Indeed, parents often name this as one of their biggest concerns with completing emotional exposure exercises. In reality, this happens only rarely during exposure exercises and is typically the result of the child not being mindfully engaged in the present. In these situations, it is helpful to stay calm and ask the child questions that turn her attention to what is going on in the present. For instance, the therapist might ask: "What does your body feel like right now?" "What do you notice your hands doing?" or "Where are your eyes focused?" Coaching the child to be mindfully aware during an exposure exercise allows her to gain a sense of mastery over her own emotional responses.

MELTDOWN OR TANTRUM DURING A HOME EXERCISE

Because avoidance of emotional experiences is the primary way in which emotional disorders are maintained, it is not surprising that an emotionally intolerant child would want to avoid engaging in exposure exercises. As therapists, we should prepare parents for the possibility that a child may have a tantrum or "meltdown" during an exposure exercise. We want to make parents feel well prepared for these reactions and remind them that they have the skills to handle any of their children's emotional responses. (Refer to chapter 3 for more details about these approaches.) First, the parent should be coached to validate the child's feelings without giving attention to the negative behavior (kicking, spitting, crying). Active ignoring strategies and positive reinforcement of appropriate reactions (in other words, "catching" the child doing something good, or displaying sadness rather than aggression when denied something he wants) are powerful tools for managing a child's emotional reactions. If the tantrum continues, it may be helpful for the parent to leave the room or have the child take a "cool down" break before reengaging him in the exercise. Finally, it is important to review with the parent and child limits within the home (for example, that it is acceptable to cry, but not to hit) and possible consequences for breaking those limits. Providing clear instructions in the office can decrease both the child's and the parent's anticipatory anxiety and set the stage for successful home-based exposure exercises.

FAILURE TO ELICIT THE DISTRESSING EMOTION

Emotional reactions to any given situation can be difficult to predict. It is possible that something that the child typically responds to with one emotion (for example, anger in response to having to do homework) may not bring about that response when conducting an exposure. Often this happens because the therapist has not accurately identified the specific trigger for a certain emotional reaction. For instance, a child may become angry when having to do homework that she does not understand (like a complicated math problem or ambiguous essay assignment). If the therapist has identified "doing homework" more generally as a trigger, an exposure exercise that involves completing easier homework assignments may not elicit the distress necessary for habituation. Thus, gathering more specific information about triggers of emotional responses will be critical for putting together the exposure hierarchy. One way to do this is to have the parent videotape exposure exercises completed at home. The therapist can then review these exercises with the child in session and query her about how she interpreted the situation and what did or did not feel distressing.

AVOIDANCE OF MENTAL ENGAGEMENT IN THE EXPOSURE

In other cases, it may be that the child is utilizing experiential avoidance even when completing an exposure exercise. For instance, a child may emotionally disengage while reading a story designed to elicit sadness. In order to increase engagement with imaginal exposures, it may be helpful to avoid having the child directly read from a script, but rather instruct him to tell the parent a story about the emotion-eliciting situation using as many sensory details as possible. The therapist may prompt the child to copy the facial and body postures consistent with the experience of that feeling. Encourage the child to identify which parts of telling the distressing story felt most uncomfortable (for example, making eye contact with the parent while talking, or including details about a specific section of the story) and then directly incorporate these elements in future exposure exercises.

Frequency, Duration, and Length of Sessions

Careful thought should be given to the structure of all exposure sessions. With regard to emotion tolerance, it is important to remember that the ultimate goal is habituation to the distress of having an emotion and recognition of coping capacity, as opposed to becoming less emotive. For example, in situations where mild or moderate anger would be expected, the goal is not to have a child feel neutral or nonresponsive, but rather to learn that anger—like all emotional experiences—is tolerable, and to learn to adaptively express that anger.

Thus, the number and length of exposure sessions should be based on the rate at which the child becomes more tolerant of experiencing various emotions. Repetition of specific exposures should be balanced with the introduction of new and more challenging activities. One specific difficulty with developing emotional tolerance relates to a core fear of many distress-intolerant youth—namely, that intense emotions will linger interminably. Ironically, once a child begins fully engaging with an emotional experience, she often finds that the feeling dissipates relatively quickly. Thus, as the child builds more tolerance for experiencing various emotions, it becomes more difficult to evoke any specific feeling for a considerable period of time. Therapists may therefore find that exposure exercises become shorter over time as the child learns to engage with her feelings and tolerate her emotional distress.

Other Considerations for Emotion Tolerance

Experiential exercises for emotional distress are common in several cognitive-behavioral-based therapeutic techniques. While this chapter largely focuses on specific exposure exercises for tolerating extreme emotional reactions, additional skills are critical for fostering distress tolerance in youth. As follows, we briefly review two other therapeutic approaches and related techniques to address mental and physical distress tolerance.

DIALECTICAL BEHAVIOR THERAPY

Dialectical Behavior Therapy (DBT; Linehan, 1993) is a form of cognitive behavioral therapy originally developed for use with clients who engage in self-harm behaviors. The therapy focuses on helping individuals learn skills for decreasing emotion dysregulation and increasing distress tolerance. The treatment is an evidence-based approach that typically involves group and individual therapy sessions, as well as skills coaching between sessions. While a comprehensive review of this treatment is outside the scope of this chapter, several DBT techniques are directly related to emotional tolerance. For instance, DBT encourages the use of specific skills for activating the parasympathetic nervous system when an individual is feeling overwhelmed by emotions, such as engaging in vigorous activity or submerging his face in cold water. DBT also encourages the use of self-soothing techniques to address emotional distress. Therapists and clients work together to create a list of calming, sensory-based activities the client can engage in when feeling upset, such as taking a bubble bath or listening to calming music. Interested clinicians are encouraged to learn more about the DBT process before implementing these techniques in their practice.

ACCEPTANCE AND COMMITMENT THERAPY

Acceptance and Commitment Therapy (ACT; Hayes et al., 1999) is another cognitive behavioral therapeutic approach that emerges from the paradox that many of the activities people engage in to feel better often serve to promote further suffering. ACT seeks to increase psychological flexibility by encouraging individuals to accept unpleasant emotional experiences as a normal and common part of the human experience. ACT clinicians often employ the metaphor of the Chinese finger trap in reference to handling distressing emotions. In a Chinese finger trap, when you pull your fingers away from each other, the material tightens around them and they get stuck. Similarly, when a child pulls away from negative emotions, she conversely ends up feeling trapped in the distress. To get out of a Chinese finger trap, you have to push your fingers together to give them room to wiggle out; to get through negative feelings, a child must stop struggling against feeling bad and accept these emotions in order to have more freedom to take action. ACT suggests a number of exercises to help an individual stop pulling away from distress and learn to accept and move through it. Techniques like mindfulness and meditation (reviewed in chapter 4) play an important role in helping children and adolescents to tolerate distress. Interested clinicians are encouraged to seek out further training and supervision in order to implement these techniques effectively.

Exposure Tasks and Activities Guide

In this section, we present a wide list of activities and ideas as a guide for clinicians' use in generating useful and creative tasks for a client's exposure hierarchy. These ideas are not organized in a sequence. Rather, the therapist should always use clinical judgment, as well as parent and child input, in determining the most effective next steps in any series of exposures, and should strive to tailor tasks to the individual needs of each child. This list can be used as a guide to help you select appropriate in-session and at-home exposure exercises.

FEELING ANGRY

Children who suppress their anger or lash out violently often do so because they experience the emotion as overwhelming. They may report a fear of losing control and hurting someone else. Alternatively, they may find the feeling of anger so distressing that they feel they need to physically release it through yelling, hitting, or kicking. When conducting these exposures, it is important that the child does not ruminate on the object of his anger, but rather focuses on the feeling he has when he feels angry. Across these exposures, ask the child to provide emotion ratings at different time-points to track changes in anger intensity. It may be helpful to also note the corresponding physiological and cognitive changes.

Visual/Auditory Exposure

Listen to recordings of insults or other things that make the child feel angry, such as another child saying that she is stupid or ugly. Bring the child's focus to the physical feelings of her anger and have her nonjudgmentally notice the thoughts in her head.

Show the child video clips of one child making fun of another (example: the scene in *A Christmas Story* in which a bully teases the main character).

Watch video clips of a parent providing an instruction to clean his room, turn off the TV or video game, start his homework, or any other command that typically elicits frustration.

Imaginal Exposures

Write about a time that she felt very angry. Make sure that she includes as many sensory details as possible. Then, have her read the story to herself over and over again, noticing how her body feels, thoughts that come to mind, and her behavioral urges.

Picture what he feels like when he's angry, focusing on each body part (such as how his hands feel, how his face feels, how his biceps feel, and so on).

Tell you about a scene in which she is not allowed to do something she wants. Have her pay attention to her angry thoughts and behavioral urges.

In Vivo Exposures

Ask the child to bring in a picture of someone who makes him feel very angry. Have him look at the picture and notice his own reactions to the photo.

Ask the child's parent or guardian to take a picture or video of the child while she is feeling overwhelmed with anger. Have the family bring the picture or video into the therapy session and have the child describe in detail what she was feeling.

Create a collage of words that make him feel angry or remind him of feeling angry. Ask the child to notice how his body feels when reading them.

Encourage the child to feel very angry, almost to the point of hitting something (or actually hitting a soft object like a pillow or mattress), and ask her to reflect on how her body feels.

Repeat the sentence *I'm so mad*, or *It's not fair*, over and over, focusing on the sensations it creates in the body.

Bring in a homework assignment that is difficult or tedious. Have him engage in completing the homework while noticing and tolerating feelings of frustration as they arise.

Transition back and forth between playing a video game for a few minutes and doing homework for a few minutes.

Ask the family to bring in materials needed to complete a chore that the child typically resists doing (examples: folding laundry, washing dishes, brushing teeth). Have the child engage in the task in session.

Play a game in which the child is intent on winning and have her lose this game.

Work on difficult brainteasers or puzzles likely to elicit frustration. Hologram puzzles in which each piece offers two different views of a picture can be particularly challenging.

Role-play the child receiving negative feedback from parents or teachers, being teased by a peer or sibling, or any other interpersonal situation that typically elicits frustration for that child.

Have the parent enter the session and provide commands or set a limit with the child (examples: "We cannot get ice cream after session," "When we get home you will need to start on your homework immediately.").

Request that the parent and child talk about a topic that they do not agree on.

FEELING SAD

Children, especially those going through a depressive episode, may develop a fear of feeling very sad. Exposures should be focused on the depression-related thoughts, physical sensations, and behaviors. As with anger, careful attention should be paid to making sure the child is not ruminating on sadness, but rather habituating to the feeling of sadness. Across these exposures, ask the child to rate his emotion intensity (or "sadness temperature") at different time-points to track changes in sadness intensity.

Visual/Auditory Exposure

Watch a very sad scene in a movie (example: the scene in *Bambi* when Bambi's mother is shot by hunters) and encourage the child to express her sadness by crying or furrowing her brow.

Show the child a picture of someone crying. Have him notice as many details about the picture as he can. Show the child a picture of someone he knows who appears sad or is crying.

Imaginal Exposures

Write or tell a story about a time the child was very sad. Have her read the story, including details about the thoughts, behavioral urges, and somatic symptoms she experienced. Have her describe what was heard, seen, tasted, touched, or smelled. Create a written script of the situation and repeatedly read the script to the child until anxiety and sadness reduce.

Ask the child to describe the saddest story he has ever heard, including as many details as possible.

In Vivo Exposure

Read the phrase *I feel sad* over and over again, focusing on the thoughts, behavioral urges, and physical symptoms this phrase brings about.

Ask the child to make a face and hold her body as if she is very sad. Have her maintain this position while she discusses how each part of her body feels.

FEELING GUILTY OR ASHAMED

It is not uncommon for children to deal with feelings of guilt or shame by attempting to suppress them. Exposures should focus on things that the child perceives (either accurately or not) to be his fault. Across these exposures, ask the child to rate his emotion intensity (or "guilt/shame temperature") at different time-points to track changes in intensity of feeling guilty or ashamed.

Visual/Auditory Exposure

Ask the child to create a story about a time she did something she felt was wrong or bad, encouraging her to include as many details as possible. Then have her listen to the recording, noticing her own reactions to the experience.

Imaginal Exposure

Come up with the worst things that the child feels he has done. Have him read the list repeatedly, focusing his attention on his feelings of shame, including his bodily reactions.

Ask the child to imagine engaging in a safe and legal activity that she feels is unethical or immoral. Have her then notice how each part of her body reacts to feeling ashamed.

In Vivo Exposures

Tell the child to purposefully make a minor mistake (example: not helping with a chore, not saying please or thank you for something given). Have him focus on what he feels in his body as this occurs.

FEELING EMBARRASSED

Different situations make different people feel embarrassed or vulnerable, so it is important to first get a sense of what elicits these feelings for the child. If she refuses to share what she finds most embarrassing, you can suggest situations that most people would feel some embarrassment about, such as nudity, being made fun of, or experiencing various bodily functions. Across these exposures, ask the child to rate her emotion intensity (or "embarrassment temperature") at different time-points to track changes in embarrassment intensity.

Visual/Auditory Exposure

Watch a very embarrassing scene in a movie (example: the scene in *Mean Girls* when the main character vomits on the object of her affection).

Look at pictures of people being made fun of or embarrassed by a situation.

Listen to sounds of flatulence or other bodily functions. Discourage the child from using laughter to avoid his feelings, and instead have him describe his internal sensations.

Draw a picture of a humiliating experience, including as many details as possible. Have the child tell you about the drawing and the details she included.

Imaginal Exposures

Imagine someone else feeling embarrassed, and ask the child to describe another child's experience with as many details as possible.

Ask the child to imagine and describe the most embarrassing thing that *could* happen, as if it were happening to him. Have him include a beginning, middle, and end; use first-person language; and talk about what he sees, hears, feels, tastes, and touches.

Write a story about the most embarrassing thing that has ever happened to the child, including what she thought, felt, and did, and have her read it out loud.

In Vivo Exposures

Role-play a humiliating or embarrassing experience with the child.

Ask the child to do something mildly embarrassing in public, such as doing jumping jacks randomly, dropping something, or speaking loudly in a quiet place. Other options include wearing an embarrassing piece of clothing in public, such as a funny hat, wig, or shoes. For an adolescent, he might practice dropping his change when paying for something in a store, or giving the cashier the wrong amount of cash. Have him notice the sensations of embarrassment and discuss these with you.

Case Example

A 14-year-old girl presented for treatment of her anxiety and depression symptoms. She reported that she would find herself becoming overwhelmed with these emotions, often engaging in crying fits in which she was not able to calm herself down for 15 to 20 minutes. She experienced many of these crying episodes as "out of the blue," and found them to be very embarrassing when they happened in front of her peers. For instance, on one occasion, she began to feel overwhelmed by sadness while at a soccer match. She started to cry loudly and felt unable to control herself, attracting the attention of many of the other students on her team. Following this experience, she began avoiding social activities, choosing instead to stay close to her mother in case she needed to be soothed.

Initially, the client voiced a preference for understanding the underlying causes of her psychological pain, rather than working on exposures to this distress. The therapist and child agreed that both of these goals could be worked on simultaneously and, after a review of the rationale for engaging in exposure therapy, she agreed to engage in these exercises. The therapist noted that while she would consistently report that she was sad, she also voiced an extreme aversion to sadness and a preference to distract herself from this feeling. For the first exposure, the client and therapist agreed that for 15 minutes they would repeatedly listen to a song that the client deemed depressing. Prior to starting the exposure, the therapist and client discussed the client's expectations for the exercise. She reported she would likely feel distressed for the entire period in which she was listening to the song. They took sadness ratings before listening to the song and at 2-minute increments throughout the exercise. While listening to the song, the therapist encouraged the client to describe her thoughts, feelings, and behavioral urges. Much to her surprise, the client found that while she was initially distressed, this feeling quickly dissipated over the course of the song. She was encouraged to continue practicing this exercise at home with other songs and stimuli that cued her sadness.

For the next set of exposures, the therapist and client focused on situations in which she had felt emotionally overwhelmed. First, the client wrote out a narrative regarding the incident at the soccer game. The therapist encouraged her to include as many details as possible about what she was thinking and how she noticed her body responding. Although initially hesitant, the client then shared the story with the therapist several times, reporting her sadness ratings during each recitation of the narrative. She also agreed to share the story with her mother, slowly habituating to the anxiety of the memory. Next, the client and the therapist completed an imaginal exposure exercise in which the client described what it would be like to go to a soccer game and feel sad. She included information from each of her senses and described in detail what it would be like to be in the situation, while the therapist recorded her talking. For homework, she was asked to listen to the recording at least five times every day, noting her sadness ratings before, during, and after each exercise.

Finally, the client and therapist compiled a list of activities she would like to take part in. The first was to go to a soccer game while her mother waited in the car (rather than on the sidelines). The client and therapist discussed when this exposure would take place and addressed possible barriers to completing the exercise, including what to do if the client felt overwhelmed and began to cry. She was then asked to complete the exposure and report back to the therapist. After completing the activity, the client stated that it went well and she enjoying taking part in the game, despite experiencing a moderate, but tolerable, level of sadness. Over the coming weeks, the client completed a number of similar exposures, in which she took part in activities she anticipated would engender feelings of sadness. By the end of treatment, the client voiced that she was able to experience being sad without having it feel overwhelming. She understood the feeling came on strongly initially and, if she did not allow herself to escape the situation, the affect would dissipate naturally over the course of 10 to 15 minutes. After treatment, her mother reported that she was able to engage in all of the activities she had struggled with prior to coming to treatment and that she was looking forward to beginning high school, knowing that she could handle any strong emotions that might come her way.

Conclusion

Emotion-intolerant children evidence significant distress in the face of intense emotions they perceive as uncontrollable and unwanted. Children may go to extreme lengths to avoid experiencing certain emotions; however, this avoidance typically has the unwanted side effect of conversely increasing the distress associated with these feelings. CBT and related behavioral approaches emphasize the importance of tolerating emotional distress and highlight the critical role that exposure therapy plays in increasing the child's ability to navigate uncomfortable feelings. This chapter reviewed modern conceptualizations of emotional intolerance, including important treatment considerations and steps for the successful implementation of exposure exercises for increasing distress tolerance. Detailed examples of hierarchy ladders and specific exposure activities were presented. Case examples were also included to highlight two common presentations of affect-related distress and real-world approaches for improving emotion tolerance.

References

Abramowitz, J. S., Deacon, B. J., & Whiteside, S. P. H. (2011). *Exposure therapy for anxiety: Principles and practice.* New York: Guilford Press.

Abramowitz, J. S., & Foa, E. B. (2000). Does comorbid depressive disorder influence outcome of exposure and response prevention for OCD? *Behavior Therapy, 31,* 795–800.

Albano, A. M., Chorpita, B. F., & Barlow, D. H. (2003). Childhood anxiety disorders. In: E. J. Mash & R. A. Barkley (Ed.), *Childhood psychopathology* (pp. 279–329). New York: Guilford Press.

Albano, A. M., & DiBartolo, P. M. (2007). *Cognitive-behavioral therapy for social phobia in adolescents: Stand up, speak out therapist guide.* New York: Oxford University Press.

Albano, A. M., & Kendall, P. C. (2002). Cognitive behavioural therapy for children and adolescents with anxiety disorders: Clinical research advances. *International Review of Psychiatry, 14*(2), 129–134.

Albano, A. M., Marten, P. A., Holt, C. S., Heimberg, R. G., & Barlow, D. H. (1995). Cognitive-Behavioral Group Treatment for Social Phobia in Adolescents A Preliminary Study. *The Journal of Nervous and Mental Disease, 183*(10), 649–656.

Ale, C. M., McCarthy, D. M., Rothschild, L. M., & Whiteside, S. P. (2015). Components of cognitive behavioral therapy related to outcome in childhood anxiety disorders. *Clinical Child and Family Psychology Review, 18*(3), 240–251.

Alfano, C. A., Ginsburg, G. S., & Kingery, J. N. (2007). Sleep-related problems among children and adolescents with anxiety disorders. *Journal of the American Academy of Child and Adolescent Psychiatry, 46*(2), 224–232.

Allan, N. P., MacPherson, L., Young, K. C., Lejuez, C. W., & Schmidt, N. B. (2014). Examining the latent structure of anxiety sensitivity in adolescents using factor mixture modeling. *Psychological Assessment, 26*(3), 741–751.

American Psychiatric Association (2013). *Diagnostic and statistical manual of mental disorders (5th ed.).* Arlington, VA: American Psychiatric Publishing.

Anderson, E. R., Veed, G. J., Inderbitzen-Nolan, H. M., & Hansen, D. J. (2010). An evaluation of the applicability of the tripartite constructs to social anxiety in adolescents. *Journal of Clinical Child and Adolescent Psychology, 39*(2), 195–207.

Andersson, G., Waara, J., Jonsson, U., Malmaeus, F., Carlbring, P., & Öst, L.-G. (2009). Internet-based self-help vs. one-session exposure in the treatment of spider phobia: A randomized controlled trial. *Cognitive Behaviour Therapy, 38,* 114–120.

Angold, A., Costello, E. J., & Erkanli, A. (1999). Comorbidity. *Journal of Child Psychology and Psychiatry, 40,* 57–87.

Antony, M. M., & Swinson, R. P. (2008). *The shyness and social anxiety workbook: proven, step-by-step strategies for overcoming your fear.* Oakland, CA: New Harbinger Publications.

Antony, M. M., & Watling, M. A. (2006). *Overcoming medical phobia: How to conquer fear of blood, needles, doctors, & dentists.* Oakland, CA: New Harbinger Publications.

Attiullah, N., Eisen, J.L., & Rasmussen, S.A. (2000). Clinical features of obsessive-compulsive disorder. *Psychiatric Clinics of North America, 23*(3), 469–491.

Baer, L. (2001). *The imp of the mind: Exploring the silent epidemic of obsessive bad thoughts.* New York: Penguin Publishing Group.

Bandura, A. (1983). Self-efficacy determinants of anticipated fears and calamities. *Journal of Personality and Social Psychology, 45*(2), 464.

Bandura, A. (1997). *Self-efficacy: The exercise of control.* New York: Macmillian.

Barkley, R. (2013). *Taking charge of ADHD: The complete, authoritative guide for parents* (3rd ed.). New York: Guildford Press.

Barkley, R. A. & Benton, C. M. (2013). *Your defiant child: Eight steps to better behavior* (2nd ed.). New York: Guilford Press.

Barlow, D. H. (1988). Office-based behavioural treatment of panic attack. In, *Panic disorder: Relative merits of pharmacotherapy and psychotherapy* (pp. 6–8). Mississauga, ON, Canada: The Medicine Group.

Barlow, D. H. (2000). Unraveling the mysteries of anxiety and its disorders from the perspective of emotion theory. *American Psychologist, 55*(11), 1247–1263.

Barlow, D. H. (2002). *Anxiety and its disorders: The nature and treatment of anxiety and panic* (2nd ed.). New York: Guilford Press.

Barlow, D. H., Farchione, T. J., Fairholme, C. P., Ellard, K. K., Boisseau, C. L., Allen, L. B., & Ehrenreich-May, J. (2011). *The unified protocol for transdiagnostic treatment of emotional disorders: Therapist guide.* New York: Oxford University Press.

Barlow, D. H., Gorman, J. M., Shear, M. K., & Woods, S. W. (2000). Cognitive-behavioral therapy, imipramine, or their combination for panic disorder: A randomized controlled trial. *Journal of the American Medical Association, 283*(19), 2529–2536.

Barlow, D. H., Raffa, S. D. & Cohen, E. M. (2002). *Psychosocial treatments for panic disorders, phobias, and generalized anxiety disorder.* In P. E. Nathan & J. M. Gorman (Eds.) A guide to treatments that work (2nd ed., pp. 301–335). New York: Oxford University Press.

Barmish, A. J., & Kendall, P. C. (2005). Should parents be co-clients in cognitive-behavioral therapy for anxious youth? *Journal of Clinical Child and Adolescent Psychology, 34*(3), 569–581.

Barrett, P. M., Dadds, M. R., & Rapee, R. M. (1996) Family treatment of childhood anxiety: A controlled trial. *Journal of Consulting and Clinical Psychology, 64*, 33–342.

Barrett, P. M., Farrell, L., Pina, A. A., Peris, T. S., & Piacentini, J. (2008). Evidence-based psychosocial treatments for child and adolescent obsessive-compulsive disorder. *Journal of Clinical Child & Adolescent Psychology, 37*(1), 131–155.

Barrett, P., Lowry-Webster, H., & Turner, G. (2000). *FRIENDS program for children: Group leaders, manual.* Brisbane, Australia: Australian Academic Press.

Baskind, S. (2007). A behavioural intervention for selective mutism in an eight-year-old boy. *Educational and Child Psychology, 24*, 87–94.

Baumrind, D. (1967). Child care practices anteceding three patterns of preschool behavior. *Genetic Psychology Monographs, 75*(1), 43–88.

Beck, A. T. (1976). *Cognitive therapy and emotional disorders*. New York: International Universities Press.

Becker, C. B., Zayfert, C., & Anderson, E. (2004). A survey of psychologists' attitudes towards and utilization of exposure therapy for PTSD. *Behaviour Research and Therapy, 42*(3), 277–292.

Beesdo, K., Bittner, A., Pine, D. S., Stein, M. B., Höfler, M., Lieb, R., & Wittchen, H. U. (2007). Incidence of social anxiety disorder and the consistent risk for secondary depression in the first three decades of life. *Archives of General Psychiatry, 64*(8), 903–912.

Beesdo, K., Knappe, S., & Pine, D. S. (2009). Anxiety and anxiety disorders in children and adolescents: Developmental issues and implications for DSM-V. *Psychiatric Clinics of North America, 32*(3), 483–524.

Beesdo K., Pine D. S., Lieb R., & Wittchen H. U. (2010). Incidence and risk patterns of anxiety and depressive disorders and categorization of generalized anxiety disorder. *Archives of General Psychiatry, 67*(1), 47–57.

Beidas, R. S., Mychailyszyn, M. P., Podell, J. L., & Kendall, P. C. (2013). Brief cognitive-behavioral therapy for anxious youth: The inner workings. *Cognitive and Behavioral Practice, 20*(2), 134–146.

Beidel, D. C., & Alfano, C. A. (2011). *Child anxiety disorders: A guide to research and treatment*. New York: Taylor & Francis Group.

Beidel, D. C., Ferrell, C., Alfano, C. A., & Yeganeh, R. (2001). The treatment of childhood social anxiety disorder. *Psychiatric Clinics of North America, 24*(4), 831–846.

Beidel, D. C., & Turner, S. M. (2007). *Shy children, phobic adults: Nature and treatment of social anxiety disorder* (pp. 11–46). Washington, DC: American Psychological Association.

Beidel, D. C., Turner, S. M., & Morris, T. L. (1995). A new inventory to assess childhood social anxiety and phobia: The Social Phobia and Anxiety Inventory for Children. *Psychological Assessment, 7*(1), 73–79.

Beidel, D. C., Turner, S. M., & Morris, T. L. (2000). Behavioral treatment of childhood social phobia. *Journal of consulting and clinical psychology, 68*(6), 1072.

Bener, A., Ghuloum, S., & Dafeeah, E. E. (2011). Prevalence of common phobias and their socio-demographic correlates in children and adolescents in a traditional developing society. *African Journal of Psychiatry, 14*(2), 140–145.

Benito, K. G., Conelea, C., Garcia, A. M., & Freeman, J. B. (2012). CBT specific process in exposure-based treatments: Initial examination in a pediatric OCD sample. *Journal of Obsessive-Compulsive and Related Disorders, 1*(2), 77–84.

Benjamin, C. L., Puleo, C. M., Settipani, C. A., Brodman, D. M., Edmunds, J. M., Cummings, C. M., & Kendall, P. C. (2011). History of cognitive-behavioral therapy in youth. *Child and Adolescent Psychiatric Clinics Of North America, 20*(2), 179–189.

Berg, I. (1997). School refusal and truancy. *Archives of Disease in Childhood, 76*, 90–91.

Berg, I., Nichols, K., & Pritchard, C. (1969). School phobia: Its classification and relationship to dependency. *Journal of Child Psychology and Psychiatry, 10*, 123–41.

Bergman, R. L. (2013). *Treatment for children with selective mutism: An integrative behavioral approach*. New York: Oxford University Press.

Bergman, R. L., Piacentini, J., & McCracken, J. T. (2002). Prevalence and description of selective mutism in a school-based sample. *Journal of the American Academy of Child and Adolescent Psychiatry, 41*(8), 938–946.

Bernstein, G. A., Mueller, B. A., Schreiner, M. W., Campbell, S. M., Regan, E. K., Nelson, P. M.,...Cullen, K. R. (2016). Abnormal striatal resting-state functional connectivity in adolescents with obsessive-compulsive disorder. *Psychiatry Research, 247*, 49–56.

Biederman, J., Faraone, S. V., Marrs, A., Moore, P., Garcia, J., Ablon, S.,...Kearns, M. E. (1997). Panic disorder and agoraphobia in consecutively referred children and adolescents. *Journal of the American Academy of Child and Adolescent Psychiatry, 36*, 214–223.

Birmaher, B., Khetarpal, S., Brent, D., Cully, M., Balach, L., Kaufman, J., & Neer, S. M. (1997). The Screen for Child Anxiety Related Emotional Disorders (SCARED): Scale construction and psychometric characteristics. *Journal of the American Academy of Child and Adolescent Psychiatry, 36*(4), 545–553.

Birmaher, B., & Ollendick, T. H. (2004). Childhood-onset panic disorder. In T. H. Ollendick & J. S. March (Eds.), *Phobic and anxiety disorders in children and adolescents* (pp. 306–333). New York: Oxford University Press.

Bittner, A., Egger, H. L., Erkanli, A., Jane Costello, E., Foley, D. L., & Angold, A. (2007). What do childhood anxiety disorders predict? *Journal of Child Psychology and Psychiatry, 48*(12), 1174–1183.

Black, B., & Uhde, T. W. (1995). Psychiatric characteristics of children with selective mutism: A pilot study. *Journal of the American Academy of Child and Adolescent Psychiatry, 34*(7), 847–856.

Blum, N. J., Kell, R. S., Starr, H. L., Lender, W. L., Bradley-Klug, K. L., Osborne, M. L., & Dowrick, P. W. (1998). Case study: Audio feedforward treatment of selective mutism. *Journal of the American Academy of Child and Adolescent Psychiatry, 37*(1), 40–43.

Boden, J. M., Fergusson, D. M., & Horwood, L. J. (2007). Anxiety disorders and suicidal behaviours in adolescence and young adulthood: Findings from a longitudinal study. *Psychological Medicine, 37*, 431–440.

Boettcher, H., Brake, C. A., & Barlow, D. H. (2016). Origins and outlook of interoceptive exposure. *Journal of Behavior Therapy and Experimental Psychiatry, 53*, 41–51.

Bögels, S. M., Snieder, N., & Kindt, M. (2003). Specificity of dysfunctional thinking in children with symptoms of social anxiety, separation anxiety and generalised anxiety. *Behaviour Change, 20*(03), 160–169.

Boisseau, C. L., Farchione, T. J., Fairholme, C. P., Ellard, K. K., & Barlow, D. H. (2010). The development of the unified protocol for the transdiagnostic treatment of emotional disorders: A case study. *Cognitive and Behavioral Practice, 17*(1), 102–113.

Bolton, D. & Perrin, S. (2008). Evaluation of exposure with response-prevention for obsessive compulsive disorder in childhood and adolescence. *Journal of Behavior Therapy and Experimental Psychiatry, 39*(1), 11–22.

Boschen, M. J. (2007). Reconceptualizing emetophobia: A cognitive-behavioral formulation and research agenda. *Journal of Anxiety Disorders, 21*, 407–419.

Boswell, J. F., Farchione, T. J., Sauer-Zavala, S., Murray, H. W., Fortune, M. R., & Barlow, D. H. (2013). Anxiety sensitivity and interoceptive exposure: A transdiagnostic construct and change strategy. *Behavior Therapy, 44*(3), 417–431.

Boswell, J. F., Thompson-Hollands, J., Farchione, T. J., & Barlow, D. H. (2013). Intolerance of uncertainty: A common factor in the treatment of emotional disorders. *Journal of Clinical Psychology, 69*(6), 630–645.

Bouchard, S. (2011). Could virtual reality be effective in treating children with phobias? *Expert Review of Neurotherapeutics, 11*(2), 207–213.

Bouchard, S., Mendlowitz, S., Coles, M., & Franklin, M. (2004). Considerations in the use of exposure with children. *Cognitive and Behavioral Practice, 11*, 56–65.

Brady, E. U., & Kendall, P. C. (1992). Comorbidity of anxiety and depression in children and adolescents. *Psychological Bulletin, 111*(2), 244–255.

Brown, T. A., Chorpita, B. F., & Barlow, D. H. (1998). Structural relationships among dimensions of the DSM-IV anxiety and mood disorders and dimensions of negative affect, positive affect, and autonomic arousal. *Journal of Abnormal Psychology, 107*(2), 179–192.

Browne, H. A., Gair, S. L., Scharf, J. M., & Grice, D. E. (2014). Genetics of Obsessive-Compulsive Disorder and Related Disorders. *Psychiatry Clinics of North America, 37*(3), 319–335.

Buhr, K., & Dugas, M. J. (2009). The role of fear of anxiety and intolerance of uncertainty in worry: An experimental manipulation. *Behaviour Research and Therapy, 47*(3), 215–223.

Bunnell, B. E., & Beidel, D. C. (2013). Incorporating technology into the treatment of a 17-year-old girl with selective mutism. *Clinical Case Studies, 12*(4), 291–306.

Burns, D. (1980). Feeling good: The new mood therapy. New York: Harper Collins.

Burstein, M., Ginsburg, G. S., & Tein, J. (2010). Parental anxiety and child symptomatology: An examination of additive and interactive effects of parent psychopathology. *Journal of Abnormal Child Psychology, 38*(7), 897–909.

Burstein, M., He, J. P., Kattan, G., Albano, A. M., Avenevoli, S., & Merikangas, K. R. (2011). Social phobia and subtypes in the National Comorbidity Survey–Adolescent Supplement: prevalence, correlates, and comorbidity. *Journal of the American Academy of Child and Adolescent Psychiatry, 50*(9), 870–880.

Carpenter, A. L., Puliafico, A. C., Kurtz, S. M. S., Pincus, D. B., & Comer, J. S. (2014). Extending parent-child interaction therapy for early childhood internalizing problems: New advances for an overlooked population. *Clinical Child and Family Psychology Review, 17*(4), 340–356.

Castle, D. J., Deale, A., & Marks, I. M. (1995). Gender differences in obsessive compulsive disorder. *Australian & New Zealand Journal of Psychiatry, 29*(1), 114–117.

Chavira, D. A., Stein, M. B., Bailey, K., & Stein, M. T. (2004). Child anxiety in primary care: Prevalent but untreated. *Depression and Anxiety, 20*, 155–164.

Chiu, A. W., Langer, D. A., McLeod, B. D., Har, K., Drahota, A., Galla, B. M.,…Wood, J. J. (2013). Effectiveness of modular CBT for child anxiety in elementary schools. *School Psychology Quarterly, 28*(2), 141–153.

Chorpita, B. F. (2007). *Modular cognitive behavioral therapy for childhood anxiety disorders.* New York: Guilford Press.

Chorpita, B. F., Albano, A. M., & Barlow, D. H. (1996). Cognitive processing in children: Relation to anxiety and family influences. *Journal of Clinical Child Psychology, 25*(2), 170–176.

Chorpita, B. F., & Barlow, D. H. (1998). The development of anxiety: The role of control in the early environment. *Psychological Bulletin, 124*, 3–21.

Christophersen, E. R., & Vanscoyoc, S. M. (2013). *Treatments that work with children: Empirically supported strategies for managing childhood problems.* Washington, DC: American Psychological Association.

Chu, B. C., Talbott Crocco, S., Arnold, C. C., Brown, R., Southam-Gerow, M. A., & Weisz, J. R. (2015). Sustained implementation of cognitive-behavioral therapy for youth anxiety and depression: Long-term effects of structured training and consultation on therapist practice in the field. *Professional Psychology: Research and Practice, 46*(1), 70–79.

Clark, D. M. (1996). Panic disorder: From theory to therapy. In P. M. Salkovskis (Ed.), *Frontiers of cognitive therapy* (pp. 318–344). New York: Guilford Press.

Clark, D.A., & Beck, A.T. (2010). *Cognitive therapy of anxiety disorders: Science and practice.* New York: Guilford Press.

Clark, L. A., & Watson, D. (1991). Tripartite model of anxiety and depression: Psychometric evidence and taxonomic implications. *Journal of Abnormal Psychology, 100*(3), 316–336.

Cohan, S. L., Chavira, D. A., & Stein, M. B. (2006). Practitioner review: Psychosocial interventions for children with selective mutism: A critical evaluation of the literature from 1990–2005. *Journal of Child Psychology and Psychiatry and Allied Disciplines, 47*(11), 1085–1097.

Cohen, J. A., Mannarino, A. P., & Deblinger, E. (2006). *Treating trauma and traumatic grief in children and adolescents.* New York: Guilford Press.

Comer, J. S., Roy, A. K., Furr, J. M., Gotimer, K., Beidas, R. S., Dugas, M. J., & Kendall, P. C. (2009). The intolerance of uncertainty scale for children: A psychometric evaluation. *Psychological Assessment, 21*(3), 402–411.

Copeland, W. E., Shanahan, L., Costello, E. J., & Angold, A. (2009). Childhood and adolescent psychiatric disorders as predictors of young adult disorders. *Archives of General Psychiatry, 66*(7), 764–772.

Coskun, M., Zoroglu, S. & Ozturk, M. (2012). Phenomenology, psychiatric comorbidity and family history in referred preschool children with obsessive-compulsive disorder. *Child and Adolescent Psychiatry and Mental Health, 6,* 1–9.

Costello, E. J., Egger, H. L., & Angold, A. (2005). The developmental epidemiology of anxiety disorders. *Child and Adolescent Psychiatric Clinics of North America, 14,* 631–648.

Costello, E. J., Mustillo, S., Erkanli, A., Keeler, G., & Angold, A. (2003). Prevalence and development of psychiatric disorders in childhood and adolescence. *Archives of General Psychiatry, 60*(8), 837–844.

Craske, M. G., & Barlow, D. H. (2006). *Mastery of your anxiety and panic* (4th ed.). New York: Oxford University Press.

Craske, M.G., Kircanski K., Zelikowsky M., et al. (2008). Optimizing inhibitory learning during exposure therapy. *Behaviour Research and Therapy, 46,* 5–27.

Craske, M. G., Treanor, M., Conway, C.C., Zbozinek, T., & Vervliet, B. (2014). Maximizing exposure therapy: An inhibitory learning approach. *Behaviour Research and Therapy, 58,* 10–23.

Creswell, C., & Cartwright-Hatton, S. (2007). Family treatment of child anxiety: Outcomes, limitations and future directions. *Clinical Child and Family Psychology Review, 10*(3), 232–252.

Cunningham, C. E., McHolm, A. E., & Boyle, M. H., (2006). Social phobia, anxiety, oppositional behavior, social skills, and self-concept in children with specific selective mutism, generalized selective mutism, and community controls. *European Child and Adolescent Psychiatry, 15,* 245–255.

Cunningham, C. E., McHolm, A., Boyle, M. H., & Patel, S. (2004). Behavioral and emotional adjustment, family functioning, academic performance, and social relationships in children with selective mutism. *Journal of Child Psychology and Psychiatry, 45*(8), 1363–1372.

Cunningham, M., Rapee, R., & Lyneham, H. (2007). Overview of the Cool Teens CD-ROM for anxiety disorders in adolescents. *The Behavior Therapist, 30*, 15–19.

Dagnan, D. & Jahoda, A. (2006). Cognitive-behavioural intervention for people with intellectual disability and anxiety disorders. *Journal and Applied Research in Intellectual Disabilities, 19*, 91–97.

Daleiden, E. L., & Vasey, M. W. (1997). An information-processing perspective on childhood anxiety. *Clinical Psychology Review, 17*(4), 407–429.

Davidson, J. R., Hughes, D. L., George, L. K., & Blazer, D. G. (1993). The epidemiology of social phobia: findings from the Duke Epidemiological Catchment Area Study. *Psychological medicine, 23*(03), 709–718.

Davis, T. E., Kurtz, P. F., Gardner, A. W., & Carman, N. B. (2007). Cognitive-behavioral treatment for specific phobias with a child demonstration severe problem behavior and developmental delay. *Research in Developmental Disabilities, 28*(6), 546–558.

Deacon, B. J., Kemp, J. J., Dixon, L. J., Sy, J. T., Farrell, N. R., & Zhang, A. R. (2013). Maximizing the efficacy of interoceptive exposure by optimizing inhibitory learning: A randomized controlled trial. *Behavior Research and Therapy, 51*(9), 588–596.

Dia, D. A., & Bradshaw, W. (2008). Cognitive risk factors to the development of anxiety and depressive disorders in adolescents. *Child and Adolescent Social Work Journal, 25*(6), 469–481.

Dixon, L. J., Kemp, J. J., Farrell, N. R., Blakey, S. M., & Deacon, B. J. (2015). Interoceptive exposure exercises for social anxiety. *Journal of anxiety disorders, 33*, 25–34.

Doerfler, L. A., Connor, D. F., Volungis, A. M., & Toscano, P. F. (2007). Panic disorder in clinically referred children and adolescents. *Child Psychiatry and Human Development, 38*, 57–71.

Donovan, C. L., Holmes, M. C., & Farrell, L. J. (2016). Investigation of the cognitive variables associated with worry in children with generalised anxiety disorder and their parents. *Journal of Affective Disorders, 192*, 1–7.

Drake, K. L., & Ginsburg, G. S. (2012). Family factors in the development, treatment, and prevention of childhood anxiety disorders. *Clinical Child and Family Psychology Review, 15*(2), 144–162.

Dugas, M. J., Laugesen, N., & Bukowski, W. M. (2012). Intolerance of uncertainty, fear of anxiety, and adolescent worry. *Journal of Abnormal Child Psychology, 40*(6), 863–870.

Dugas, M. J., & Robichaud, M. (2007). *Cognitive-behavioral treatment for generalized anxiety disorder: From science to practice.* New York: Taylor & Francis.

Ebesutani, C., Okamura, K., Higa-McMillan, C., & Chorpita, B. F. (2011). A psychometric analysis of the Positive and Negative Affect Schedule for Children–Parent Version in a school sample. Psychological Assessment, 23, 406–416. Effective Child Therapy. DataCore, n.d. http://effectivechildtherapy.org/

Egger, H.L., Costello, E.J., & Angold, A. (2003). School refusal and psychiatric disorders: A community study. *Journal of the American Academy of Child and Adolescent Psychiatry, 42*, 797–807.

Ehrenreich, J. T., Santucci, L. C., & Weiner, C. L. (2008). Separation anxiety disorder in youth: Phenomology, assessment, and treatment. *Psicol Conductual, 16*(3), 389–412.

Ehrenreich-May, J., & Bilek, E. L. (2011). Universal prevention of anxiety and depression in a recreational camp setting: An initial open trial. *Child & Youth Care Forum, 40*(6) 435–455.

Eisen, A. R., Raleigh, H., & Neuhoff, C. C. (2008). The unique impact of parent training for separation anxiety disorder in children. *Behavior Therapy, 39*, 195–206.

Eisen, A.R., & Schaefer, C.E. (2005). *Separation anxiety in children and adolescents.* New York: Guilford Press.

Eisenstadt, T.H., Eyberg, S.M., McNeil, C.B., Newcomb, K., & Funderburk, B. (1993). Parent-Child Interaction Therapy with behavior problem children: Relative effectiveness of two stages and overall treatment outcome. *Journal of Clinical Child Psychology, 22*, 42–51.

Eley, T. C., Rijsdijk, F. V., Perrin, S., O'Connor, T. G., & Bolton, D. (2008). A multivariate genetic analysis of specific phobia, separation anxiety and social phobia in early childhood. *Journal of Abnormal Child Psychology, 36*, 839–848.

Elizur, Y., & Perednik, R. (2003). Prevalence and description of selective mutism in immigrant and native families: A controlled study. *Journal of the American Academy of Child and Adolescent Psychiatry, 42*, 1451–1459.

Ellard, K. K., Fairholme, C. P., Boisseau, C. L., Farchione, T. J., & Barlow, D. H. (2010). Unified protocol for the transdiagnostic treatment of emotional disorders: Protocol development and initial outcome data. *Cognitive and Behavioral Practice, 17*(1), 88–101.

Ellis, D. M., & Hudson, J. L. (2010). The metacognitive model of generalized anxiety disorder in children and adolescents. *Clinical Child and Family Psychological Review, 13*, 151–163.

Essau, C. A., Conradt, J., & Petermann, F. (1999). Frequency of panic attacks and panic disorder in adolescents. *Depression and Anxiety, 9*, 19–26.

Essau, C. A., Lewinsohn, P. M., Olaya, B., & Seeley, J. R. (2014). Anxiety disorders in adolescents and psychosocial outcomes at age 30. *Journal of Affective Disorders, 163*, 125–132.

Esbjørn, B. H., Normann, N., & Reinholdt-Dunne, M. L. (2015). Adapting Metacognitive Therapy to Children with Generalised Anxiety Disorder: Suggestions for a Manual. *Journal of Contemporary Psychotherapy, 45*(3), 159–166.

Fairburn, C. G. (2008). *Cognitive behavioral therapy and eating disorders.* New York: Guilford Press.

Fang, A., Sawyer, A. T., Asnaani, A., & Hofmann, S. G. (2013). Social mishap exposures for social anxiety disorder: An important treatment ingredient. *Cognitive and behavioral practice, 20*(2), 213–220.

Fialko, L., Bolton, D., & Perrin, S. (2012). Applicability of a cognitive model of worry to children and adolescents. *Behaviour Research and Therapy, 50*(5), 341–349.

Fisak, B. J., Oliveros, A., & Ehrenreich, J. T. (2006). Assessment and behavioral treatment of selective mutism. *Clinical Case Studies, 5*, 382–402.

Flannery-Schroeder, E., Suveg, C., Safford, S., Kendall, P. C. & Webb, A. (2004). Comorbid externalising disorders and child anxiety treatment outcomes. *Behaviour Change, 21*(1), 14–25.

Foa, E. B., & Kozak, M. J. (1986). Emotional processing of fear: Exposure to corrective information. *Psychological Bulletin, 99*(1), 20–35.

Ford, M. A., Sladesczek, I. E., Carlson, J., & Krochwell, T. R. (1998). Selective mutism: Phenomenological characteristics. *School Psychology Quarterly, 13*, 192–227.

Forehand, R. & Long, N. (1996). *Parenting the Strong-Willed Child.* New York, NY: McGraw Hill.

Forsyth, J. P., Fusé, T. M., & Acheson, D. A. (2008). Interoceptive exposure for panic disorder. In W. O'Donohue, J. Fisher, & S. C. Hayes (Eds.), *Cognitive behavior therapy: Applying empirically supported techniques in your practice, 2nd ed.* (pp. 296–308). New York: Wiley.

Franklin, M. E., Kratz, H. E., Freeman, J.B., Ivarsson, T., Heyman, I., Sookman, D.,...March, J. (2015). Cognitive-behavioral therapy for pediatric obsessive-compulsive disorder: Empirical review and clinical recommendations. *Psychiatry Research, 227*(1), 78–92.

Freeman, J., Garcia, A., Frank, H., Benito, K., Conelea, C., Walther, M., & Edmunds, J. (2014). Evidence base update for psychosocial treatments for pediatric obsessive-compulsive disorder. *Journal of Clinical Child & Adolescent Psychology, 43*(1), 7–26.

Fremont, W.P. (2003). School refusal in children and adolescents. American Family Physician, 68, 1555– 1560, 1563–1564.

Furr, J. M., Comer, J. S., Wilner, J., Kerns, C., Feinberg, L., Wilson, L., et al. (2012, November). The Boston University Brave Buddies Program: A replication of the Brave Buddies intensive, outpatient treatment program for children with selective mutism. In H. Sacks & P.T. Chan (Chairs), *Breaking the sound barrier: Exploring effective CBTs for childhood selective mutism.* Symposium conducted at the meeting of the Association for Behavioral and Cognitive Therapies, National Harbor, MD.

Garcia, A., Freeman, J., Francis, G., Miller, L. M., & Leonard, H. L. (2004). Selective mutism. In: T. Ollendick (Ed.), *Phobic and anxiety disorders in children and adolescents: A clinician's guide to effective psychosocial and pharmacological interventions* (pp. 443–455). London: Oxford University Press.

García-López, L. J., Olivares, J., & Hidalgo, M. D. (2005). A pilot study on sensitivity of outcome measures for treatments of generalized social phobia in Spanish adolescents. *International Journal of Clinical and Health Psychology, 5*(2), 385–392.

García-López, L. J., Olivares, J., Turner, S. M., Beidel, D. C., Albano, A. M., & Sánchez-Meca, J. (2002). Results at long-term among three psychological treatments for adolescents with generalized social phobia (II): clinical significance and effect size. *Psicología Conductual, 10*(2), 371–388.

Geller, D., Biederman, J., Faraone, S. V., Frazier, J., Coffey, B. J., Kim, G., & Bellordre, C. A. (2000). Clinical correlates of obsessive compulsive disorder in children and adolescents referred to specialized and non-specialized clinical settings. *Depression and Anxiety, 11*(4), 163–168.

Geller, D.A., March, J., & The AACAP Committee on Quality Issues (CQI). (2012). Practice Parameter for the assessment and treatment of children and adolescents with obsessive-compulsive disorder. *Journal of the American Academy of Child and Adolescent Psychiatry, 51*(1), 98–113.

Ginsburg, G. S., Siqueland, L., Masia-Warner, C., & Hedtke, K. A. (2004). Anxiety disorders in children in children: Family matters. *Cognitive and Behavioral Practice, 11*(1), 28–43.

Giorgio, J. M., Sanflippo, J., Kleiman, E., Reilly, D., Bender, R. E., Wagner, C. A.,...Alloy, L. B. (2010). An experiential avoidance conceptualization of depressive rumination: Three tests of the model. *Behaviour Research and Therapy, 48*(10), 1021–1031.

Goldstein, A. J., & Chambless, D. L. (1978). A reanalysis of agoraphobia. *Behavior Therapy, 9,* 47–59.

Gouze, K. R., Hopkins, J., Bryant, F. B., & Lavigne, J. V. (2016). Parenting and anxiety: Bidirectional relations in young children. *Journal of Abnormal Child Psychology,* 1–12.

Grayson, J. B. (2010). OCD and the intolerance of uncertainty: Treatment issues. *Journal of Cognitive Psychotherapy: An International Quarterly, 24*(1), 3–15.

Greco, L. A., Lambert, W., & Baer, R. A. (2008). Psychological inflexibility in childhood and adolescence: development and evaluation of the Avoidance and Fusion Questionnaire for Youth. *Psychological Assessment, 20*, 93–102.

Gregory, A. M., Caspi, A., Moffitt, T. E., Koenen, K., Eley, T. C., & Poulton, R. (2007). Juvenile mental health histories of adults with anxiety disorders. *American Journal of Psychiatry, 164*(2), 301–308.

Grover, R. L., Hughes, A. A., Bergman, R. L., & Kingery, J. N. (2006). Treatment modifications based on childhood anxiety diagnosis: Demonstrating the flexibility in manualized treatment. *Journal of Cognitive Psychotherapy, 20*(3), 275–286.

Gryczkowski, M. R., Tiede, M. S., Dammann, J. E., Jacobsen, A. B., Hale, L. R., & Whiteside, S. P. H. (2013). The timing of exposure in clinic-based treatment for childhood anxiety disorders. *Behavior Modification, 37*(2), 211–225.

Hadley, N. H. (1994). *Elective mutism: A handbook for educators, counselors, and health care professionals.* Dordrecht, The Netherlands: Kluwer Academic Publishers.

Hadwin, J. A., Garner, M., & Perez-Olivas, G. (2006). The development of information processing biases in childhood anxiety: A review and exploration of its origins in parenting. *Clinical Psychology Review, 26*(7), 876–894.

Hagopian, L. P., & Slifer, K. J. (1993). Treatment of separation anxiety disorder with graduated exposure and reinforcement targeting school attendance. *Journal of Anxiety Disorders, 7*, 271–280.

Halldorsdottir, T. & Ollendick, T. H. (2014). Comorbid ADHD: Implications for the treatment of anxiety disorders in children and adolescents. *Cognitive and Behavioral Practice, 21*(3), 310–322.

Halldorsdottir, T., Ollendick, T. H., Ginsburg, G., Sherrill, J., Kendall, P. C., Walkup, J., & Piacentini, J. (2014). Treatment outcomes in anxious youth with and without comorbid ADHD in the CAMS. *Journal of Clinical Child & Adolescent Psychology, 44*(6), 985–991.

Hamm, A. O. (2009). Specific phobias. *Psychiatric Clinics of North America, 32*(3), 577–591.

Hargett, M. Q. (1996). Treatment integrity and acceptability with families: A case study of a child with school refusal. *Psychology in the Schools, 33*(4), 319–324.

Hayes, S. C., Strosahl, K., & Wilson, K. G. (1999). *Acceptance and Commitment Therapy: An experiential approach to behavior change.* New York: Guilford Press.

Hayward, C., Killen, J. D., Kraemer, H. C., & Taylor, C. B. (2000). Predictors of panic attacks in adolescents. *Journal of the American Academy of Child and Adolescent Psychiatry, 39*(2), 207–214.

Hayward, C., Varady, S., Albano, A. M., Thienemann, M., Henderson, L., & Schatzberg, A. F. (2000). Cognitive-behavioral group therapy for social phobia in female adolescents: results of a pilot study. *Journal of the American Academy of Child and Adolescent Psychiatry, 39*(6), 721–726.

Hembree, E.A., Rauch, S.A.M., & Foa, E.B. (2003). Beyond the manual: The insider's guide to prolonged exposure therapy for PTSD. *Cognitive and Behavioral Practice, 10*, 22–30.

Hoffman, E. C., & Mattis, S. G. (2000). A developmental adaptation of panic control treatment for panic disorder in adolescence. *Cognitive and Behavioral Practice, 7*, 253–261.

Hofmann, S. G. (2007). Cognitive factors that maintain social anxiety disorder: A comprehensive model and its treatment implications. *Cognitive behaviour therapy, 36*(4), 193–209.

Hollon, S. & Beck, A. T. (2013). Cognitive and cognitive-behavioral therapies. In M. Lambert (Ed.), *Handbook of psychotherapy and behavior change* (pp.393–442). New York: Wiley.

Honjo, S., Nishide, T., Niwa, S., Sasaki, Y., Kaneko, H., Inoko, K., et al. (2001). School refusal anddepression with school nonattendance in children and adolescents: Comparative assessment between the Children's Depression Inventory and somatic complaints. *Psychiatry and Clinical Neurosciences, 55*, 629–634.

Houlihan, D. D., & Jones, R. N. (1989). Treatment of a boy's school phobia with in vivo systemic desensitization. *Professional School Psychology, 4*, 285–293.

Hoza, B., Pelham Jr., W. E., Dobbs, J., Owens, J. S., & Pillow, D. R. (2002). Do boys with attention deficit/hyperactivity disorder have positive illusory self-concepts? *Journal of Abnormal Psychology, 111*, 268–278.

Hudson, J. I., Hiripi, E., Pope Jr., H. G., & Kessler, R. C. (2007). The prevalence and correlates of eating disorders in the National Comorbidity Survey Replication. *Biological Psychiatry, 61*(3), 348–358.

Hudson, J. L., & Rapee, R. M. (2004). From Anxious Temperament to Disorder: An Etiological Model.

Hudson, J. L., Rapee, R. M., Deveney, C., Schniering, C. A., Lyneham, H. J., & Bovopoulos, N. (2009). Cognitive-behavioral treatment versus an active control for children and adolescents with anxiety disorders: A randomized trial. *Journal of the American Academy of Child and Adolescent Psychiatry, 48*(5), 533–544.

Ivarsson, T., Skarphedinsson, G., Kornør, H., Axelsdottir, B., Biedilæ, S., Heyman, I., & March, J. (2015). The place of and evidence for serotonin reuptake inhibitors (SRIs) for obsessive compulsive disorder (OCD) in children and adolescents: Views based on a systematic review and meta-analysis. *Psychiatry Research, 227*(1), 93–103.

Jensen, T. K., Holt, T., Ormhaug, S. M., Egeland, K., Granly, L., Hoaas, L. C.,…Wentzel-Larsen, T. (2014). A randomized effectiveness study comparing trauma-focused cognitive behavioral therapy with therapy as usual for youth. *Journal of Clinical Child and Adolescent Psychology, 43*(3), 356–369.

Johnstone, K.A. & Page, A.C. (2004). Attention to phobic stimuli during exposure: The effect of distraction on anxiety reduction, self-efficacy and perceived control. *Behaviour Research and Therapy, 42*, 249–275.

Kabat-Zinn, J. (1994). *Wherever you go, there you are.* London: Hyperion.

Kaufman, J., Birmaher, B., Brent, D., & Rao, U. (1997). Schedule for Affective Disorders and Schizophrenia for School-Age Children-Present and Lifetime version (K-SADS-PL): Initial reliability and validity data. *Journal of the American Academy of Child and Adolescent Psychiatry, 36*(7), 980–988.

Kazdin, A. E., & Weisz, J. R. (1998). Identifying and developing empirically supported child and adolescent treatments. *Journal of Consulting and Clinical Psychology, 66*(1), 19–36.

Kearney, C. A (2008). An interdisciplinary model of school absenteeism in youth to inform professional practice and public policy. *Education Psychology Review, 20*(3), 257–282.

Kearney, C.A., & Albano, A.M. (2004). The functional profile of school refusal behavior: Diagnostic aspects. *Behavior Modification, 28*, 147–161.

Kearney, C.A., & Albano, A.M. (2007). *When children refuse school: A cognitive-behavioral therapy approach/Therapist's guide* (2nd ed.). New York: Oxford University Press.

Kearney, C. A., Albano, A. M., Eisen, A. R., Allan, W. D., & Barlow, D. H. (1997). The phenomenology of panic disorder in youngsters: An empirical study of a clinical sample. *Journal of Anxiety Disorders, 11*, 49–62.

Kearney, C. A., Haight, C., & Day, T. L. (2011). Selective mutism. In D. McKay & E. Storch (Eds.), *Handbook of child and adolescent anxiety disorders* (pp. 275–287). New York: Springer.

Kearney, C. A., & Silverman, W. K. (1999). Functionally based prescriptive and nonprescriptive treatment for children and adolescents with school refusal behavior. *Behavior Therapy, 30*, 673–695.

Keeton, C. P., Kolos, A. C., & Walkup, J. T. (2009). Pediatric generalized anxiety disorder: Epidemiology, diagnosis, and management. *Pediatric Drugs, 11*(3), 171–183.

Kendall, P. C. (1994). Treating anxiety disorders in children: Results of a randomized clinical trial. *Journal of Consulting and Clinical Psychology, 62*(1), 100–110.

Kendall, P. C., Choudhury, M., Hudson, J., & Webb, A. (2002). The CAT project workbook for the cognitive-behavioral treatment of anxious adolescents. *Ardmore PA: Workbook.*

Kendall, P. C., Compton, S. N., Walkup, J. T., Birmaher, B., Albano, A. M., Sherrill, J.,… Keeton, C. (2010). Clinical characteristics of anxiety disordered youth. *Journal of Anxiety Disorders, 24*(3), 360–365.

Kendall, P. C., Cummings, C. M., Villabo, M. V., Narayanan, M. K., Treadwell, K., Baron, K.,…Albano, A. M. (2016). Mediators of change in the Child/Adolescent Multimodal Study. *Journal of Consulting and Clinical Psychology, 84*(1), 1–14.

Kendall, P. C., Flannery-Schroeder, E., Panichelli-Mindel, S., Southam-Gerow, M., Henin, A., & Warman, M. (1997). Therapy for youths with anxiety disorders: A second randomized clinical trial. *Journal of Consulting and Clinical Psychology, 65*, 366–380.

Kendall, P. C., & Hedtke, K. (2006). *Cognitive-behavioral therapy for anxious children: Therapist manual* (3rd ed.). Ardmore, PA: Workbook Publishing.

Kendall, P. C., Hudson, J. L., Gosch, E., Flannery-Schroder, E., & Suveg, C. (2008). Cognitive-behavioral therapy for anxiety disorder youth: A randomized clinical trial evaluating child and family modalities. *Journal of Consulting and Clinical psychology, 76*, 282–297.

Kendall, P. C., Peterman, J. S., & Cummings, C. M. (2015). Cognitive-behavioral therapy, behavioral therapy, and related treatments in children. In A. Thapar, D. S. Pine, J. F. Leckman, S. Scott, M. J. Snowling, & E. A. Taylor (Eds.), Rutter's child and adolescent psychiatry (6th ed.) (pp. 496–509). Hoboken, NJ: Wiley-Blackwell.

Kendall, P. C., & Pimentel, S. S. (2003). On the physiological symptom constellation in youth with generalized anxiety disorder (GAD). *Journal of Anxiety Disorders, 17*(2), 211–221.

Kendall, P. C., Robin, J. A., Hedtke, K. A., Suveg, C., Flannery-Schroeder, E., & Gosch, E. (2005). Considering CBT with anxious youth? Think exposures. *Cognitive and Behavioral Practice, 12*(1), 136–150.

Kendall, P. C., Safford, S., Flannery-Schroeder, E., & Webb, A. (2004). Child anxiety treatment: Outcomes in adolescence and impact on substance use and depression at 7.4-year follow-up. *Journal of Consulting and Clinical Psychology, 72*(2), 276–287.

Kennedy, S. J., Rapee, R. M., & Edwards, S. L. (2009). A selective intervention program for inhibited preschool-aged children of parents with an anxiety disorder: Effects on current anxiety disorders and temperament. *Journal of the American Academy of Child and Adolescent Psychiatry, 48*(6), 602–609.

Kessler, R. C., Berglund, P., Demler, O., Jin, R., Merikangas, K. R., & Walters, E. E. (2005). Lifetime prevalence and age-of-onset distributions of DSM-IV disorders in the National Comorbidity Survey Replication. *Archives of General Psychiatry, 62*(6), 593–602.

Kessler, R. C., Chiu, W. T., Demler, O., & Walters, E. E. (2005). Prevalence, severity, and comorbidity of twelve-month DSM-IV disorders in the National Comorbidity Survey Replication (NCSR-R). *Archives of General Psychiatry, 62*(6), 617–627.

Khalid-Khan, S., Santibanez, M. P., McMicken, C., & Rynn, M. A. (2007). Social anxiety disorder in children and adolescents. *Pediatric Drugs, 9*(4), 227–237.

Khanna, M. S., & Kendall, P. C. (2008). Computer-assisted CBT for child anxiety: The Coping Cat CD-ROM. *Cognitive and Behavioral Practice, 15*(2), 159–165.

Kim, S. J., Kim, B. N., Cho, S. C., Kim, J. W., Shin, M. S., Yoo, H. J., & Kim, H. W. (2010). The prevalence of specific phobia and associated co-morbid features in children and adolescents. *Journal of Anxiety Disorders, 24*(6), 629–634.

King, N.J., & Bernstein, G.A. (2001). School refusal in children and adolescents: A review of the past 10 years. *Journal of the American Academy of Child and Adolescent Psychiatry, 40,* 197–205.

King, N.J., Gullone, E., Tonge, B. J., & Ollendick, T. H. (1993). Self-reports of panic attacks and manifest anxiety in adolescents. *Behaviour Research and Therapy, 31,* 111–116.

King, N. J., Ollendick, T. H., Mattis, S. G., Yang, B. & Tonge, B. (1997). Nonclinical panic attacks in adolescents: Prevalence, symptomatology and associated features. *Behaviour Change, 13,* 171–183.

King, N. J., Tonge, B. J., Heyne, D., Pritchard, M., Rollings, S., Young, D.,…Ollendick, T. H. (1998). Cognitive-behavioral treatment of school-refusing children: A controlled evaluation. *Journal of the American Academy of Child and Adolescent Psychiatry, 37,* 395–403.

Knapp, A. A., Blumenthal, H., Mischel, E. R., Badour, C. L., & Leen-Feldner, E. W. (2016). Anxiety sensitivity and its factors in relation to generalized anxiety disorder among adolescents. *Journal of Abnormal Child Psychology, 44*(2), 233–244.

Kolko, D. J., Ayllon, T., & Torrence, C. (1987). Positive practice routines in overcoming resistance to the treatment of school phobia: A case study with follow-up. *Journal of Behavior Therapy and Experimental Psychiatry, 18,* 249–257.

Kurtz, S. (2009). Camp Brave Buddies, 2009: Summer day treatment program for children with selective mutism. Retrieved from http://childmind.org/center/brave-buddies/.

Kurtz, S. M. S. (2012, April). Brave Buddies: An intensive group treatment for SM in an analog classroom setting. In S. Sung (Chair), *Recent advances in the assessment and treatment of children with selective mutism.* Symposium conducted at the meeting of the Anxiety Disorders Association of America, Arlington, VA.

Kristensen, H. (2000). Multiple informants' report of emotional and behavioural problems in a nation-wide sample of selective mute children and controls. *European Child and Adolescent Psychiatry, 10*(2), 135–142.

Lader, M.H., and Matthews A.M. (1968). A physiological model of phobic anxiety and desensitization. (1968). *Behaviour Research and Therapy, 6,* 411–421.

Lamdin, D. J. (1996). Evidence of student attendance as an independent variable in education production functions. *Journal of Educational Research, 89,* 155–162.

Lang, P. J. (1968). Fear reduction and fear behavior: Problems in treating a construct. Research in Psychotherapy 3rd Conference, Chicago, IL, May–June 1968. American Psychological Association.

Lang, R., Regester, A., Mulloy, A., Rispoli, M., & Botout, A. (2011). Behavioral intervention to treat selective mutism across multiple social situations and community settings. *Journal of Applied Behavior Analysis, 44*(3), 623–628.

Langley, A. K., Falk, A., Peris, T., Wiley, J. F., Kendall, P. C., Ginsburg, G.,…Piacintini, J. (2014). The child anxiety impact scale: Examining parent- and child-reported impairment in child anxiety disorders. *Journal of Clinical Child and Adolescent Psychology, 43*(4), 579–591.

Langley, A. K., Lewin, A. B., Bergman, R. L., Lee, J. C., & Piacentini, J. (2010). Correlates of comorbid anxiety and externalizing disorders in childhood obsessive compulsive disorder. *European Child and Adolescent Psychiatry, 19*(8), 637–645.

Last, C. G., Hansen, C., & Franco, N. (1998). Cognitive-behavioral treatment of school phobia. *Journal of the American Academy of Child and Adolescent Psychiatry, 37*, 404–411.

Leahy, R. (1996). *Cognitive therapy: Basic principles and applications.* Lanham, Maryland: Rowman & Littlefield.

Lebowitz, E. R., Shic, F., Campbell, D., Basile, K., & Silverman, W. K. (2015). Anxiety sensitivity moderates behavioral avoidance in anxious youth. *Behaviour research and therapy, 74*, 11–17.

Lebowitz, E. R., Woolston, J., Bar-Haim, Y., Calvocoressi, L., Dauser, C., Warnick, E., &… Leckman, J. F. (2013). Family accommodation in pediatric anxiety disorders. *Depression and Anxiety, 30*(1), 47–54.

Lewin, A. B., Storch, E. A., Merlo, L. J., Adkins, J. W., Murphy, T., & Geffken, G. A. (2005). Intensive cognitive behavioral therapy for pediatric obsessive compulsive disorder: A treatment protocol for mental health providers. *Psychological Services, 2*(2), 91–104.

Lewinsohn, P. M., Gotlib, I. H., Lewinsohn, M., Seeley, J. R., & Allen, N. B. (1998). Gender differences in anxiety disorders and anxiety symptoms in adolescents. *Journal of Abnormal Psychology, 107*(1), 109.

Lewinsohn, P. M., Hops, H., Roberts, R. E., Seeley, J. R., & Andrews, J. A. (1993). Adolescent psychopathology: I. Prevalence and incidence of depression and other DSM-III-R disorders in high school students. *Journal of Abnormal Psychology, 102*, 133–144.

Lind, C., & Boschen, M. J. (2009). Intolerance of uncertainty mediates the relationship between responsibility beliefs and compulsive checking. *Journal of Anxiety Disorders, 23*(8), 1047–1052.

Linehan, M. M. (1993). *Skills training manual for treating borderline personality disorder.* New York: Guilford Press.

Lipsitz, J. D., Barlow, D. H., Mannuzza, S., Hofmann, S. G., & Fyer, A. J. (2002). Clinical features of four DSM-IV-specific phobia subtypes. *The Journal of Nervous and Mental Disease, 190*(7), 471–478.

Lipsitz, J. D., Fyer, A. J., Paterniti, A., & Klein, D. F. (2001). Emetophobia: Preliminary results of an Internet survey. *Depression and Anxiety, 14*, 149–152.

Lynas, C. M. T., Kurtz, S. M. S., & Brandon, A. (2012, October). *Adventure camp intensive treatment for selective mutism: A replication of Brave Buddies.* Paper presented at the meeting of the Selective Mutism Group, Child Anxiety Network, Orlando, FL.

Maack, D. J., Deacon, B. J., & Zhao, M. (2013). Exposure therapy for emetophobia: A case study with three-year follow up. *Journal of Anxiety Disorders, 27*, 527–534.

Mahoney, A. E. J., & McEvoy, P. M. (2012). A transdiagnostic examination of intolerance of uncertainty across anxiety and depressive disorders. *Cognitive Behaviour Therapy, 41*(3), 212–222.

Manassis, K., Fung, D., Tannock, R., Sloman, L., Fiksenbaum, L., & McInnes, A. (2003). Characterizing selective mutism: Is it more than social anxiety? *Depression & Anxiety, 18*(3), 153–161.

Manassis, K., Lee, T. C., Bennett, K., Zhao, X. Y., Mendlowitz, S., Duda, S.,…Barrett, P. (2014). Types of parental involvement in CBT with anxious youth: A preliminary meta-analysis. *Journal of Consulting and Clinical Psychology, 82*(6), 1163–1172.

Manassis, K., Tannock, R., Garland, E. J., Minde, K., & McInnes, A. (2007). The sounds of silence: Language, cognition, and anxiety in selective mutism. *Journal of the American Academy of Child and Adolescent Psychiatry, 46*(9), 1187–1195.

Mancebo, M. C., Garcia, A. M., Pinto, A., Freeman, J. B., Przeworski, A., Stout, R,…Rasmussen, S. A. (2008). Juvenile-onset OCD: Clinical features in children, adolescents and adults. *Acta Psychiatrica Scandinavica, 118*(2), 149–159.

March, J., Foa, E., Gammon, P., Chrisman, A., Curry, J., Fitzgerald, D.,…Freeman, J. (2004). Cognitive-behavior therapy, sertraline, and their combination for children and adolescents with obsessive-compulsive disorder: The Pediatric OCD Treatment Study (POTS) randomized controlled trial. *Journal of the American Medical Association, 292*, 1969–1976.

March, J. S., Parker, J. D., Sullivan, K., Stallings, P., & Conners, C. K. (1997). The Multidimensional Anxiety Scale for Children (MASC): factor structure, reliability, and validity. *Journal of the American Academy of Child and Adolescent Psychiatry, 36*(4), 554–565.

Marques, T., Pereira, A. I., Barros, L., & Muris, P. (2013). Cognitive vulnerability profiles of highly anxious and non-anxious children. *Child Psychiatry and Human Development, 44*(6), 777–785.

Masi, G., Favilla, L., Mucci, M., & Millepiedi, S. (2000). Panic disorder in clinically referred children and adolescents. *Child Psychiatry and Human Development, 31*, 139–151.

Masi, G., Millepiedi, S., Mucci, M., Bertini, N., Milantoni, L., & Arcangeli, F. (2005). A naturalistic study of referred children and adolescents with obsessive-compulsive disorder. *Journal of the American Academy of Child and Adolescent Psychiatry, 44*(7), 673–681.

Masi, G., Millepiedi, S., Mucchi, M., Poli, P., Bertini, N., & Milantoni, L. (2004). Generalized anxiety disorder in referred children and adolescents. *Journal of the American Academy of Child and Adolescent Psychiatry, 43*(6), 752–760.

Masi, G., Mucci, M., Favilla, L., Romano, R., & Poli, P. (1999). Symptomatology and comorbidity of generalized anxiety disorder in children and adolescents. *Comprehensive Psychiatry, 40*(3): 210–215.

McEvoy, P. M., & Mahoney, A. E. (2011). Achieving certainty about the structure of intolerance of uncertainty in a treatment-seeking sample with anxiety and depression. *Journal of Anxiety Disorders, 25*(1), 112–122.

McFayden, M., & Wyness, J. (1983). You don't have to be sick to be a behavior therapist but it can help! Treatment of a "vomit" phobia. *Behavioral Psychotherapy, 11*, 173–176.

McGlynn, F. D., Smitherman, T. A., & Gothard, K. D. (2004). Comment on the status of systematic desensitization. *Behavior modification, 28*(2), 194–205.

McGuire, J. F., Piacentini, J., Lewin, A. B., Brennan, E. A., Murphy, T. K., & Storch, E. A. (2015). A meta-analysis of cognitive behavior therapy and medication for child obsessive-compulsive disorder: Moderators of treatment efficacy, response, and remission. *Depression and Anxiety, 32*(8), 580–593.

McLaughlin, K. A., Borkovec, T. D., & Sibrava, N. J. (2007). The effects of worry and rumination on affect states and cognitive activity. *Behavior Therapy, 38*(1), 23–38.

McLean, C. P., & Anderson, E. R. (2009). Brave men and timid women? A review of the gender differences in fear and anxiety. *Clinical Psychology Review, 29*(6), 496–505.

McLeod, B. D. (2007). Examining the association between parenting and childhood anxiety: A meta-analysis. *Clinical Psychology Review, 27,* 155–172.

McLeod, B.D., Wood, J.J., & Weisz, J.R. (2007). Examining the association between parenting and childhood anxiety: a meta-analysis. *Clinical Psychology Review, 27,* 155–172.

McShane, G., Walter, G., & Rey, J.M. (2001). Characteristics of adolescents with school refusal. *Australian and New Zealand Journal of Psychiatry, 35,* 822–826.

Mele, C. M., & Kurtz, S. M. S. (2013, April). *Parent-child interactions in behavioral treatment of selective mutism: A case study.* Poster session presented at the meeting of the Anxiety Disorders Association of America, La Jolla, CA.

Menzies, R. G., & Clarke, J. C. (1995). The etiology of phobias: A nonassociative account. *Clinical Psychology Review, 15,* 23–48.

Merikangas, K. R., He, J., Burstein, M., Swanson, S. A., Avenevoli, S., Cui, L.,…Swendsen, J. (2010). Lifetime prevalence of mental disorders in U.S. adolescents: Results from the National Comorbidity Study-Adolescent Supplement (NCS-A). *Journal of the American Academy of Child and Adolescent Psychiatry, 49*(10), 980–989.

Merlo, L. J., Lehmkuhl, H. D., Geffken, G. R., & Storch, E. A. (2009). Decreased family accommodation associated with improved therapy outcome in pediatric obsessive-compulsive disorder. *Journal of Consulting and Clinical Psychology, 77*(2), 355–360.

Miller, P. R., Dasher, R., Collins, R., Griffiths, P., & Brown, F. (2001). Inpatient diagnostic assessments: 1. Accuracy of structured vs. unstructured interviews. *Psychiatry Research, 105*(3), 255–264.

Miller, W.R. & Rollnick, S. (2002). *Motivational interviewing: Preparing people for change: 2nd Edition.* New York: Guilford Press.

Mineka, S., Watson, D., & Clark, L. A. (1998). Comorbidity of anxiety and unipolar mood disorders. *Annual Review of Psychology, 49*(1), 377–412.

Moffitt, C. E., Chorpita, B. F., & Fernandez, S. N. (2003). Intensive cognitive-behavioral treatment of school refusal behavior. *Cognitive and Behavioral Practice, 10,* 51–60.

Mowrer, O. (1947). On the dual nature of learning—A re-interpretation of "conditioning" and "problem-solving." *Harvard Educational Review, 17,* 102–148.

Mowrer, O.H. (1960). Basic research methods, statistics, and decision theory. *American Journal of Occupational Therapy, 14,* 199–205.

Muris, P., & Field, A. P. (2008). Distorted cognition and pathological anxiety in children and adolescents. *Cognition and Emotion, 22*(3), 395–421.

Nakamura, B. J., Pestle, S. L., & Chorpita, B. F. (2009). Differential sequencing of cognitive-behavioral techniques for reducing child and adolescent anxiety. *Journal of Cognitive Psychotherapy, 23*(2), 114–135.

Newhouse-Oisten, H. K., Kestner, K. M., & Frieder, J. E. (2016). An evaluation of modified exposure therapy for a child diagnosed with obsessive compulsive disorder and pervasive developmental disorder- not otherwise specified. *Behavior Analysis: Research and Practice, 16*(3), 147–155.

Newman, M. G., Llera, S. J., Erickson, T. M., Przeworski, A., & Castonguay, L. G. (2013). Worry and generalized anxiety disorder: a review and theoretical synthesis of evidence on nature, etiology, mechanisms, and treatment. *Annual Review of Clinical Psychology, 9,* 275–297.

Noël, V. A., & Francis, S. E. (2011). A meta-analytic review of the role of child anxiety sensitivity in child anxiety. *Journal of Abnormal Child Psychology, 39*(5), 721–733.

Nolen-Hoeksema, S., & Morrow, J. (1993). Effects of rumination and distraction on naturally occurring depressed mood. *Cognition and Emotion, 7*(6), 561–570.

Nuttall, C., & Woods, K. (2013). Effective intervention for school refusal behavior. *Educational Psychology in Practice, 29*(4), 347–366.

Olatunji, B. O., Smits, J. A., Connolly, K., Willems, J., & Lohr, J. M., (2007). Examination of the decline in fear and disgust during exposure to threat-relevant stimuli in blood-injection-injury phobia. *Journal of Anxiety Disorders, 21*(3), 445–455.

Olivares, J., & Garcia-Lopez, L. J. (1998). Therapy for Adolescents with Social Phobia Generalized: A new cognitive-behavioral treatment protocol for social phobia in adolescence. *Unpublished manuscript.*

Ollendick, T. H. (1995). Cognitive-behavioral treatment of panic disorder with agoraphobia in adolescents: A multiple baseline design analysis. *Behavior Therapy, 26,* 517–531.

Ollendick, T. H., & Davis III, T. E. (2013). One-session treatment for specific phobias: A review of Öst's single-session exposure with children and adolescents. *Cognitive Behavior Therapy, 42*(4), 275–283.

Ollendick, T. H., & King, N. J. (1994). Fears and their level of interference in adolescents. *Behaviour Research and Therapy, 32,* 635–638.

Ollendick, T. H., King, N. J., & Muris, P. (2002). Fears and phobias in children: Phenomenology, epidemiology, and aetiology. *Child and Adolescent Mental Health, 7*(3), 98–106.

Ollendick, T. H., & March, J. S. (Eds.) (2004). *Phobic and anxiety disorders in children and adolescents: A clinician's guide to effective psychosocial and pharmacological interventions.* New York: Oxford University Press.

Ollendick, T. H., Öst, L. G., Reuterskiöld, L., Costa, N., Cederlund, R., Sirbu, C.,…Jarrett, M. A. (2009). One-session treatment of specific phobias in youth: A randomized clinical trial in the United States and Sweden. *Journal of Consulting and Clinical Psychology, 77*(3), 504–516.

Ollendick, T. H., Yang, B., Dong, Q., Xia, Y., & Lin, L. (1995). Perceptions of fear in other children and adolescents: The role of gender and friendship status. *Journal of Abnormal Child Psychology, 23,* 439–452.

Ollendick, & L. G. Öst (Eds.), *Intensive one-session treatment of specific phobias* (pp. 59–96). New York: Springer Science and Business Media, LLC.

O'Neill, J., Piacentini J. C., Change, S., Levitt, J. G., Rozenman, M., Bergman, L., Salamon, N., Algre, J. R., & McCracken, J. T. (2012). MRSI correlates of cognitive-behavioral therapy in pediatric obsessive-compulsive disorder. *Progress in Neuro-Psychopharmacology & Biological Psychiatry, 36,* 161–186.

Öst, L. G. (2012). One-session treatment: Principles and procedures with adults. In T. E. Davis III, T. H. Öst, L. G., & Ollendick, T. H. (2001). Manual for one-session treatment of specific phobias. *Unpublished manuscript.*

Öst, L. G., Riise, E. N., Wergeland, G. J., Hansen, B., & Kvale, G. (2016). Cognitive behavioral and pharmacological treatments of OCD in children: A systematic review and meta-analysis. *Journal of Anxiety Disorders, 43,* 58–69.

Öst, L. G., & Sterner, U. (1987). Applied tension: A specific behavioural method for treatment of blood phobia. *Behaviour Research and Therapy, 25,* 25–29.

Öst, L., Svensson, L., Hellström, K., & Lindwall, R. (2001). One-session treatment of specific phobias in youths: A randomized clinical trial. *Journal of Consulting and Clinical Psychology, 69*(5), 814–824.

Owens, J. S., Goldfine, M. E., Evangelista, N. M., Hoza, B. & Kaiser, N. M. (2007). A critical review of self-perceptions and the positive illusory bias in children with ADHD. *Clinical Child and Family Psychology Review, 10*, 335–351.

Pellegrini, D.W. (2007). School non-attendance: Definitions, meanings, responses, interventions. *Educational Psychology in Practice, 23*, 63–77.

Peris, T., Compton, S., Kendall, P., Birmaher, B., Sherrill, J., March, J.,…Piacentini, J. (2014). Trajectories of change in youth anxiety during cognitive behavior therapy. *Journal of Consulting and Clinical Psychology, 83*, 239–252.

Peterman, J. S., Read, K. L., Wei, C., & Kendall, P. C. (2015). The art of exposure: putting science into practice. *Cognitive and Behavioral Practice, 22*(3), 379–392.

Phillips, N. K., Hammen, C. L., Brennan, P. A., Najman, J. M., & Bor, W. (2005). Early adversity and the prospective prediction of depressive and anxiety disorders in adolescents. *Journal of Abnormal Child Psychology, 33*(1), 13–24.

Piacentini, J., Bergman, R.L., Keller, M., & McCracken, J. (2003). Functional impairment in children and adolescents with obsessive-compulsive disorder. *Journal of Child and Adolescent Psychopharmacology, 13*(Suppl 2), S61–S69.

Pina, A. A., Zerr, A. A., Gonzales, N. A., & Ortiz, C. D. (2009). Psychosocial interventions for school refusal behavior in children and adolescents. *Child Development Perspectives, 3*(1), 11–20.

Pina, A. A., Silverman, W. K., Weems, C. F., Kurtines, W., & Goldman, M. L. (2003). A comparison of completers and noncompleters of exposure-base cognitive and behavioural treatment for phobic and anxiety disorders in youth. *Journal of Consulting and Clinical Psychology, 71*(4), 701–705.

Pincus, D. B., Ehrenreich, J. T., & Mattis, S. G. (2008). *Mastery of anxiety and panic for adolescents: Riding the wave. Therapist guide.* New York: Oxford University Press.

Pincus, D. B., Ehrenreich May, J., Whitton, S. W., Mattis, S. G., & Barlow, D. H. (2010). Cognitive-behavioral treatment of panic disorder in adolescence. *Journal of Clinical Child and Adolescent Psychology, 39*(5), 638–649.

Pincus, D., Santucci, L. C., Ehrenreich, J. T., & Eyberg, S. M. (2008). The implementation of modified parent child interaction therapy for youth with separation anxiety disorder. *Cognitive and Behavioral Practice, 15*, 118–125.

Pine, D. S., Cohen, P., Gurley, D., Brook, J., & Ma, Y. (1998). The risk for early-adulthood anxiety and depressive disorders in adolescents with anxiety and depressive disorders. *Archives of General Psychiatry, 55*(1), 56–64.

Puliafico, A. C., & Kendall, P. C. (2006). Threat-related attentional bias in anxious youth: A review. *Clinical Child and Family Psychology Review, 9*(3–4), 162–180.

Puleo C. M., Conner, B. T., Benjamin, C. L., & Kendall, P. C. (2011). CBT for childhood anxiety and substance use at 7.4-year follow-up: A reassessment controlling for known predictors. *Journal of Anxiety Disorders, 25*(5), 690–696.

Quirk, G.J. (2004). Learning not to fear, faster. *Learning and Memory, 11*, 125–126.

Rahman, O., Reid, J. M., Parks, A. M., McKay, D. & Storch, E. A. (2011). Obsessive-Compulsive Disorder. In D. McKay and E. A. Storch (Eds.), *Handbook of Child and Adolescent Anxiety Disorders* (323–338). New York: Springer.

Rapee, R., Lyneham, H., Schniering, C., Wuthrich, V., Abbott, M., Hudson, J., & Wignall, A. (2006). Cool Kids therapist manual: For the Cool Kids child and adolescent anxiety programs. Sydney, Australia: Centre for Emotional Health, Macquarie University:

Rapee, R. M., Schniering, C. A., & Hudson, J. L. (2009). Anxiety disorders during childhood and adolescence: Origins and treatment. *Annual Review of Clinical Psychology, 5,* 311–341.

Rapee, R. M., & Spence, S. H. (2004). The etiology of social phobia: Empirical evidence and an initial model. *Clinical Psychology Review, 24*(7), 737–767.

Rapoport, J. L., Inoff-Germain, G., Weissman, M. M., Greenwald, S., Narrow, W. E., Jensen, P.,…Canino, G. (2000). Childhood obsessive-compulsive disorder in the NIMH MECA study: parent versus child identification of cases. Methods for the Epidemiology of Child and Adolescent Mental Disorders. *Journal of Anxiety Disorders, 14*(6), 535–548.

Read, K. L., Comer, J. S., & Kendall, P. C. (2013). The Intolerance of Uncertainty Scale for Children (IUSC): Discriminating principal anxiety diagnoses and severity. *Psychological Assessment, 25*(3), 722–729.

Reiss, S., & McNally, R. J. (1985). The expectancy model of fear. In S. Reiss & R. R. Bootzin (Eds.), *Theoretical issues in behavior therapy* (pp. 107–122). New York: Academic Press.

Reiss, S., Peterson, R. A., Gursky, D. M., & McNally, R. J. (1986). Anxiety sensitivity, anxiety frequency and the prediction of fearfulness. *Behaviour Research and Therapy, 24*(1), 1–8.

Reuther, E. T., Davis, T. E., Moree, B. N., & Matson, J. L. (2011). Treating selective mutism using modular CBT for child anxiety: A case study. *Journal of Clinical Child Psychology and Psychiatry, 40*(1), 156–163.

Richburg, M. L., & Cobia, D. C. (1994). Using behavioral techniques to treat elective mutism: A case study. *Elementary School Guidance and Counseling, 28*(3), 214–219.

Ritz, T., Meuret A. E., & Alvord, M. K. (2014). Blood-injection-injury phobia. In L. Grossman, & S. Walfish (Eds.), *Translating psychological research into practice,* (pp. 295–301). New York: Springer.

Rothbart, M. K., & Rueda, M. R. (2005). The development of effortful control. In U. Mayr, E. Awh, & S. Keele (Eds.), *Developing individuality in the human brain: A tribute to Michael I. Posner* (pp. 167–188) Washington, DC: American Psychological Association.

Rudy, B. M., Lewin, A. B., Geffken, G. R., Murphy, T. K., & Storch, E. A. (2014). Predictors of treatment response to intensive cognitive-behavioral therapy for pediatric obsessive-compulsive disorder. *Psychiatry Research, 220*(1–2), 433–440.

Rumberger, R. W. (1995). Dropping out of middle school: A multilevel analysis of students and schools. *American Educational Research Journal, 32*(3), 583–625.

Ruscio, A. M., Brown, T. A., Chiu, W. T., Sareen, J., Stein, M. B., & Kessler, R. C. (2008). Social fears and social phobia in the USA: results from the National Comorbidity Survey Replication. *Psychological Medicine, 38*(01), 15–28.

Santucci, L. C., & Ehrenreich-May, J. (2010, November). A one-week summer treatment program for children with separation anxiety disorder: Results of a randomized controlled trial. In K. P. Gallo & D. B. Pincus (Chairs), *Innovative formats of CBT for child anxiety: Efficacy, feasibility, and acceptability* (pp. 471–498). Symposium conducted at the 44th annual convention of the Association for Behavioral and Cognitive Therapies, San Francisco.

Santucci, L. C., Ehrenreich, J. T., Trosper, S. E., Bennett, S. M., & Pincus, D. B. (2009). Development and preliminary evaluation of a one-week summer treatment program for separation anxiety disorder. *Cognitive and Behavioral Practice, 16*(3), 317–331.

Scahill, L., Riddle, M. A., McSwiggin-Hardin, M., Ort, S. I., King, R. A., Goodman, W. K.,...Leckman, J. F. (1997). Children's Yale-Brown Obsessive Compulsive Scale: Reliability and validity. *Journal of the American Academy of Child and Adolescent Psychiatry, 36*(6), 844–852.

Seager, I., Rowley, A. M., & Ehrenreich-May, J. (2014). Targeting common factors across anxiety and depression using the unified protocol for the treatment of emotional disorders in adolescents. *Journal of Rational-Emotive & Cognitive-Behavior Therapy, 32*(1), 67–83.

Sharp, W. G., Sherman, C., & Gross, A. M. (2007). Selective mutism and anxiety: A review of the current conceptualization of the disorder. *Journal of Anxiety Disorders, 21*, 568–579.

Shear, K., Jin, R., Ruscio, A. M., Walters, E. E., & Kessler, R. C. (2006). Prevalence and correlates of estimated DSM-IV child and adult separation disorder in the National Comorbidity Survey Replication. *American Journal of Psychiatry, 163*(6), 1074–1083.

Silveria, R., Jainer, A., & Bates, G. (2004). Fluoxetine treatment of selective mutism in pervasive developmental disorder. *International Journal of Psychiatry in Clinical Practice, 8*, 179–180.

Silverman W, & Albano A. (1996). The Anxiety Disorders Interview Schedule for Children–IV (child and parent versions) San Antonio, TX: Psychological Corporation.

Silverman, W. K., Kurtines, W. M., Ginsburg, G. S., Weems, C. F., Lumpkin, P. W., & Carmichael, D. H. (1999). Treating anxiety disorders in children with group cognitive-behavior therapy: A randomized clinical trial. *Journal of Consulting and Clinical Psychology, 76*, 995–1003.

Sisemore, T. A. (2012). The clinician's guide to exposure therapies for anxiety spectrum disorders: Integrating techniques and applications from CBT, DBT, and ACT. Oakland, CA: New Harbinger.

Spence, S. H. (1998). A measure of anxiety symptoms among children. *Behaviour Research and Therapy, 36*(5), 545–566.

Spence, S. H., Donovan, C., & Brechman-Toussaint, M. (2000). The treatment of childhood social phobia: The effectiveness of a social skills training-based, cognitive-behavioural intervention, with and without parental involvement. *Journal of Child Psychology and Psychiatry, 41*(6), 713–726.

Spence, S. H., & Rapee, R. M. (2016). The etiology of social anxiety disorder: an evidence-based model. *Behaviour Research and Therapy, 86*, 50–67.

Spencer, E. D., Dupont, R. L., & Dupont, C. M. (2003). *The anxiety cure for kids: A guide for parents.* Hoboken, NJ: John Wiley & Sons.

Spinhoven, P., Drost, J., de Rooij, M., van Hemert, A. M., & Penninx, B. H. (2016). Is experiential avoidance a mediating, moderating, independent, overlapping, or proxy risk factor in the onset, relapse and maintenance of depressive disorders? *Cognitive Therapy and Research, 40*(2), 150–163.

Stampfl, T. G., & Levis, D. J. (1967). Essentials of implosive therapy: a learning-theory-based psychodynamic behavioral therapy. *Journal of Abnormal Psychology, 72*(6), 496.

Stassen Berger, Kathleen (2011). *The developing person through the life span* (8th ed.). New York: Worth.

Steinhausen, H. S., Wachter, M., Laimbock, K., & Metzke, C. W. (2006). A long-term outcome study of selective mutism in childhood. *Journal of Child Psychology and Psychiatry, 47*(7), 751–756.

Stinson, F., S., Dawson, D. A., Chou, S. P., Smith, S., Goldstein, R. B., Ruan, W. J., & Grant, B. F. (2007). The epidemiology of DSM-IV specific phobia in the USA: Results from the National Epidemiologic Survey on Alcohol and Related Conditions. *Psychological Medicine, 37,* 1047–1059.

Storch, E. A., Geffken, G. R., Merlo, L. J., Mann, G., Duke, D., Munson, M.,…Goodman, W. K. (2007). Family-based cognitive-behavioral therapy for pediatric obsessive-compulsive disorder: comparison of intensive and weekly approaches. *Journal of the American Academy of Child and Adolescent Psychiatry, 46,* 469–478.

Storch, E. A., Merlo, L. J., Bengtson, M., Murphy, T. K., Lewis, M. H., Yang, M. C.,… Goodman, W. K. (2007). D-cycloserine does not enhance exposure-response prevention therapy in obsessive-compulsive disorder. *International Clinical Psychopharmacology, 22*(4), 230–237.

Strauss, C. C., Last, C. G., Hersen, M., & Kazdin A. E. (1988). Association between anxiety and depression in children and adolescents with anxiety disorders. *Journal of Abnormal Child Psychology, 16*(1), 57–68.

Sung, S. C., & Smith, H. L. (2009). Cognitive-behavioral therapy for refractory selective mutism. In D. McKay & E. A. Storch (Eds.), *Cognitive behavioral therapy for children: Treating complex and refractory cases* (pp. 141–170). New York: Springer.

Suveg, C., Aschenbrand, S.G., & Kendall, P.C. (2005). Separation anxiety disorder, panic disorder, and school refusal. *Child and Adolescent Psychiatric Clinics of North America, 14,* 773–795.

Suveg, C., Hoffman, B., Zeman, J. L., & Thomassin, K. (2009). Common and specific emotion-related predictors of anxious and depressive symptoms in youth. *Child Psychiatry and Human Development, 40*(2), 223–239.

Suveg, C., Sood, E., Comer, J. S., & Kendall, P. C. (2009). Changes in emotion regulation following cognitive-behavioral therapy for anxious youth. *Journal of Clinical Child and Adolescent Psychology, 38*(3), 390–401.

Thompson-Hollands, J., Kerns, C. E., Pincus, D. B., & Comer, J. S. (2014). Parental accommodation of child anxiety and related symptoms: Range, impact, and correlates. *Journal of Anxiety Disorders, 28*(8), 765–773.

Tiwari, S., Kendall, P. C., Hoff, A. L., Harrison, J. P., & Fizur, P. (2013). Characteristics of exposure sessions as predictors of treatment response in anxious youth. *Journal of Clinical Child and Adolescent Psychology, 42*(1), 34–43.

Topolski, T. D., Hewitt, J. K., Eaves, L. J., Silberg, J. L., Meyer, J. M., Pickles, A., & Simonff, E. (1997). Genetic and environmental influences on child reports of manifest anxiety and symptoms of separation anxiety and overanxious disorders: A community-based twin study. *Behavior Genetics, 27*(1), 15–28.

Torp, N. C., Dahl, K., Skarphedinsson, G., Thomsen, P. H., Valderhaug, R., Weidle, B.,… Ivarsson, T. (2015). Effectiveness of cognitive behavior treatment for pediatric obsessive-compulsive disorder: Acute outcomes from the Nordic Long-term OCD Treatment Study (NordLOTS). *Behaviour Research and Therapy, 64,* 15–23.

Tryon, W.W. (2005). Possible mechanisms for why desensitization and exposure therapy work. *Clinical Psychology Review, 25,* 67–94.

Valderhaug, R., & Ivarsson, T. (2005). Functional impairment in clinical samples of Norwegian and Swedish children and adolescents with obsessive-compulsive disorder. *European Child and Adolescent Psychiatry, 14*(3), 164–173.

Vecchio, J. L., & Kearney, C. A. (2009). Treating youths with selective mutism with an alternating design of exposure-based practice and contingency management. *Behavior Therapy Journal, 40*, 380–392.

Viana, A. G., Beidel, D. C., & Rabian, B. (2009). Selective mutism: A review and integration of the last 15 years. *Clinical Psychology Review, 29*(1), 57–67.

Voort, J.L., Svecova, J., Jacobsen, A.B., & Whiteside, S.P. (2010). A retrospective examination of the similarity between clinical practice and manualized treatment for childhood anxiety disorders. *Cognitive and Behavioral Practice, 17*(3), 322–328.

Walkup, J. T., Albano, A. M., Piacentini, J., Birmaher, B., Compton, S. N., Sherrill, J. T.,… Waslick, B. (2008). Cognitive behavioral therapy, sertraline, or a combination in childhood anxiety. *New England Journal of Medicine, 359*(26), 2753–2766.

Watson J.P., Gaind, R., and Marks, I.M. (1972). Physiological habituation to continuous phobic stimulation. *Behaviour Research and Therapy, 10*, 269–278.

Watson, H. J., & Rees, C. S. (2008). Meta-analysis of randomized, controlled treatment trials for pediatric obsessive-compulsive disorder. *Journal of Child Psychology and Psychiatry, 49*, 489–498.

Weems, C. F., & Costa, N. M. (2005). Developmental differences in the expression of childhood anxiety symptoms and fears. *Journal of the American Academy of Child and Adolescent Psychiatry, 44*(7): 656–663.

Weems, C. F., Silverman, W. K., Rapee, R. M., & Pina, A. A. (2003). The role of control in childhood anxiety disorders. *Cognitive Therapy and Research, 27*(5), 557–568.

Weissman, M. M., Klerman, G. L., Markowitz, J. S., & Quellette, R. (1989). Suicidal ideation and suicide attempts in panic disorder and attacks. *New England Journal of Medicine, 321*, 1209–1214.

Weisz, J. R., Kuppens, S., Eckshtain, D., Ugueto, A. M., Hawley, K. M., & Jensen-Doss, A. (2013). Performance of evidence-based youth psychotherapies compared with usual clinical care: a multilevel meta-analysis. *JAMA Psychiatry, 70*(7), 750–761.

Wells, A. (2009). *Metacognitive therapy for anxiety and depression*. New York, NY: Guilford Press.

Whiteside, S. H., Deacon, B. J., Benito, K., & Stewart, E. (2016). Factors associated with practitioners' use of exposure therapy for childhood anxiety disorders. *Journal of Anxiety Disorders, 40*, 29–36.

Whitton, S. W., Luiselli, J. K., & Donaldson, D. L. (2006). Cognitive-behavioral treatment of generalized anxiety disorder and vomiting phobia in an elementary-age child. *Clinical Case Studies, 5*(6), 477–487.

Willemsen, H., Chowdhury, U., & Briscall, L. (2002). Needle phobia in children: A discussion of aetiology and treatment options. *Clinical Child Psychology and Psychiatry, 7*(4), 609–619.

Wittchen, H. U., & Fehm, L. (2003). Epidemiology and natural course of social fears and social phobia. *Acta Psychiatrica Scandinavica, 108*(s417), 4–18.

Wittchen, H. U., Lecrubier, Y., Beesdo, K., & Nacon, A. (2003). Relationships among anxiety disorders: Patterns and implications. In D. J. Nutt & J. C. Ballenger (Eds.), *Anxiety disorders* (pp. 25–37). Oxford, UK: Blackwell Science.

Wolpe, J. (1958). *Behavior therapy by reciprocal inhibition*. Stanford, CA: Stanford University Press.

Wolpe, J. & Lazarus, A.A. (1966). *Behavior therapy techniques: A guide to the treatment of neuroses.* Elmsford, NY: Pergamon Press.

Wood, J.J. (2006). Parental Intrusiveness and children's separation anxiety in a clinical sample. *Child Psychiatry and Human Development, 37,* 73–87.

Wood, J. J., McLeod, B. D., Hiruma, L. S., & Phan, A. Q. (2008). *Child anxiety disorders: A family-based treatment manual for practitioners.* New York: W W Norton & Company.

Woodward, L. J. & Fergusson, D. M. (2001). Life course outcomes of young people with anxiety disorders in adolescence. *Journal of the American Academy of Child and Adolescent Psychiatry. 40*(9), 1086–1093.

Yeganeh, R., Beidel, D. C., Turner, S. M., Pina, A. A., & Silverman, W. K. (2003). Clinical distinctions between selective mutism and social phobia: An investigation of childhood psychopathology. *Journal of the American Academy of Child and Adolescent Psychiatry, 42,* 1069–1075.

Young, B. J., Bunnell, B. E., & Beidel, D. C. (2012). Evaluation of children with selective mutism and social phobia: A comparison of psychological and psychophysiological arousal. *Behavior Modification, 36,* 525–544.

Zohar, A. H. (1999). The epidemiology of obsessive-compulsive disorder in children and adolescents. *Child and Adolescent Psychiatric Clinics of North America, 8*(3), 445–460.

Zucker, B. (2011). *Take control of OCD: The ultimate guide for kids with OCD.* Waco, TX: Prufrock Press.

Author Biographies

Veronica L. Raggi, PhD, is a licensed clinical psychologist who has specialized in treating children and adolescents for the past ten years in private practice, school, hospital, and outpatient medical settings, including New York University (NYU) Child Study Center, Children's National Medical Center, and the University of Maryland, College Park. She presents, consults, and trains mental health professionals in utilizing cognitive behavioral therapy (CBT), and has published in numerous scholarly journals on evidence-based treatment approaches for mental health disorders in youth. She has developed *CBT Tools for Kids*, an iPhone application to help youth monitor their thoughts and feelings, and utilize CBT skills (available at itunes.apple.com).

Jessica G. Samson, PsyD, is a licensed clinical psychologist with expertise in treating children and adolescents using evidence-based treatment interventions. She has clinical research experience from her work on two large National Institute of Mental Health-funded randomized-controlled trials at Johns Hopkins. She has eight years of experience in a private practice setting, and focuses her clinical work on treating anxiety, depression, tic disorders, and body-focused repetitive behaviors.

Julia W. Felton, PhD, is a licensed clinical psychologist, and assistant professor in the division of public health at Michigan State University. In addition to her clinical work with children and young adults, she has received a number of grants to research the development of anxiety, depression, and risky behaviors across adolescence.

Heather R. Loffredo, PsyD, is a licensed clinical psychologist with over a decade of experience in treating children and adolescents in hospital, community, school, and private practice settings. Her areas of expertise include assessment and treatment of anxiety disorders, and modification of evidenced-based treatments for special populations.

Lisa H. Berghorst, PhD, is a licensed clinical psychologist with expertise in using evidence-based treatments to address mood and anxiety disorders in children, adolescents, and young adults. In addition, she teaches at Northwestern University Feinberg School of Medicine, and has clinical research experience from the National Institute of Mental Health, Harvard University, and the Center for Depression, Anxiety and Stress Research at McLean Hospital. She has published numerous journal articles and book chapters related to mood and anxiety disorders, and resilience.

At the time of this writing, all authors were clinicians at Alvord, Baker & Associates, LLC in Montgomery County, MD.

List of Contributors

Betsy Carmichael, LCSW

Colleen Cummings, PhD

Michelle Gryczkowski, PhD

Nina Shiffrin, PhD

Index

B

Barkley, Russell, 104
behaviors: accommodating, 25, 28–30; assessing the function of, 95; modeling desired, 175; overprotective, 29; shaping approximations of, 174–175. *See also* avoidance behaviors; safety behaviors
beliefs: change in maladaptive, 82; evaluating anxious, 21–22
bias, 4, 102
blood-related exposures, 190–193
boundaries, maintaining, 35–36
Bravery Goal Chart, 92
bravery reward systems, 89–90
breathing: diaphragmatic, 62, 122; retraining technique, 122

C

camp-based programs, 11
case examples: of emotion intolerance, 312–314; of generalized anxiety disorder, 241–242; of obsessive-compulsive disorder, 294–296; of panic disorder, 129–130; of school phobia, 165–167; of selective mutism, 218; of separation anxiety disorder, 150–151; of social phobia, 264–266
catastrophic thinking, 51–52, 110, 221, 253
causal factors: for generalized anxiety disorder, 221; for obsessive-compulsive disorder, 269; for panic disorder, 109; for school phobia, 153; for selective mutism, 201; for separation anxiety disorder, 132; for social phobia, 245; for specific phobias, 169
CBT for Depression in Children and Adolescents (Kennard, Hughes, and Foxwell), 101
Child Anxiety Multimodal Study (CAMS), 13
child-directed interaction (CDI), 208
childhood anxiety: age of onset for, 1–2; clinical assessment of, 15–26; conditions co-occurring with, 98–107; developmental vs. pathological, 2–3; effectively responding to, 33–38; exposure therapy for, 8–9; gender differences in, 2; maintenance of, 6–8; nature and course of, 1–2; parental

behavior and, 6, 27–39; prevalence of, 1; risk factors for, 3–6
children and adolescents: course of anxiety in, 2; preparing for exposure work, 40–66; validating the experience of, 34
Children's Yale-Brown Obsessive Compulsive Scale (CY-BOCS), 18
Chinese finger trap metaphor, 307
choking-related exposures, 177–178
Chorpita, B. F., 45
clinical assessment of child anxiety, 15–26; diagnostic assessment, 15–18; functional behavioral assessment, 18–26
clinical interviews, 16–17
clinical presentation: of emotion intolerance, 299; of generalized anxiety disorder, 220–222; of obsessive-compulsive disorder, 268–269; of panic disorder, 108–109; of school phobia, 152–153; of selective mutism, 200–201; of separation anxiety disorder, 131–132; of social phobia, 244–245; of specific phobia, 168–169
clinically relevant factors: in emotion intolerance, 300–302; in generalized anxiety disorder, 222–225; in obsessive-compulsive disorder, 271–280; in panic disorder, 111–114; in school phobia, 154–157; in selective mutism, 202–204; in separation anxiety disorder, 133–136; in social phobia, 246–249; in specific phobias, 170–173
cloud image task, 228
cognitive behavioral therapy (CBT): exposure within the context of, 10–11; historical development of, 9; negative thought patterns challenged in, 48–60; relaxation skills taught in, 61–66; research on exposure with, 12–14; risk factors and exposure-based, 11–12; skills related to exposure work, 44–46; thought awareness skills in, 46–48; trauma-focused, 12
cognitive biases, 4
cognitive considerations: for generalized anxiety disorder, 227–230; for obsessive-compulsive disorder, 283–284; for panic disorder, 121; for school phobia, 160–161; for selective mutism, 213–214; for

MORE BOOKS *from*
NEW HARBINGER PUBLICATIONS

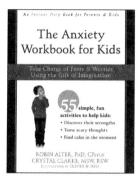
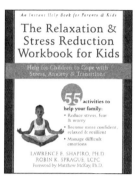
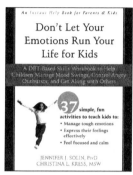
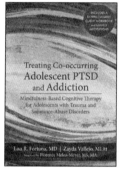
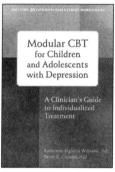
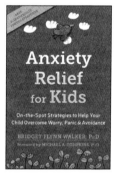

Register your **new harbinger** titles for additional benefits!

When you register your **new harbinger** title—purchased in any format, from any source—you get access to benefits like the following:

- Downloadable accessories like printable worksheets and extra content

- Instructional videos and audio files

- Information about updates, corrections, and new editions

Not every title has accessories, but we're adding new material all the time.

Access free accessories in 3 easy steps:

1. Sign in at NewHarbinger.com (or **register** to create an account).

2. Click on **register a book**. Search for your title and click the **register** button when it appears.

3. Click on the **book cover or title** to go to its details page. Click on **accessories** to view and access files.

That's all there is to it!

If you need help, visit:

NewHarbinger.com/accessories

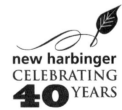

new harbinger
CELEBRATING
40 YEARS